Merlino's

# Pathology For Massage Therapy

## Second Edition

David Merlino, LMT

*Merlino's Pathology for Massage Therapy, Second Edition*


To obtain written permission to reproduce select portions of this book, email the author directly at david@wandererstudios.us.

Bulk order discounts are available for academic institutions. To obtain a written estimate or place an order, please email the author directly at david@wandererstudios.us.

**wandererstudios.us**

ISBN-13: 978-1-7328356-5-8

Photo credits: Amanda Merlino, Desmond Merlino, Steven Merlino, Starrisa Reyna, Ashley Capone, TJ Wilson, Rose Matthews, Mike Escobar, Frank Butler, Kayla Jean Madsen, Andrew Briggs, Shawn James, Heather Southwick.
Stock photos via Shutterstock.

Special Thanks: Every school and student who has used any of my guides, everyone who has supported me in my endeavors, my family, friends, Ross Tucker, Shawn James, Colin Moriarty, Rhiannon Box, Rocky McCahan, Melissa Leonhard, The Bodhi Tree Center, and Tim Ferriss.

**PUBLISHER'S DISCLAIMER**

The material presented in this study guide is for informational purposes only. Any information regarding Medications, CPR, First Aid, and Contraindications should be researched by the reader to obtain the most up-to-date requirements, as these subjects are ever-changing.

**INSTRUCTOR RESOURCES**

To request downloadable instructor resources, including PowerPoint presentations and test banks, email david@wandererstudios.us.

**ALSO AVAILABLE**

Subscribe to the MBLEx Test Prep Podcast on iTunes, Spotify, Soundcloud, Stitcher, and anywhere else you get podcasts!
Follow us on Facebook at facebook.com/mblextestprep

**Published by**

WANDERER STUDIOS

**2019**

# Table of Contents

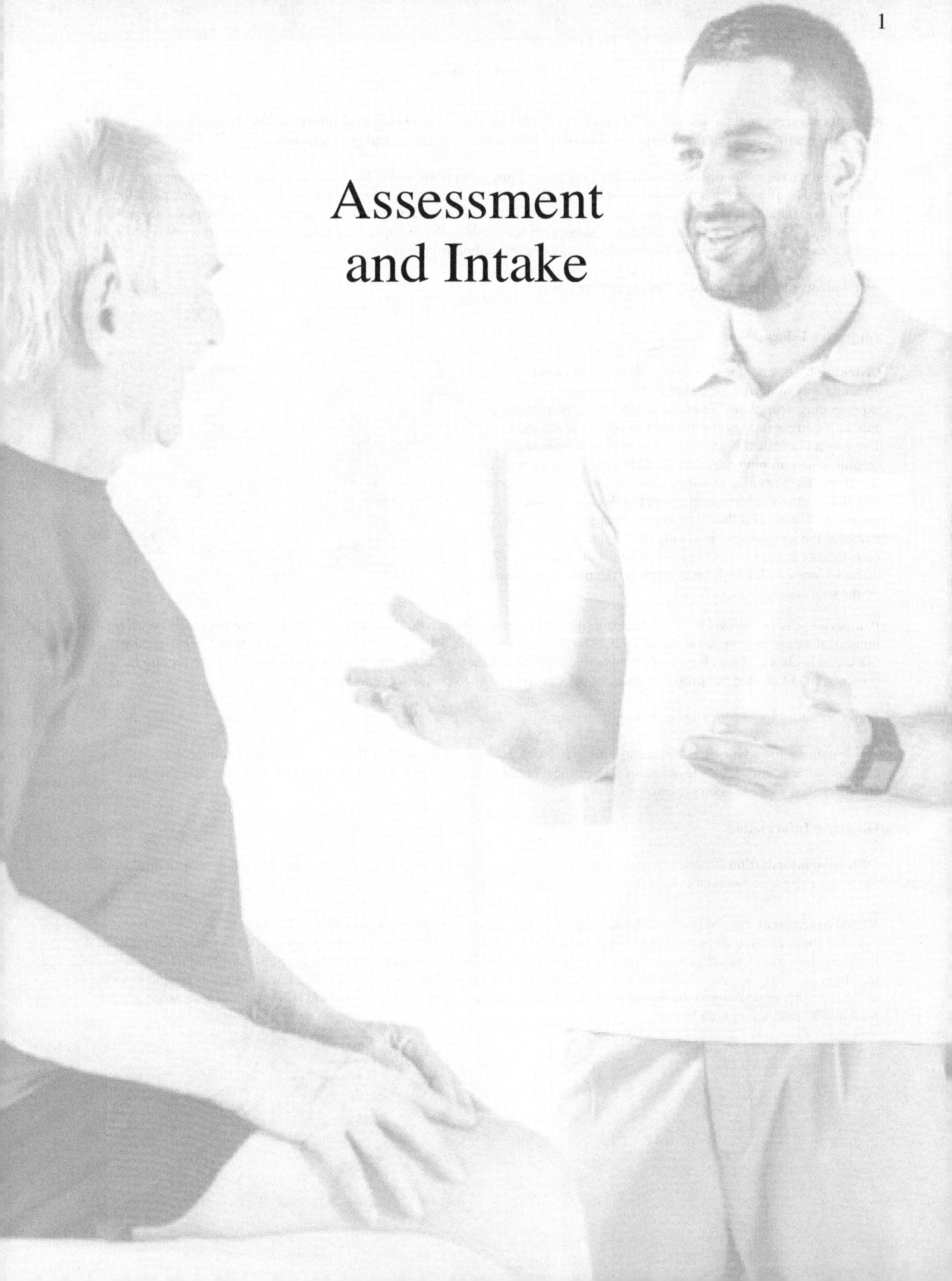

# Assessment and Intake

## Assessment

Assessments are a vital component of any massage treatment. Assessments are **evaluations** of the client primarily done before a massage, but the therapist is constantly assessing, even during and after a treatment.

Assessments have many different uses, from determining any contraindications the client may have, to tailoring a massage session specifically for that client and what they need. An example could be, if a client complains of low back pain, the therapist could then do visual assessment, range-of-motion exercises, and palpation to determine what the possible cause of the low back pain could be. Then, after the assessment is complete, the therapist may tailor the session to work specifically on the areas of concern(possibly the hamstrings, quadratus lumborum, psoas major, or rectus femoris).

Assessments may be performed in many different ways:

### Subjective Information

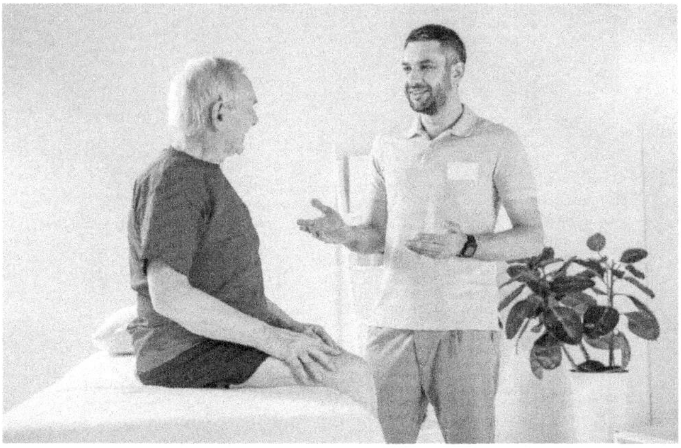

**Listening** to the client and their complaints is the most effective way to determine issues a client may be experiencing. Anything the client details about themselves and their current state is considered subjective information. The way a client details areas of concern may be extremely helpful in determining the cause of their issues. An example, if a client begins stating that they have pain in the lower back, and also pain in the hamstrings, then the therapist might inquire as to activities the client is performing that may put strain on the hamstrings. Knowing that tightness in the hamstrings can lead to pain in the low back can help the therapist work with the client to alleviate the pain by working on the root cause.

Pain levels may be utilized by the therapist to determine exactly how painful an area is. A pain scale is usually based on numerical value, ranging from 1-5 or 1-10. The higher the number a client states, the more pain they are experiencing. In the scenario above, if the client were to state that their back pain was at a 6 out of 10, then the pain they are feeling is present and noticeable, but probably does not affect their ability to perform every day actions.

Some questions to consider when dealing with pain:

Is this pain acute and localized in one specific area, such as sprained ankles? Is the pain widespread and more chronic, such as with Multiple Sclerosis? Does the pain come and go, or is it persistent? What does the pain feel like? How long has the pain been present?

### Objective Information

**Objective information** is anything that the therapist can physically see or observe. This information is measurable, and is not up to a client or therapist's interpretation of the information.

**Visual assessment** may be performed, focusing on alignment of specific bony landmarks to determine areas of concern. Some of these areas to compare bilaterally include the ears(possible neck tension), acromion processes (shoulder/back/chest tension), iliac crests(back/hip/thigh tension), anterior superior iliac spines(back/hip/thigh tension), and head of fibulae(back/hip/thigh tension). Visual assessment also includes how a client presents themselves while doing things as simple as talking to the therapist or walking to the massage room. A therapist may be able to tell if a client is limping, or is in some sort of pain just by interacting with them.

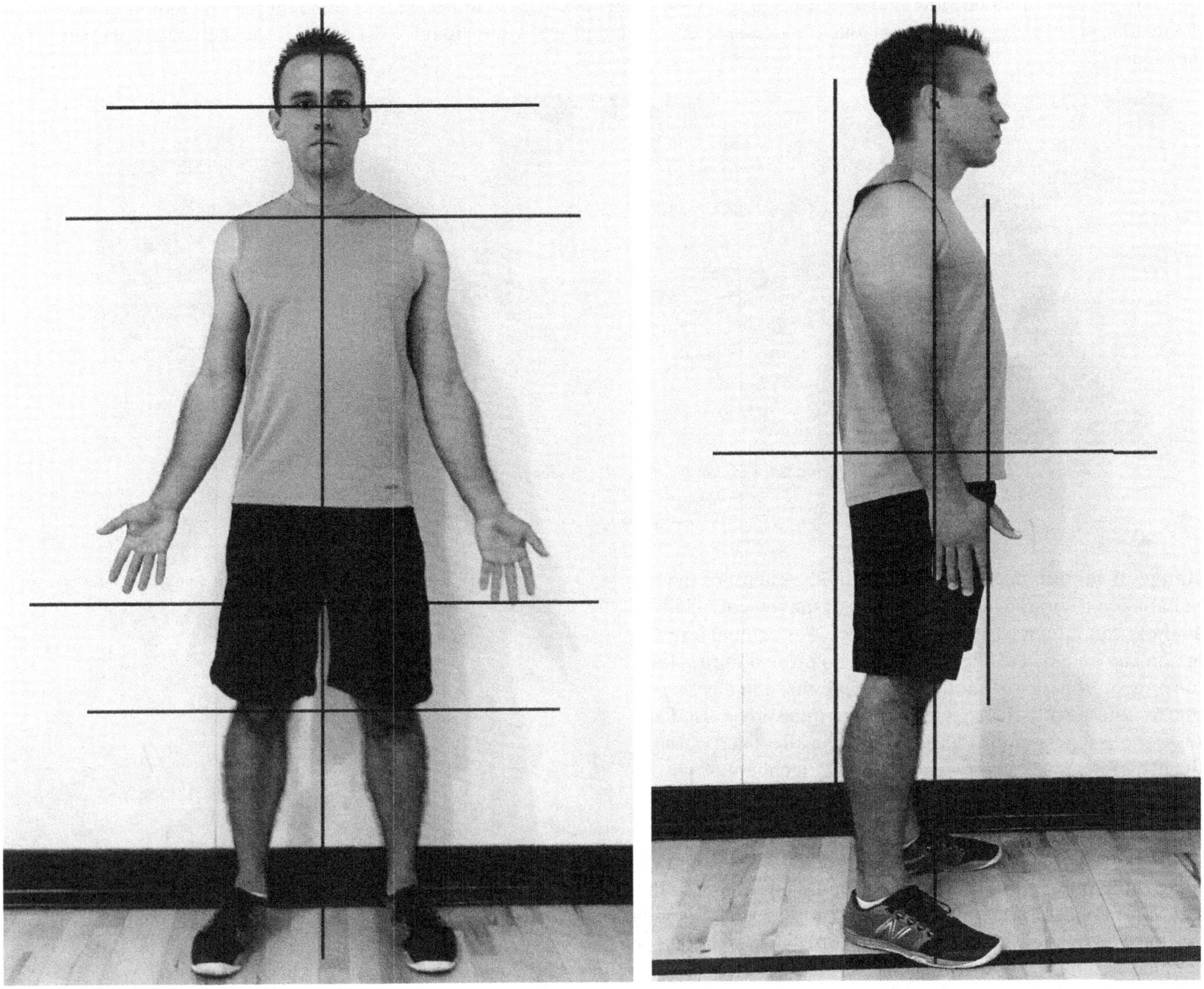

Common areas of visual assessment. These areas can be observed while standing, in addition to the client performing range-of-motion or gait analysis. This allows the therapist to observe any abnormalities between standing and performing an action.

The therapist may be able to see certain things in a person's skin, such as inflammation or pallor. Edema and skin infections are physically observable. Scars may be a sign of past trauma that could be causing pain or discomfort. Physical disabilities can often be observed in people with conditions such as cerebral palsy or paralysis.

**Gait analysis** may help determine hypertonic muscles unilaterally, and injuries. When observing a client walking, the therapist should pay attention to any imbalances the client has. This may indicate structural issues, pain, muscle weakness, or neurological issues. Observing the feet and their position while walking can give the therapist an idea of muscle tightness or previous injuries if the foot is over-pronated or over-supinated. Pain may be expressed on the face while walking.

**Palpation** is useful in feeling for adhesions or restrictions in muscles, localized ischemia, and inflammation. Ischemia, which is the lack of blood flow into an area, will feel cool to the touch. Inflammation, due to an increased amount of blood in the area, should feel warm to the touch. Assessing edema and pitting edema(page 138) requires the therapist to palpate the area.

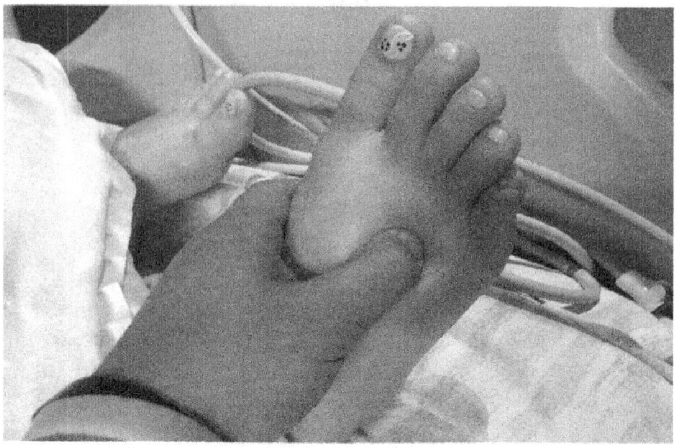
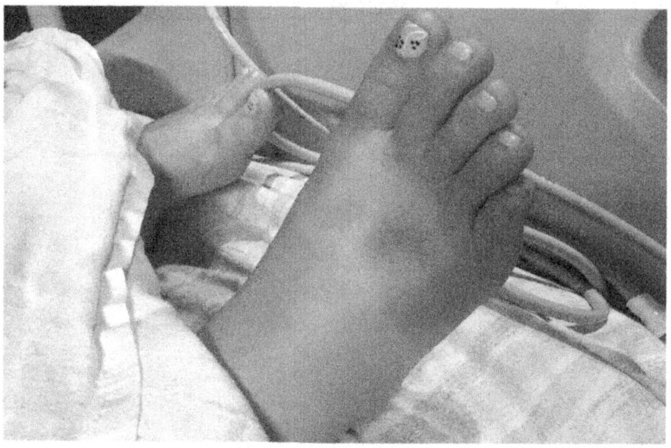

Palpation helps to assess pitting edema, seen above.

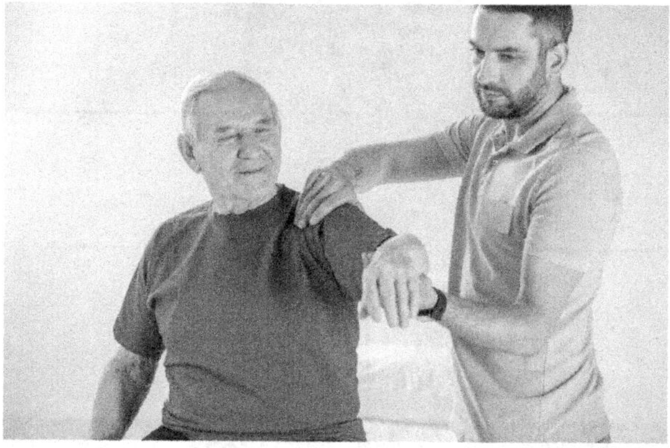

**Range-of-motion** may be performed by the client for the therapist to determine any restrictions of movement. Gait analysis can fall under range-of-motion. Performing any action can help determine if there is pain present during the movement, if range-of-motion is compromised in any way due to injuries or imbalances, or to determine any muscular restrictions a person may have that can be alleviated through the use of massage therapy and stretching techniques.

**Breathing** may be observed visually and via listening to the client's breathing rate and pattern. Shortness of breath may be cause for concern if there is no known cause, such as exercise. Increased respiration may be the result of the sympathetic response being activated and indicates stress. Watching a person breathe and how their body moves during respiration can help determine if there are any structural issues affecting breathing. Wheezing and coughing may indicate some sort of infection, or that the client is in the acute stage of a condition such as asthma.

**Precautions**

During a massage, certain precautions need to be adhered to in order to prevent injury or complications to the client.

**Endangerment sites** are areas of the body that, while massage may be performed on, need to be treated with **extra caution**. These are commonly due to insufficient tissues in the area to support, cushion, and protect important structures like blood vessels and nerves. Endangerment sites include the anterior triangle of the neck, the axilla, the anterior elbow, and the popliteal region.

**Local contraindications** are areas of the body that must be **avoided** when performing a massage. While endangerment sites allow for massage to be performed, local contraindications do not permit massage on localized areas. Reasons for a part of the body to be considered a local contraindication vary, from inflammation and trauma to infections(such as athlete's foot). The rest of the body may receive massage, but these specific areas must be avoided.

**Absolute contraindications prohibit** the use of massage. Massage on a person with an absolute contraindication, such as when a person is infected by a virus like influenza, can worsen the condition for the client, cause damage to the body, or even spread an infection or condition to the massage therapists. Do not perform a massage on a client with an absolute contraindication!

## Endangerment Sites

Common endangerment sites on the anterior body

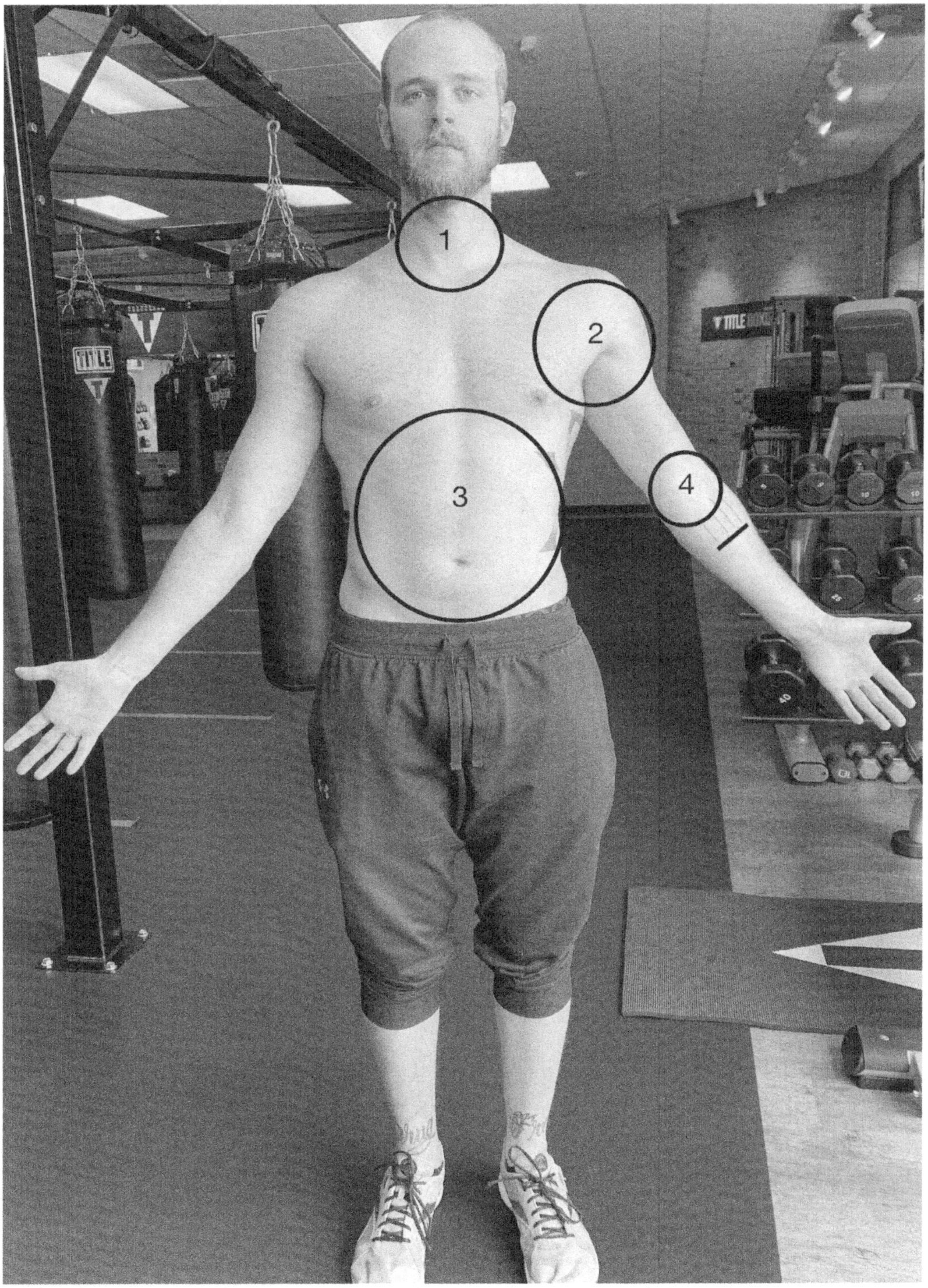


1. Anterior Triangle of the Neck
2. Axilla
3. Abdomen
4. Antecubital Region

Common endangerment sites on the posterior body

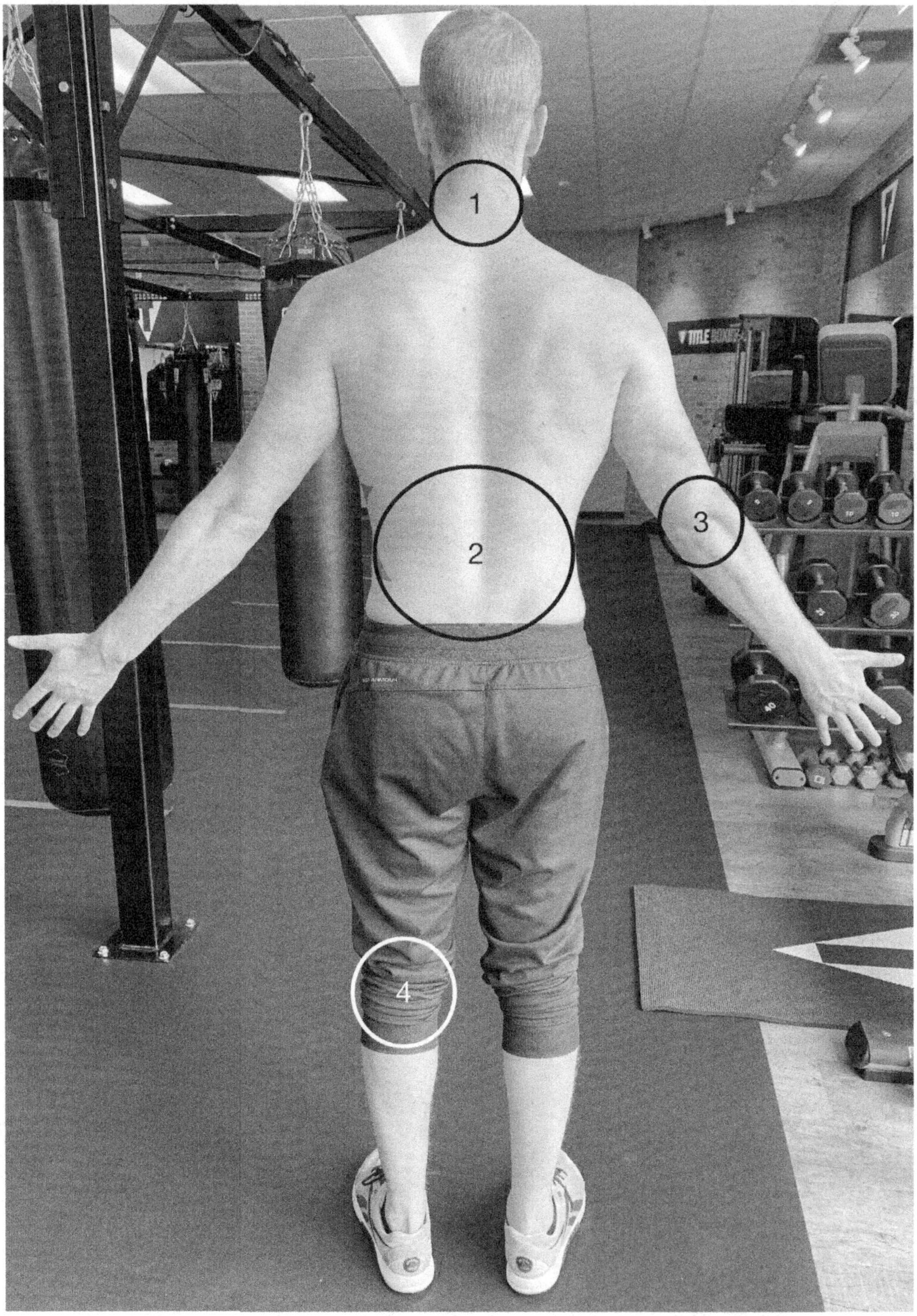


1. Posterior Neck
2. Lower Back/Floating Ribs
3. Olecranon Process
4. Popliteal Region

# Intake Forms

One of the primary ways a massage therapist can assess a client is by utilizing an intake form. These forms give the massage therapist the ability to ask numerous questions relating to the client and their well-being, which can give the therapist important insights into the client's physical and emotional states.

Intake forms should be constructed neatly, keeping similar information and questions together. This is mainly done to minimize client confusion and to speed up the time it takes for the client to fill out the form.

### Medical History

Medical history is one of the primary sections detailed on an intake form. Medical history is important because it can help determine any contraindications before the massage even begins. It may also assist the therapist in developing an effective treatment plan, even if the treatment only lasts one session. The therapist needs to be aware of any past surgeries, current injuries, illnesses, and medications the client may be taking. All of these factors can determine the appropriate type of massage to perform, the appropriate session length, etc.

An intake form should always have a section to detail any allergies a client may have. Clients may be allergic to many different types of chemicals or plants, which may be used during the massage treatment. Nut-based massage oils should be avoided. A hypo-allergenic massage lubricant should be sought to avoid any complications. Essential oils should not be automatically added to massage lubricant, as clients may be sensitive to them. Perfume scents should be avoided. Any allergies a client has should be documented by the client on the intake form.

### Informed Consent

Informed consent refers to the client authorizing services provided by the massage therapist based on all information provided by the massage therapist regarding the services. The client agreeing to these services allows the massage therapist to perform the services. An example, if the client is booked for a hot stone massage, they need to be notified of what the treatment entails, potential benefits, and potential risks. Once the client has all of the information regarding the hot stone massage, they can either approve of the service, or deny the service and book a different type of massage.

The client also needs to be made aware of the massage therapist's training, experience, and credentials in regards to the treatment being offered. This is provided so that the client is aware of the level of training provided by the massage therapist. A client may feel uneasy with a recently licensed massage therapist performing the treatment, and may instead opt for a more experienced massage therapist. Providing training information regarding specific modalities, such as hot stone massage, helps to assure the client that the therapist is knowledgeable in that modality and able to perform the treatment.

### HIPAA

The Health Insurance Portability and Accountability Act, also known as **HIPAA**, was enacted August 21st, 1996. It was created by the US Department of Health and Human Services. Inside HIPAA lies the **Privacy Rule**, which is used to **protect** all **individually identifiable** health information. The Privacy Rule ensures client/patient information is kept private. It does, however, allow this information to be transferred between healthcare providers when necessary, which allows high-quality health care. Assessments and diagnoses do not need to be re-done, as the information is already present. HIPAA should be outlined with the client intake form.

### Signature and Date

Signatures and dates should always be signed by the client at the time of the intake form being filled out. This allows for a massage therapist to have added protection in case of malpractice or negligence lawsuits.

An example of a client intake form can be found on the following page.

## Wanderer Studios Client Intake Form

Name: ______________________________ Date of Birth: ______________________

Telephone: ______________________ Email: ______________________________

Emergency Contact: ______________________ Relationship: ____________________

Emergency Contact Phone: __________________________

Occupation: _____________________ Hobbies: ______________________________

Reason for Visit: ____________________________________________________

---

### Health History

Check all that apply:

| | | |
|---|---|---|
| ____ Allergies | ____ Cancer | ____ Pregnant |
| ____ Arthritis | ____ Diabetes | ____ Psoriasis |
| ____ Asthma | ____ Headaches | ____ Scoliosis |
| ____ Back Pain | ____ High Blood Pressure | ____ Seizures |
| ____ Blood Clots | ____ Numbness/Tingling | ____ Skin Conditions |
| ____ Bruise Easily | ____ Osteoporosis | ____ Varicose Veins |

Are you taking medications? If so, please list: ___________________________________
__________________________________________________________________

Any past surgeries? If so, please list: _____________________________________

Do you exercise: Y/N If so, how frequently?: _________________________________

Have you received massage therapy before: Y/N

Are there any areas you would like the massage therapist to avoid: Y/N

If so, please list: ___________________________________________________
__________________________________________________________________
__________________________________________________________________

Please highlight any areas on the body you would like the massage therapist to concentrate on during the session

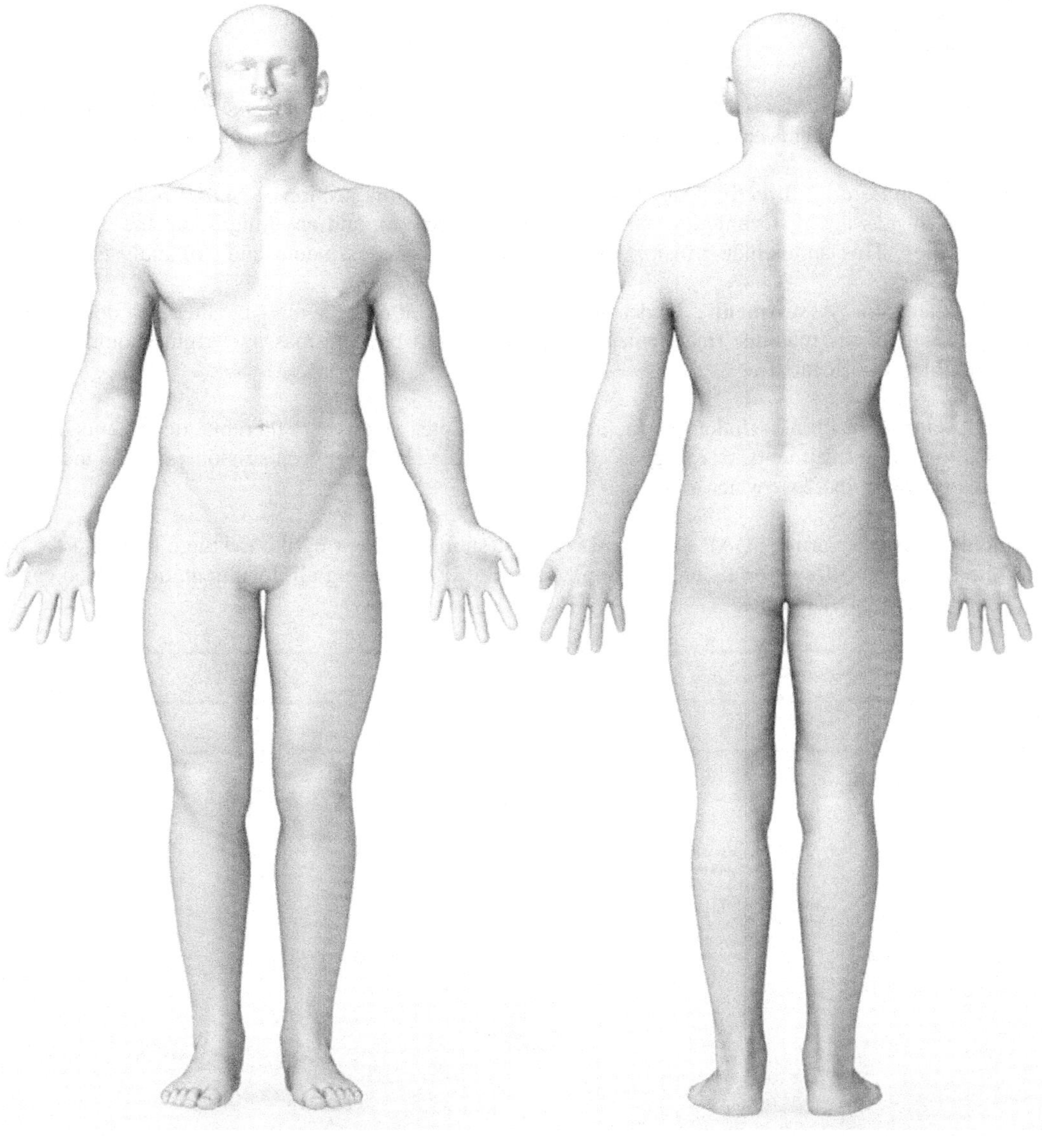

Please explain the areas highlighted: ____________________________________________
________________________________________________________________________
________________________________________________________________________
________________________________________________________________________

Print Name: ______________________________________

Signature: ______________________________________

Date: ______________________________________

## SOAP Notes

**SOAP notes** are the most common form of post-massage documentation. SOAP notes help a massage therapist **document** everything that happened or was said during a massage session. Documenting this information can be helpful in many different ways, from tailoring future massage treatments to protecting the therapist from any malpractice or negligence lawsuits that may arise.

The "**S**" of SOAP stands for "**Subjective**". Under this section of SOAP notes, a massage therapist documents anything the client details about themselves. This can include where they experience pain, their job or hobbies, etc.

The "**O**" of SOAP stands for "**Objective**" or "**Observation**". Under this section of SOAP notes, a massage therapist documents the type of massage or techniques being performed(objective), and anything about the client the therapist can physically see(observe). This can include bruising, inflammation, visual assessments, and gait analysis.

The "**A**" of SOAP stands for "**Assessment**". Under this section of SOAP notes, a massage therapist documents any changes in the client as a result of the massage treatment. An example could be "Pre-massage, right shoulder elevated. Post-massage, right shoulder less elevated".

The "**P**" of SOAP stands for "**Plan**". Under this section of SOAP notes, a massage therapist documents any recommendations for future treatments, or exercises suggested for the client between sessions(such as increase stretching in a specific muscle or area, or increase water intake).

**Client files**, including intake forms, SOAP notes, and receipts, should be kept by the massage therapist for a minimum of **six** years, per the IRS. This allows for audits to take place by the IRS. Having all documentation stored can help prevent any possible penalties issued by the IRS.

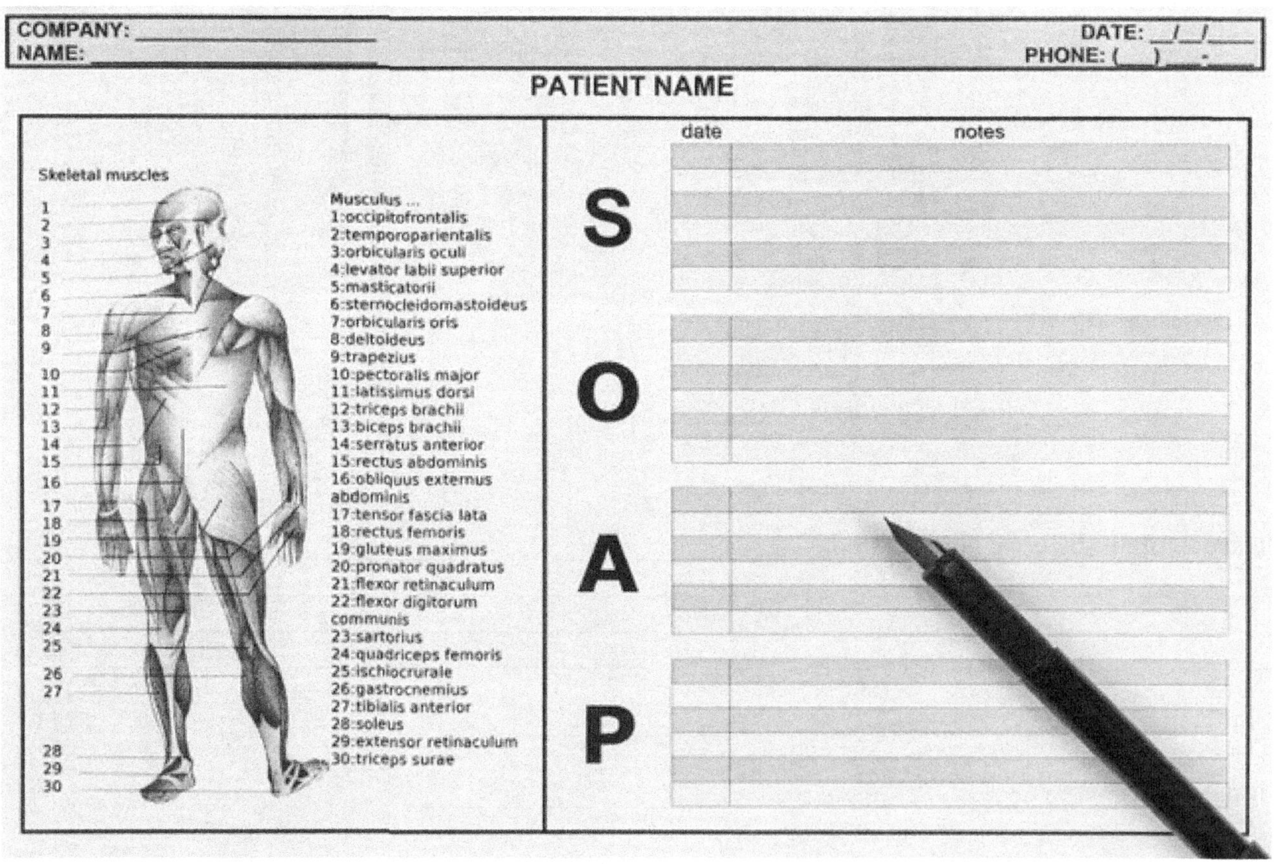

# Assessment and Intake

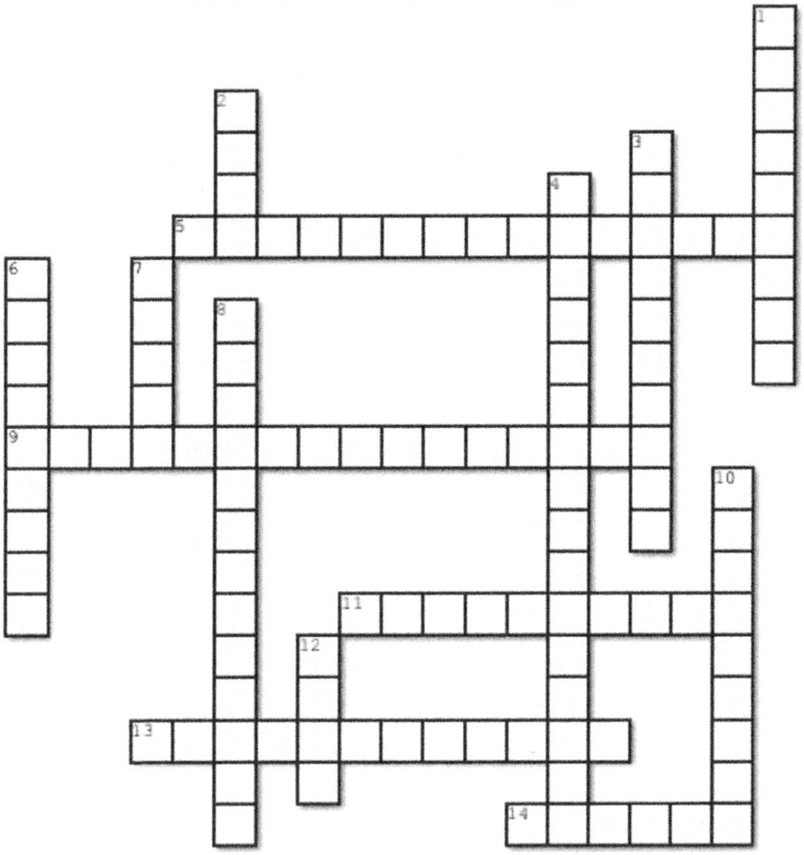

**Across**

5. The client authorizing treatment based on being provided all available information about the treatment
9. A location on the body that warrants caution while performing a massage on the area
11. Information the client details about themselves and their state of being
13. Observing a person's walking pattern
14. Form used to determine a client's expectations, medical history, contraindications, and overall well-being

**Down**

1. Touching an area to feel for things like inflammation, edema, and adhesions
2. Section on SOAP notes where any future recommendations the therapist has given are detailed
3. An evaluation of the client primarily before the massage begins
4. A condition or situation that prevents a massage from being performed on one part of the body or in totality
6. The most effective way to determine a client's needs, expectations, and issues
7. Act that ensures a client's information is kept private and protected
8. The amount of movement that is able to be performed at a specific joint or by a specific muscle
10. Information that is observable and measurable
12. Documentation of the massage session is most commonly performed by using this form

Answer Key on Page 286

## Assessment and Intake Quiz

1. Plan information is
A. Information the client shares about themselves
B. Measurable information visible to the massage therapist
C. Medical conditions the client has been assessed with
D. Recommendations for future massage sessions

2. A client comes in for a massage, complaining of pain in the right upper trapezius and neck. The first thing a massage therapist should do in this situation is
A. Ask the client if they are taking any medications for the pain
B. Ask the client to perform range-of-motion on the affected area
C. Palpate the area to locate any adhesions present
D. Determine any causes of the pain

3. The client authorizing services based on all available information being provided to the client by the massage therapist
A. Informed consent
B. Validation
C. HIPAA
D. Boundaries

4. Medical conditions the client has been assessed with are documented on which section of SOAP notes
A. Subjective
B. Objective
C. Assessment
D. Plan

5. A glove should be worn by the massage therapist if
A. The client has an open wound on the back
B. The client has an open wound on the arm
C. The massage therapist has an open wound on the leg
D. The massage therapist has an open wound on the hand

6. Information the client shares about themselves is documented under which section of SOAP notes
A. Objective
B. Subjective
C. Assessment
D. Plan

7. HIPAA ensures client information remains
A. Confidential
B. In the government's possession
C. With the client's spouse
D. Unimportant

8. A condition that prohibits the use of massage in any fashion
A. Endangerment site
B. Indifferent contraindication
C. Local contraindication
D. Absolute contraindication

9. Gait analysis is observation and interpretation of a person's
A. Walking pattern
B. Somatic holding pattern
C. Sitting pattern
D. Range of motion

10. An assessment is performed
A. Only before and after a massage
B. Only before a massage
C. Only after a massage
D. Before, during, and after the massage

11. The best way to assess a client is by
A. Asking them to fill out an intake form
B. Palpating their hamstrings while standing
C. Reviewing SOAP notes
D. Analyzing the client's gait

12. Section of an intake form that contains past surgeries
A. Name
B. Medical history
C. Informed consent
D. Occupation

13. Common endangerment sites include all of the following except
A. Anterior triangle of the neck
B. Popliteal region
C. Abdomen
D. Anterior thigh

14. Client files should be kept by the therapist for
A. One year
B. Six years
C. Five years
D. Ten years

15. A massage condition that prohibits massage being performed in a specific area only
A. Local contraindication
B. Endangerment site
C. Absolute contraindication
D. Total contraindication

Answer Key on Page 289

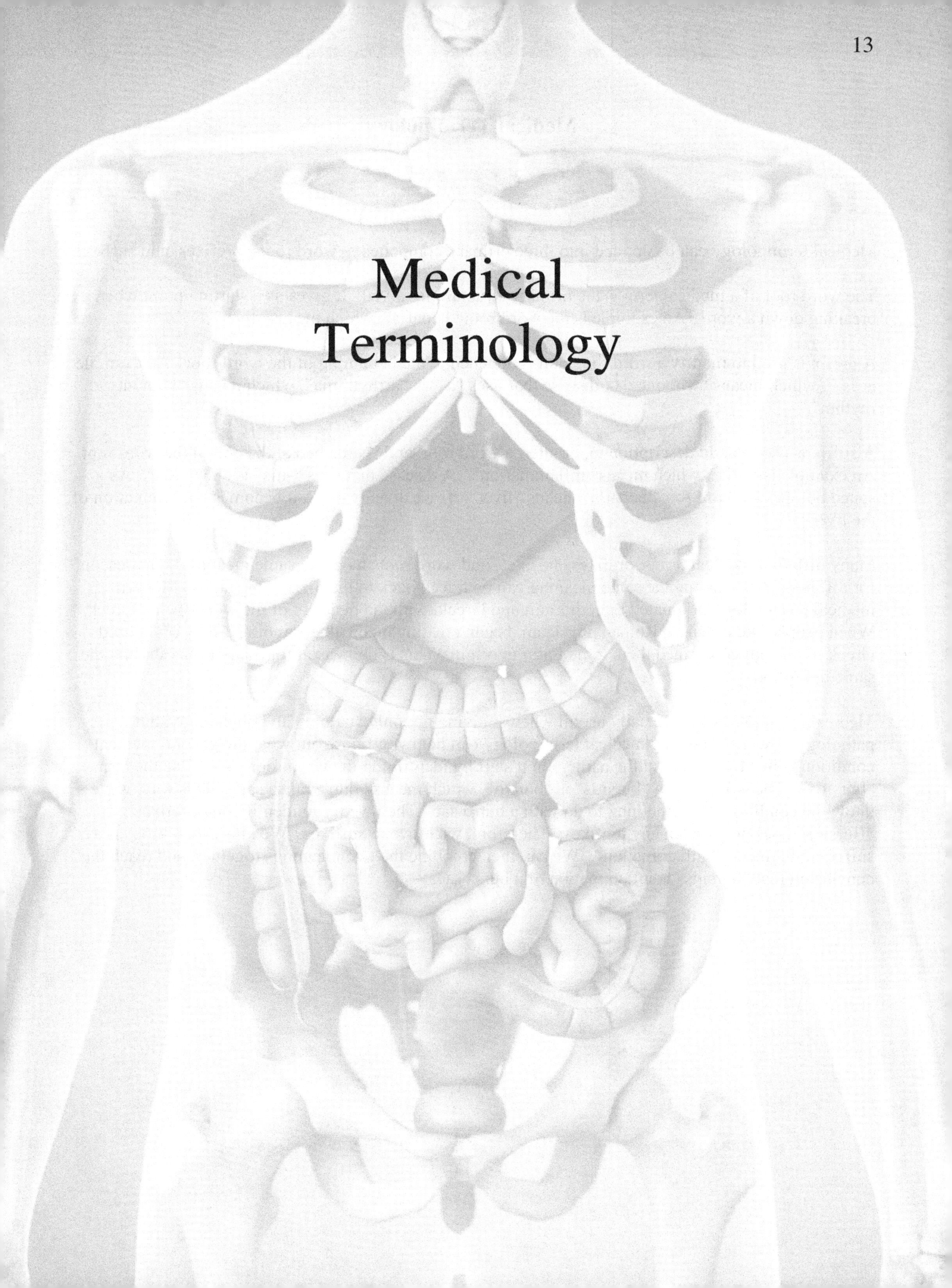

# Medical Terminology

# Medical Terminology

Medical terminology can be divided into three primary components: word roots, prefixes, and suffixes.

The word root of a medical term is the primary structure involved. It gives us a starting point when breaking down a word. An example is the word root "hepat/o", which means "liver".

A prefix is used to modify a word root, and is attached at the beginning of the word root. An example is "a-", which means "without". A disease that uses "a-" is "arrhythmia", which means "without rhythm".

A suffix is used to add description to, or alter, a word root, and is attached at the end of the word root. An example is "-itis", which means "inflammation". A disease that uses "-itis" is "hepatitis". As stated before, the word root "hepat/o" means "liver". If we attach "-itis", it becomes "inflammation of the liver".

Many different medical terms, prefixes, suffixes, and word roots have the same meaning. The reason for different terms having the same meaning can be traced back to the origin languages. Modern medical terminology originated in both Latin and Greek, with the majority of the words being Greek. When people like Celsus, a Roman physician, began creating medical terminology, they often used Greek terms, but conformed them to be Latin in origin. This is the reason for many terms sharing the same definition.

Medical terminology is especially useful when studying not only anatomy and physiology, but pathology as well. Knowing medical terminology can help you figure out what the general medical condition is just by looking at the name. First start by identifying the word root. We'll use the term "bursitis". The word root in "bursitis" is "burs/o", which means "bursa/bursa sac". This way, we know the condition has something to do with a bursa sac. Then we try to identify any prefixes. "Bursitis" does not contain any prefixes. Therefore, we move to suffixes. We know that "-itis" is a suffix, and it means "inflammation". We can then combine the two meanings together, and reach the conclusion that "bursitis" is inflammation of a bursa sac.

# Medical Terminology

### Cardiovascular Word Roots

angi/o: vessel
aort/o: aorta
arteriol/o: arteriole
arteri/o: artery
ather/o: fatty plaque
atri/o: atrium
bas/o: alkaline
cardi/o: heart
chrom/o: color
eosin/o: rose colored
granul/o: granule
hemangi/o: blood vessel
hem/o: blood
kary/o: nucleus
leuk/o: white
lymph/o: lymph
morph/o: form
myel/o: canal
nucle/o: nucleus
phag/o: eat
phleb/o: vein
poikil/o: irregular
reticul/o: mesh
scler/o: hard
sider/o: iron
sphygm/o: pulse
thromb/o: clot
vascul/o: vessel
ven/o: vein
ventricul/o: ventricle

### Digestive Word Roots

append/o: appendix
appendic/o: appendix
bucc/o: cheek
cheil/o: lip
chol/e: bile
cholangi/o: bile vessel
cholecyst/o: gallbladder
choledoch/o: bile duct
col/o: large intestine
colon/o: large intestine
dont/o: teeth
duoden/o: duodenum
enter/o: small intestine
esophag/o: esophagus
gastr/o: stomach
gingiv/o: gums
gloss/o: tongue
hepat/o: live
ile/o: ileum
jejun/o: jejunum
labi/o: lip
lingu/o: tongue
odont/o: teeth
or/o: mouth
pancreat/o: pancreas
pharyng/o: pharynx
proct/o: anus
pylor/o: pylorus
rect/o: rectum
sial/o: saliva
sigmoid/o: sigmoid colon
stomat/o: mouth

### Endocrine Word Roots

aden/o: gland
adren/o: adrenal glands
adrenal/o: adrenal glands
calc/o: calcium
gluc/o: sugar
glyc/o: sugar
gonad/o: gonads
home/o: same
kal/i: potassium
pancreat/o: pancreas
thym/o: thymus gland
thyr/o: thyroid
thyroid/o: thyroid
toxic/o: poison
thalam/o: thalamus

### Integumentary Word Roots

adip/o: fat
albin/o: white
carcin/o: cancer
cirrh/o: yellow
cutane/o: skin
cyan/o: blue
derm/o: skin
dermat/o: skin
erythem/o: red
erythemat/o: red
erythr/o: red
hidr/o: sweat
histi/o: tissue
hist/o: tissue
ichthy/o: scaly
jaund/o: yellow
kerat/o: hard
leuk/o: white
lip/o: fat
melan/o: black
myc/o: fungi
onych/o: nail
pil/o: hair
scler/o: hard
seb/o: sebum
squam/o: scale
sudor/o: sweat
trich/o: hair
ungu/o: nail
xanth/o: yellow
xer/o: dry

### Lymphatic Word Roots

aden/o: gland
adenoid/o: adenoids
immun/o: immune
leuk/o: white
lymph/o: lymph
lymphaden/o: lymph gland
lymphangi/o: lymph vessel
myel/o: canal
phag/o: eat
splen/o: spleen
thym /o: thymus
tonsill/o: tonsils

### Muscular Word Roots

adhes/o: stick to
aponeur/o: aponeurosis
duct/o: carry
erg/o: work
fasci/o: fascia
fibr/o: fiber
fibros/o: fiber
flex/o: bend
is/o: same
kinesi/o: movement
lei/o: smooth
lev/o: lift
levat/o: lift
metr/o: length
quadr/i: four
quadr/o: four
rect/o: straight
rhabd/o: rod-shaped
ten/o: tendon
tend/o: tendon
tendin/o: tendon
tens/o: strain
ton/o: tension
tort/i : twisted

### Nervous Word Roots

astr/o: star
ax/o: axon
cephal/o: head
cerebell/o: cerebellum
clon/o: clonus
cortic/o: cortex
crani/o: skull
dendr/o: tree
dur/o: dura mater
encephal/o: brain
esthesi/o: sensation
gangli/o: ganglion
gli/o: glue
kinesi/o: movement
lex/o: word
lob/o: lobe
medull/o: medulla
mening/o: meninges
ment/o: mind
mot/o: move
myel/o: canal
narc/o: stupor
neur/o: nerve
olig/o: few
phas/o: speech
phren/o: mind
psych/o: mind
spin/o: spine

synapt/o: point of contact
tax/o: order
thalam/o: thalamus
thec/o: sheath

### Reproductive Word Roots

amni/o: amnion
andr/o: male
cervic/o: neck
colp/o: vagina
vagin/o: vagina
embry/o: embryo
epididym/o: epididymis
episi/o: vulva
fet/o: fetus
galact/o: milk
genit/o: genitalia
gynec/o: woman
hyster/o: uterus
hymen/o: hymen
lact/o: milk
leiomy/o: smooth muscle
mamm/o: breast
mast/o: breast
men/o: menstruation
metr/o: uterus
nat/o: birth
o/o: egg
oophor/o: ovary
orch/o: testicle
ovari/o: ovary
pen/o: penis
perine/o: perineum
prostat/o: prostate
salping/o: fallopian tube
sperm/o: sperm
spermat/o: sperm
test/o: testicle
uter/o: uterus
vagin/o: vagina
vas/o: vessel
vesicul/o: seminal vesicle
vulv/o: vulva

### Respiratory Word Roots

alveol/o: alveolus
anthrac/o: black
atel/o: incomplete
bronch/o: bronchus
bronchi/o: bronchus
coni/o: dust
cyan/o: blue
embol/o: plug
emphys/o: inflate
epiglott/o: epiglottis
hem/o: blood
laryng/o: larynx
lob/o: lobe
muc/o: mucous
nas/o: nose
or/o: mouth
orth/o: straight
ox/o: oxygen
pector/o: chest
pharyng/o: pharynx
phon/o: sound
phren/o: diaphragm
pleur/o: pleura
pneum/o: lung
pneumon/o: lung
pulm/o: lung
rhin/o: nose
sinus/o: sinus
spir/o: breathe
steth/o: chest
thorac/o: chest
trache/o: trachea

### Skeletal Word Roots

acr/o: extremity
acromi/o: acromion
ankyl/o: crooked
arthr/o: joint
brachi/o: arm
calcane/o: calcaneus
carp/o: carpals
cephal/o: head
cervic/o: neck
chondr/o: cartilage
clavicul/o: clavicle
cleid/o: clavicle
condyl/o: condyle
cost/o: ribs
crani/o: cranium
dactyl/o: fingers/toes
femor/o: femur
fibul/o fibula
humer/o: humerus
ili/o: ilium
ischi/o: ischium
kyph/o: hill
lamin/o: lamina
lord/o: curve
metacarp/o: metacarpals
metatars/o: metatarsals
myel/o: canal
orth/o: straight
oste/o: bone
patell/o: patella
ped/i: foot
pelv/i: pelvis
pelv/o: pelvis
phalang/o: phalanges
pod/o: foot
pub/o: pubis
rachi/o: spine
radi/o: radius
sacr/o: sacrum
scapul/o: scapula
scoli/o: crooked
spondyl/o: vertebrae
synov/o: synovium
tal/o: talus
tars/o: tarsals
thorac/o: chest
uln/o: ulna
vertebr/o: vertebrae

### Urinary Word Roots

albumin/o: albumin
azot/o: nitrogenous
cyst/o: bladder
glomerul/o: glomerulus
kal/i: potassium
ket/o: ketone bodies
meat/o: opening
nephr/o: kidney
pyel/o: renal pelvis
ren/o: kidney
trigon/o: trigone
ur/o: urine
ureter/o: ureter
urethr/o: urethra
urin/o: urine
vesic/o: bladder

### Oncology Word Roots

aden/o: gland
blast/o: germ cell
carcin/o: cancer
cauter/o: burn
chem/o: chemical
cry/o: cold
hist/o: tissue
immun/o: immunity
leiomy/o: smooth muscle
leuk/o: white
mut/a: genetic change
myel/o: canal
onc/o: tumor
rhabdomy/o: skeletal muscle
sarc/o: connective tissue

### Miscellaneous Word Roots

aur/i: ear
bi/o: life
burs/o: bursa
cerat/o: horn
chir/o: hand
corac/o: crow-like
coron/o: crown
dextr/o: right
dors/o: back
dynam/o: power
ect/o: outside
faci/o: face
glauc/o: gray
hydr/o: water
irid/o: iris
kerat/o: cornea
lacrim/o: tear
lapar/o: abdominal wall
myring/o: eardrum
omphal/o: navel
opthalam/o: eye
phot/o: light
py/o: pus
pyr/o: heat
therm/o: heat
tympan/o: eardrum
viscer/o: internal organs
zo/o: animal
zym/o: fermentation

**Prefixes**

a-: without
ab-: away
ad-: towards
af-: towards
allo-: other
an-: without
ana-: against
aniso-: unequal
ante-: before
anti-: against
auto-: self
bi two
brady-: slow
cine-: movement
circum-: around
contra-: against
de-: cessation
di-: double
dia-: through
dipl-: double
dys-: difficult
ec-: out
echo-: repeated sound
ecto-: outside
ef-: away
en-: within
end-: within
endo-: within
epi-: above
eso-: inward
eu-: good
ex-: outside
exo-: outside
extra-: outside
hemi-: half
hetero-: different
homo-: same
hyper-: excessive
hypo-: below
im-: not
in-: in
infra-: below
inter-: between
intra-: inside
iso-: same
macro-: large
mal-: bad
meso-: middle
meta-: change
micro-: small
mono-: one
multi-: many
neo-: new
nulli-: none
oxy-: sharp
pan-: all
para-: beside
per-: through
peri-: around
poly-: many
post-: after
pre-: before
primi-: first
pro-: before
pseudo-: false
quadri-: four
retro-: behind
semi-: half
sub-: under
super-: above
supra-: above
sym-: together
syn-: together
tachy-: rapid
trans-: through
tri-: three
ultra-: excessive
uni-: one

**Suffixes**

-ac: referring to
-acusis: hearing
-al: referring to
-algia: pain
-ar: referring to
-ary: referring to
-ate: form of
-ation: process
-asthenia: weakness
-blast: germ cell
-capnia: carbon dioxide
-cele: hernia
-centesis: puncture
-clasis: break
-clast: break
-crine: secrete
-cusis: hearing
-cyte: cell
-desis: binding
-derma: skin
-duction: bringing
-dynia: pain
-eal: referring to
-ectasis: dilation
-ectomy: removal
-edema: swelling
-emesis: vomiting
-emia: blood
-esis: condition
-esthesia: sensation
-ferent: to carry
-gen: produce
-genesis: produce
-globin: protein
-gnosis: knowing
-gram: record
-graph: recording
-graphy: recording
-ia: condition
-iasis: abnormal condition
-iatry: medicine
-ic: referring to
-ical: referring to
-ician: specialist
-icle: small
-ile: referring to
-ine: referring to
-ism: condition
-ist: specialist
-itis: inflammation
-kinesia: movement
-lalia: speech
-lampsia: shine
-lepsy: seizure
-lith: stone
-logist: specializing in
-logy: study of
-lucent: clear
-lysis: dissolve
-malacia: soften
-mania: frenzy
-megaly: enlargement
-meter: measuring tool
-metry: measuring
-oid: resembling
-oma: tumor
-orexia: appetite
-ory: referring to
-ose: referring to
-osis: condition
-ous: referring to
-paresis: partial paralysis
-pathy: disease
-penia: deficiency
-pexy: fixation
-phasia: speech
-philia: attraction
-phobia: fear
-phoria: feeling
-phylaxis: protection
-physis: growth
-plasia: formation
-plasm: growth
-plasty: repair
-plegia: paralysis
-pnea: breathing
-poiesis: formation
-porosis: porous
-rrhage: bursting forth
-rrhaphy: suture
-rrhea: discharge
-rrhexis: rupture
-scope: examining
-spasm: twitch
-scopy: visual exam
-stenosis: narrowing
-stomy: opening
-tension: stretch
-thorax: chest
-thymia: emotion
-tic: referring to
-tomy: incision
-toxic: poison
-tripsy: crushing
-trophy: nourishment
-uria: urine
-y: condition

## General Medical Terms

### A

ABC: References things to check before administering resuscitation efforts, Airway, Breathing, Circulation.
Abscess: A localized collection of pus.
Acute: Sudden, severe onset of a medical condition or disease.
Adhesion: Stuck together.
Ambulant/Ambulatory: The ability to walk.
Arrest: Cessation of bodily activity or function.
Aseptic: Sterile.
Autonomy: Being self-governed.

### B

Benign: Does not spread.
Biopsy: Surgically removing tissue to examine microscopically.

### C

Cachexia: Loss of appetite, weight, with muscle atrophy, usually associated with a serious medical condition such as cancer.
Carcinogen: A substance that may cause cancer.
Chronic: A disease or condition that persists over a period of time.

### D

Diagnosis: Determination of the cause of a disease.

### E

Edema: An excessive accumulation of fluid in an area.
Etiology: The study of the cause of a disease.
Excision: Surgically removing a structure or tissue.

### F

Febrile: Presence of a fever.
Fistula: Location where an organ has developed an opening into another organ.

### I

Idiopathic: An unknown cause of disease.
Incision: Cutting into, typically with a scalpel.
Incontinence: Loss of control of the bladder and/or bowels.
In Situ: "In original place", commonly references cancer that is still in its place of origin, such as the epithelium of the skin.
Intravenous: Inside a vein, usually referencing injections.
Ischemia: Lack of blood flow to an area, which may result in necrosis.

### M

Malaise: General unwell feeling or discomfort.
Malformation: A structure that is not formed properly.
Malignant: Spreading of cancer from one area to another.

### N

Necrosis: Death of tissue.
Neopathy: A new disease.

### P

Pallor: General paleness.
Palsy: Paralysis.
Peptic: Referring to the stomach.
Phlegm: Secretions expelled from the lungs, also known as sputum.
Phobia: Fear of a person, thing, or situation.
Prognosis: Predicted outcome of a disease and recovery rate.
Pulse: Expansion of an artery as blood passes through.
Pyrogenic: Producing fever.

### S

Sepsis: An infection.
Sign: Observable indications of an illness.
Sinus: A cavity.
Sputum: Secretions expelled from the lungs, also known as phlegm.
Symptom: A physical manifestation of an illness.
Syndrome: Groups of symptoms caused by a disease.

### T

Transient: Short duration.

# Anatomy and Physiology

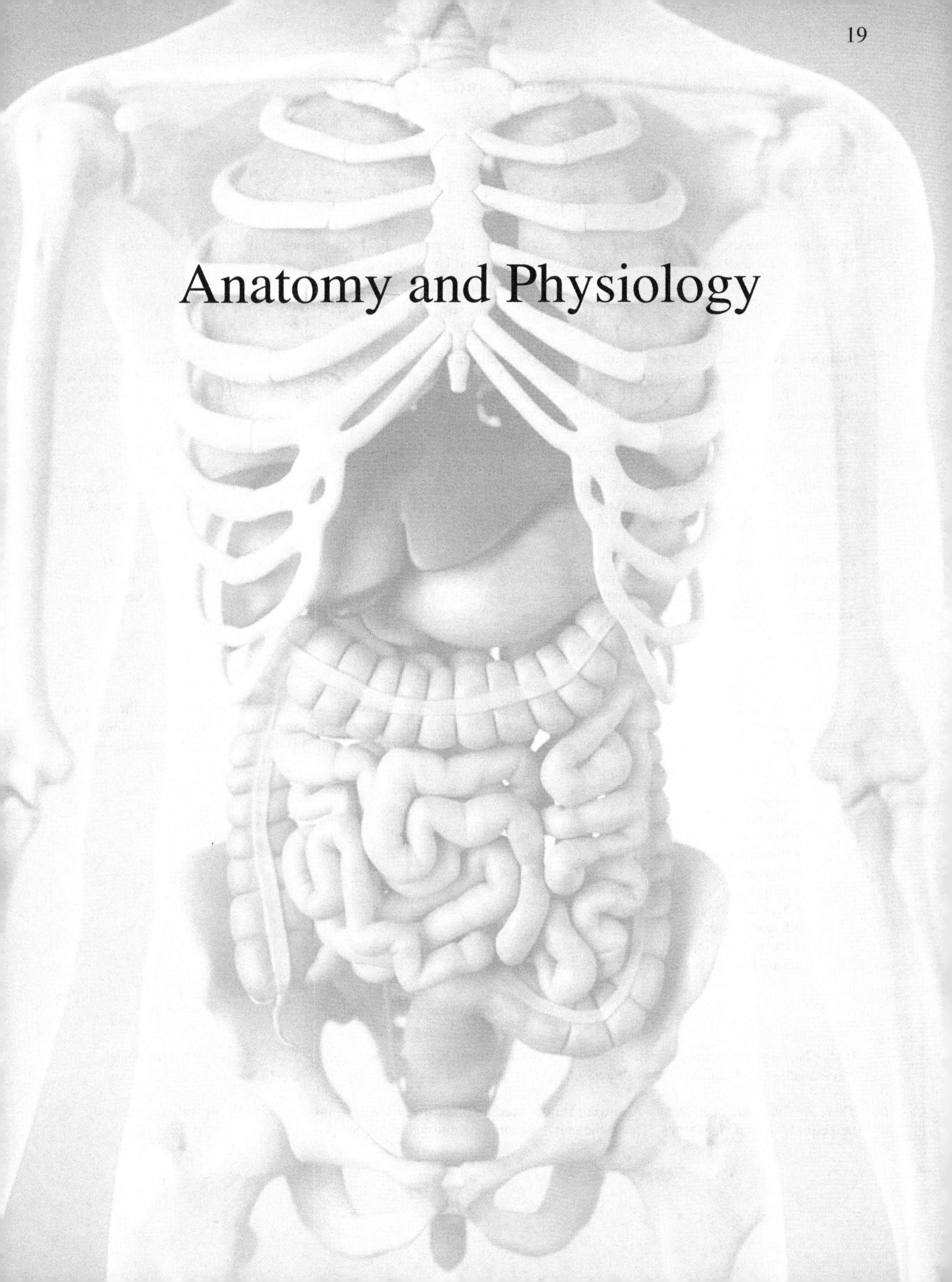

# Anatomy and Physiology

Anatomy and Physiology, two extremely important aspects of the human body. **Anatomy**, simply put, is the study of the **structure** of the human body. All of the parts that make up the body constitute anatomy, from bones, muscles, and nerves, to cells, tendons, ligaments, and everything in between.

**Physiology** is the study of the **function** of the body. How do the parts of the body that make up the body's anatomy function? What do they do? This is physiology. Anatomy and Physiology go hand-in-hand.

## Homeostasis

**Homeostasis** is the existence and maintenance of a **constant internal environment**. The body's internal environment is constantly changing and responding to various stimuli. Examples of stimuli are temperature, hormones, diet, and the body's pH level. These stimuli that change the body's internal environment in some way are known as **homeostatic variables**. As the variables change, so too does the internal environment.

How does the body respond to these changes? Using **homeostatic mechanisms**, such as sweating and shivering. An example, when your body temperature gets too high, your body mechanically(physically) responds by sweating. Sweat evaporates off the skin, which cools the body down, lowering body temperature. When the body becomes too cold, the body responds by mechanically increasing the amount of twitching in the skeletal muscles. This increased twitching, which is normally undetectable, results in shivering, which produces body heat, raising body temperature.

The body's internal environment is constantly changing, and the body constantly adjusts certain aspects of itself to respond to these changes. If temperature is an example, the **set point**(normal range) of a body's temperature is 98.6 degrees Fahrenheit. The internal body temperature is never set right at 98.6 degrees. It is constantly fluctuating around the set point, maintaining a normal range of optimal body function.

## Regional Anatomy

Regional Anatomy is the study of the structures of the body, broken down into different parts. When describing the position of one structure in the body in relation to another structure or structures, we use **directional terms**. An example, using the term "medial condyle" instead of just "condyle" lets us communicate effectively which condyle is being discussed.

The main directional terms are:

- **Superior**: Above.
- **Inferior**: Below.
- **Anterior**: Front.
- **Posterior**: Back.
- **Proximal**: Closer to the midline.
- **Distal**: Further from the midline.
- **Medial**: Middle.
- **Lateral**: Side.
- **Deep**: More internal.
- **Superficial**: Towards the surface.

## Body Planes

Body planes are important for viewing structures from different aspects. These can be used when doing simple visual assessment, or in instances such as surgery or cadaver dissection.

There are four main body planes: A **midsagittal**, or **median** plane, runs down the **midline** of the body, splitting the body into **equal left and right sides**. This is the only location for a midsagittal plane.

A **sagittal** plane also splits the body into left or right sides, but **not equally**. It can be located anywhere along the body except down the midline.

A **transverse**, or **horizontal** plane, splits the body into **superior and inferior** portions. It does not have to be at the waist. It can split the body into superior and inferior at any point along the body.

A **frontal**, or **coronal** plane, as the name suggests, splits the body into front and back, or **anterior and posterior**. If a person wanted to dissect the heart and make all four chambers visible, they would cut the heart into a frontal or coronal plane. See photo on page 48.

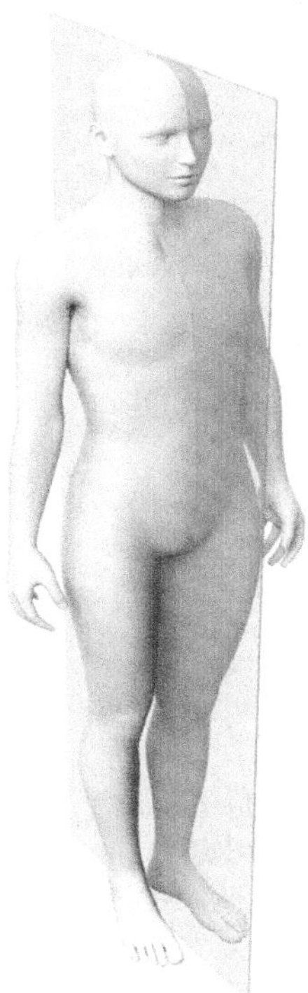

Midsagittal Plane

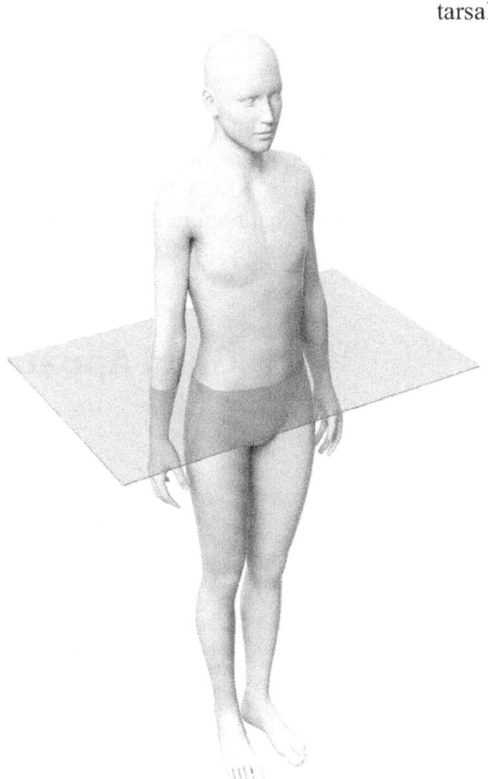

Transverse/Horizontal Plane

**Body Regions**

The body, as stated earlier, can be broken down into different parts, or regions. There are three main body regions: the **central** body region, the **upper limb**, and the **lower limb**.

The **central** body region contains all of the structures located in the center of the body: the **head**, the **neck**, and the **trunk**. Take away the arms and legs, and you're left with the central body region.

The **trunk** can be further divided into three regions: the **thorax**, or chest, the **abdomen**, and the **pelvis**. The thorax contains the heart, lungs, esophagus, thymus, and major blood vessels connecting to the heart. The abdomen contains the majority of our digestive organs, including the stomach, liver, gallbladder, pancreas, small intestine, and large intestine. It also contains the kidneys and ureters. The pelvis contains the urinary bladder, urethra, and reproductive organs.

The **upper limb** can be broken down into four regions: the **arm**, **forearm**, **wrist**, and **hand**. The arm contains the humerus. The forearm contains the radius and ulna. The wrist contains the carpals. The hand contains the metacarpals and phalanges.

The **lower limb** can also be broken down into four regions: the **thigh**, **leg**, **ankle**, and **foot**. The thigh contains the femur. The leg contains the tibia and fibula. The ankle contains the tarsals. The foot contains the metatarsals and phalanges.

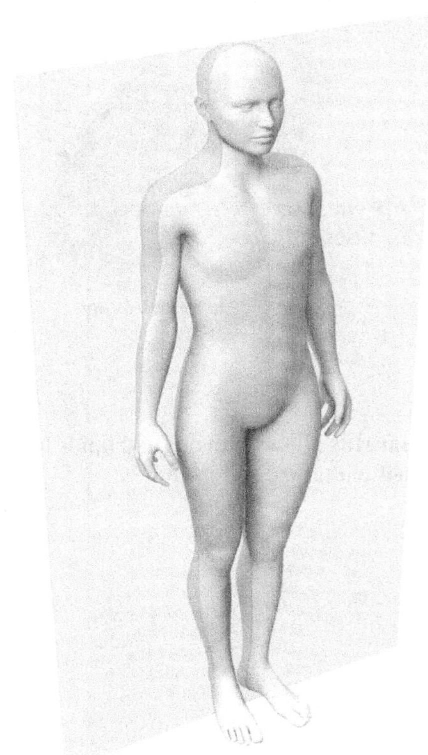

Frontal/Coronal Plane

## Cells

**Cells** are the functional **units** of all tissues. Cells are responsible for performing all essential life functions, from synthesizing nutrients to destroying pathogens and debris. Cells **divide** via a process known as **mitosis**. During mitosis, the cell splits from one single mother cell into two separate daughter cells. These daughter cells then divide further into daughter cells of their own, and the cycle repeats until enough cells are present to form a tissue.

Inside each cell are **organelles**, structures that help regulate function of the cell.

**Cytoplasm** is found inside the cell, and is a **gel-like substance**. It allows organelles, nutrients, and waste products to move throughout the cell.

CELL NUCLEUS

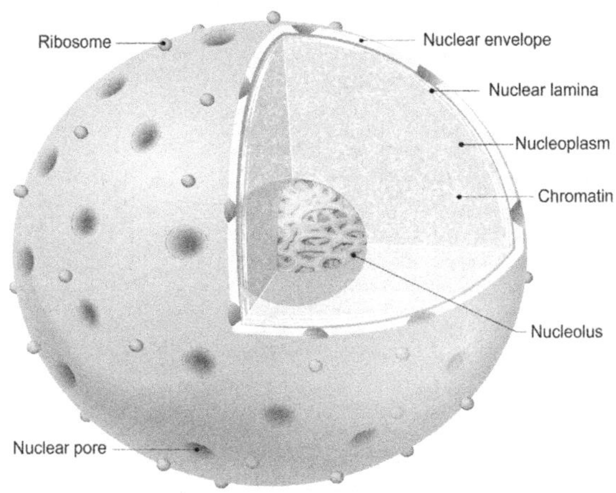


The **nucleus** regulates the **overall function** of the cell. Inside the nucleus is **DNA**(deoxyribonucleic acid), which is the building block for life. Also inside the nucleus is the **nucleolus**, which contains **RNA**(ribonucleic acid). RNA is vital in transmitting signals from DNA to ribosomes for protein synthesis.

## Mitochondrion

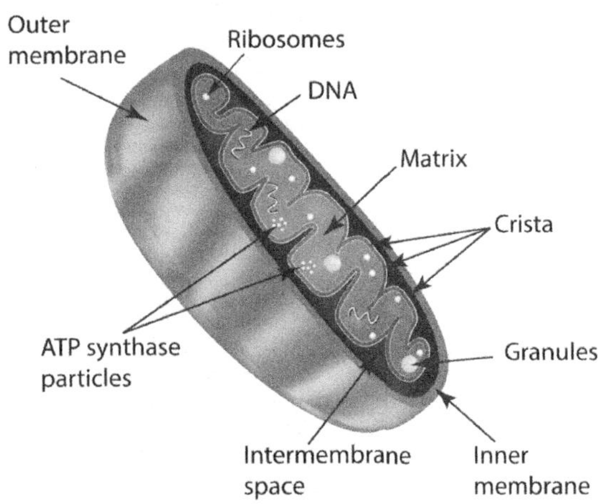


**Mitochondria** are responsible for the production of **adenosine triphosphate**(ATP), the molecule that provides **energy** to the body by transporting chemical energy to parts of the body that require it.

## Golgi Apparatus

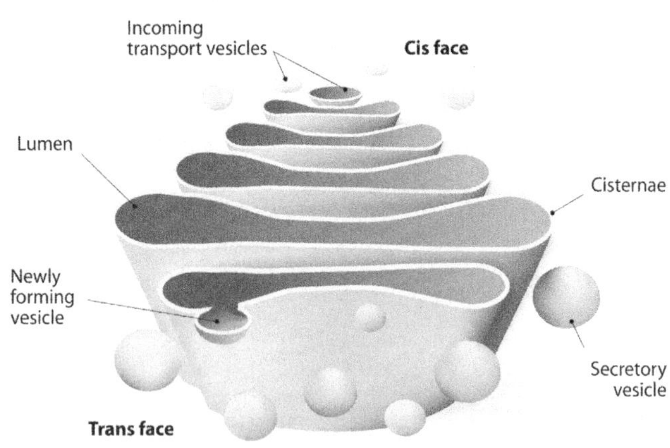


**Golgi apparatus** allows proteins and lipids to be bundled and **transported** within the cell itself.

# Endoplasmic reticulum

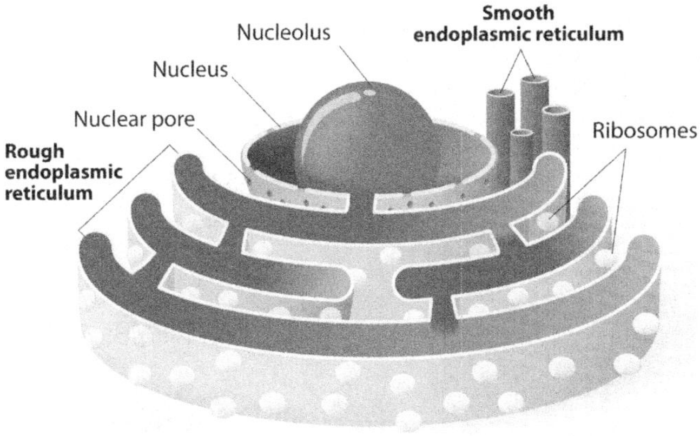


The **smooth endoplasmic reticulum** is responsible for synthesizing **carbohydrates** and **lipids** for use in producing new cell membranes. The **rough endoplasmic reticulum** is studded with **ribosomes**, and is primarily responsible for **protein** production.

# LYSOSOME

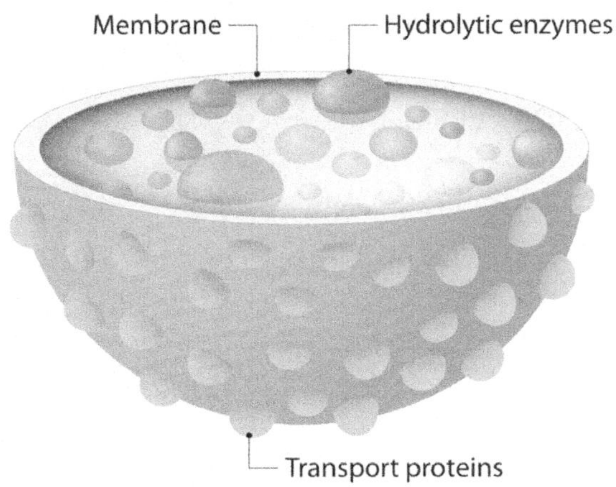


**Lysosomes** are responsible for **breaking down** several different substances inside the cell, including protein and waste products.

# Ribosome

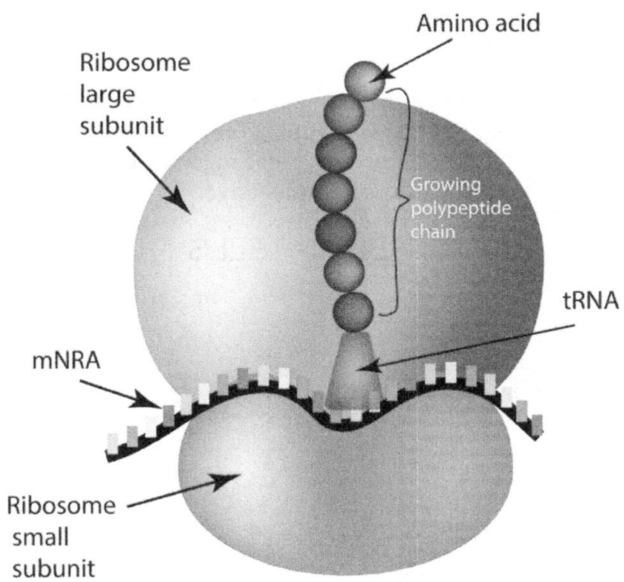


**Ribosomes**, which contain protein and RNA, are responsible for **synthesizing cell proteins**.

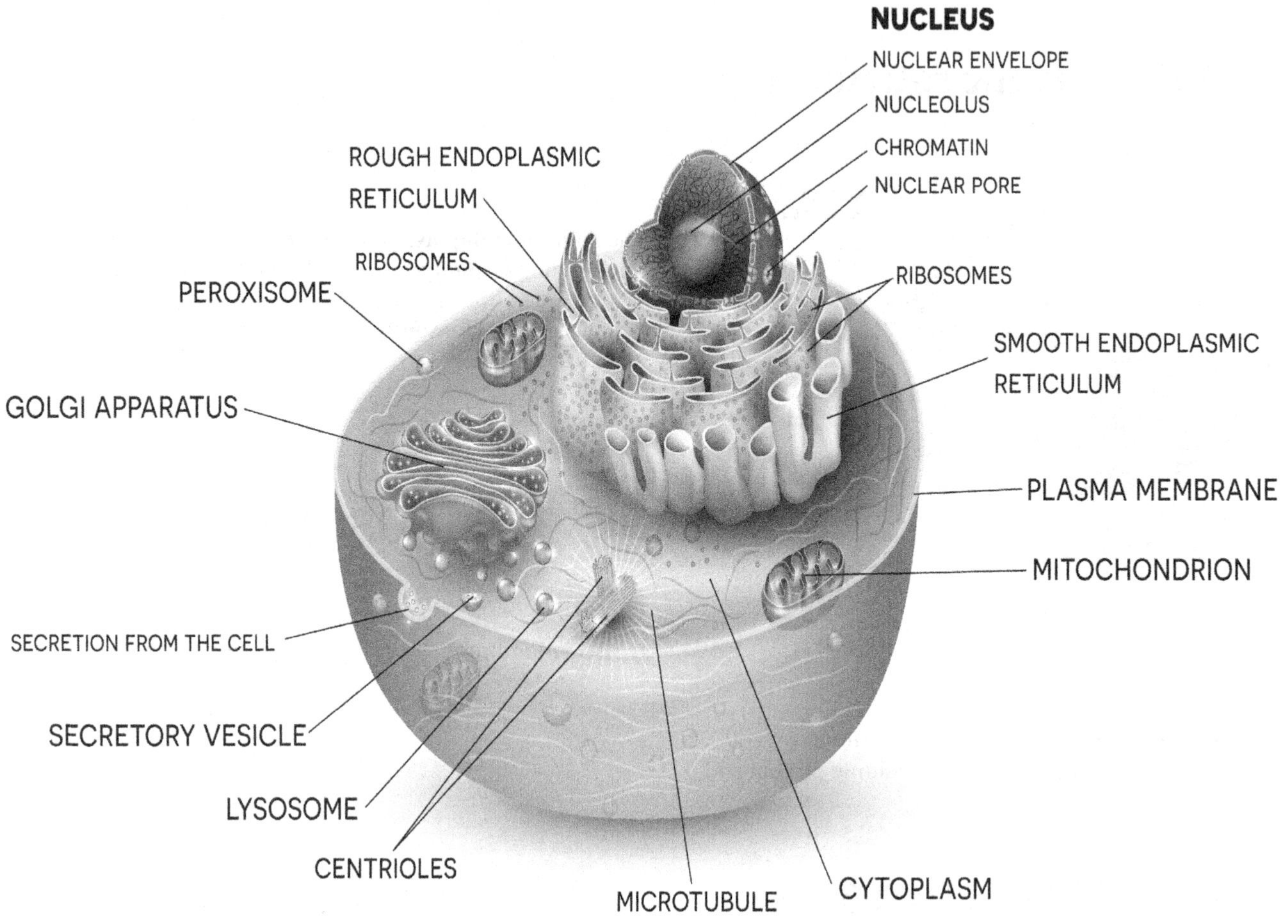


## Tissue

The body is constructed by smaller parts making bigger parts, until we have an organism. The organization of the body is: cells > tissues > organ > organ system > organism. A **tissue** is made of a group of **cells** with **similar function and structure**. When these cells, all formed roughly the same way, which perform the same action, come together, they form a tissue. There are **four** types of tissue in the human body: **epithelial**, **muscular**, **nervous**, and **connective**.

• **Epithelial** tissue forms most **glands**, the **digestive tract**, the **respiratory tract**, and the **epidermis**. Anywhere there is a mucous membrane, there is epithelium. Epithelial tissue is responsible for **protection**(the epidermis protects the body from pathogens and trauma), **secretion**(glands secrete substances, from hormones to mucous), and **absorption** of nutrients(the linings of the small intestine are made of epithelium, which allows nutrients to be absorbed into the blood stream). Epithelial tissue is also **avascular**, which means there is no direct blood supply to the tissue. This is what allows layers of the epidermis to be peeled away without any bleeding.

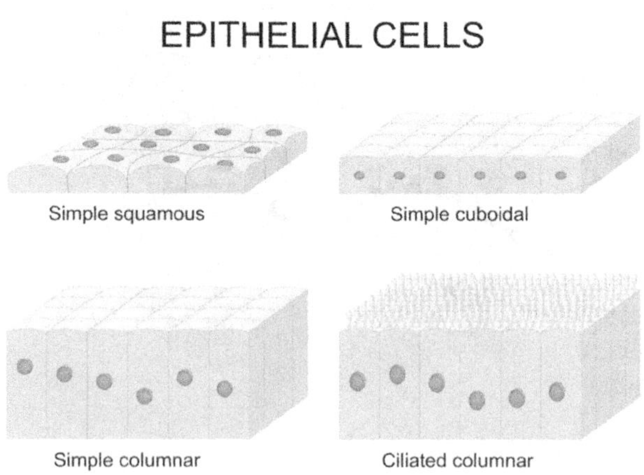

• **Muscular** tissue creates **muscles**. There are three types of muscles: **skeletal** muscles, so named because they connect to the skeleton, **cardiac** muscles, which create the heart, and **smooth** muscles, which are abundant in several locations in the body.

**Skeletal** muscles, as the name implies, attach to the **skeleton**. Another name for skeletal muscle is "**striated**" muscle, due to its appearance under a microscope. These muscles are **voluntary**, meaning you can control them. When these muscles contract, they pull on the bones they attach to, which allows movement.

Skeletal muscles are always in a state of **twitching**, even if you can't feel it. It's this twitching, very fine contractions, that produces **body heat**. When body temperature drops, the skeletal muscles increase the amount of contraction, which produces high body temperature, with the twitching of the muscles becoming more apparent. This is what happens when you shiver!

**Cardiac** muscle is the muscle that makes the **heart**. Another name for cardiac muscle is "**branching**" muscle, due to its appearance under a microscope. Cardiac muscle is **involuntary**, meaning you can't control it. Cardiac muscle is powerful, shooting **blood** out of the heart with each contraction. The only function of cardiac muscle is to send blood from one place to another.

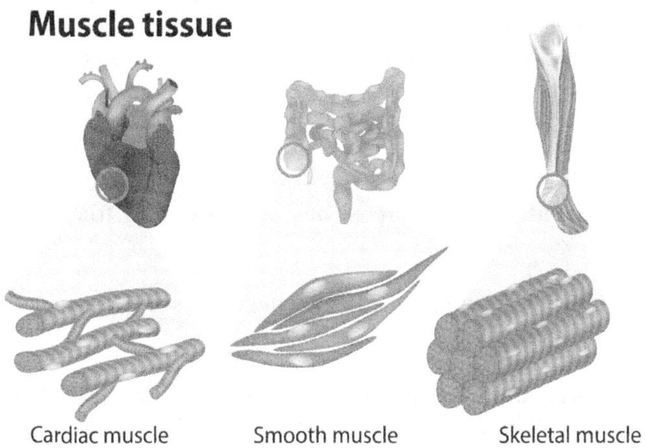


**Smooth** muscle is found in several locations throughout the body. Another name for smooth muscle is "**non-striated**" muscle, due to its appearance under a microscope. Smooth muscle is **involuntary**, meaning you can't control it. Smooth muscle, because it is found in several different regions of the body, has several different functions. Smooth muscle can be found in the **walls** of **hollow organs** such as the stomach and intestines. When these muscles contract, they force food through the Digestive System, which is known as **peristalsis**.

Other locations smooth muscle can be found are in the skin, and in the eyes. In the skin, smooth muscle attaches to hair. When these muscles contract, they stand hair up, producing goosebumps. These muscles are known as the arrector pili muscles. In the eyes, smooth muscles help to dilate the iris and pupil.

• **Nervous** tissue forms the **brain**, **spinal cord**, and **nerves**. The primary cell of nervous tissue is known as a **neuron**. Neurons process nervous impulses, sending these impulses to other tissues, such as muscles, or between other neurons.

Neurons receive **action potentials**(electric impulses), which are brought into the cell by **dendrites**, branch-like projections coming off the cell body of the neuron. Once the nucleus processes the information coming into the cell, it sends the impulse out of the cell to its destination by way of the **axon**, a long projection coming off the cell body. The axons terminate at other neurons, or help innervate muscles.

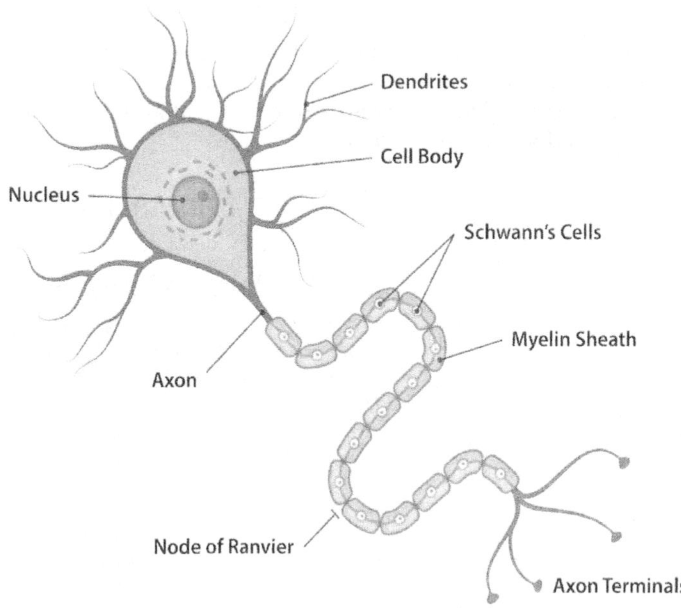

# CONNECTIVE TISSUES

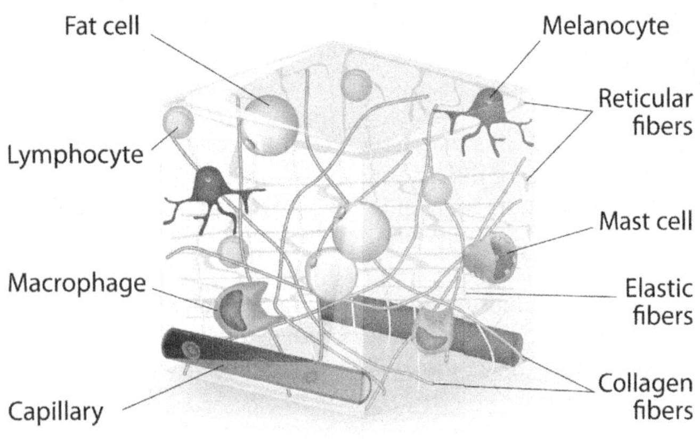


• **Connective** tissue is the most abundant form of tissue in the body. There are several different structures made by connective tissue, including **tendons**, **ligaments**, **fascia**, **bones**, **lymph**, **cartilage**, and **blood**. Connective tissue, as the name suggests, is responsible for **connecting** tissues. In addition to connecting tissues, it helps to **separate** tissues, as seen in serous membranes and cartilage.

Connective tissue contains two specific types of cells known as **blast** cells and **clast** cells. These cells play a very important role in the health of connective tissue. Blast cells are germ cells that are responsible for **building** connective tissue. Blast cells divide and build tissue until the structure is complete. Once the structure is complete, the blast cells mature, and stop dividing. Clast cells are responsible for **breaking down** tissue, which is very important in keeping the tissue healthy. If a person suffers an injury to connective tissue such as a fracture or sprain, clast cells will enter the area and destroy the dead tissue, cleaning the area, which allows blast cells a clean surface to build new tissue on.

**Serous Membranes**

**Serous membranes** are forms of connective tissue that are used to **separate** organs from one another, preventing friction. They accomplish this by **surrounding** the organ or body cavity.

Inside the thorax, there are two serous membranes: the **pericardium**, which surrounds the **heart**, and the **pleural** membranes, which surround the **lungs**. These membranes help protect these organs from injury.

Inside the abdomen and pelvis, there is one serous membrane: the **peritoneum**. This membrane keeps the organs inside the abdomen and pelvis from being injured, and provides a pathway for many blood vessels, lymph vessels, and nerves to travel. The peritoneum is commonly utilized to filter waste from the body in a person with kidney failure, a procedure known as peritoneal dialysis(page 247).

Inside of a serous membrane is a thick fluid, known as **serous fluid**. This fluid helps the membranes absorb shock. Holding the fluid in place are two walls. The inner wall, which comes into contact with the organs, is known as the **visceral serous membrane**. The outer wall, which comes into contact with other structures such as bones or other organs, is known as the **parietal serous membrane**.

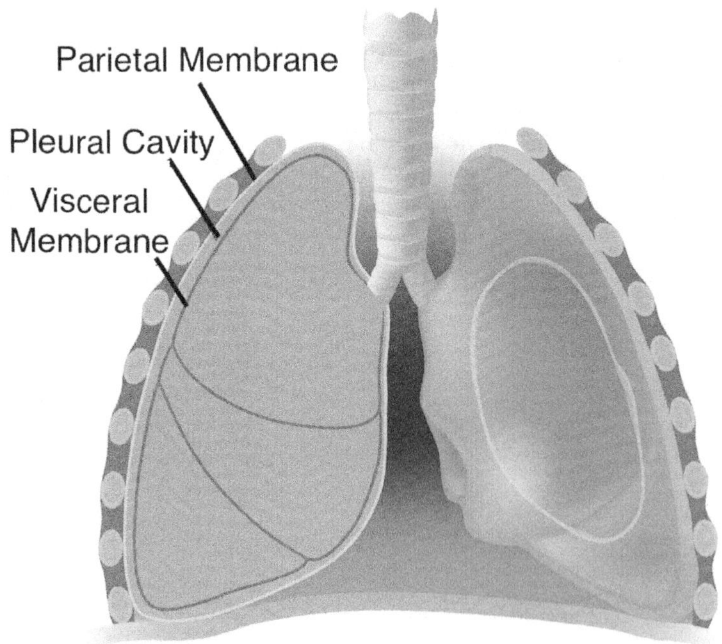

# Anatomy and Physiology

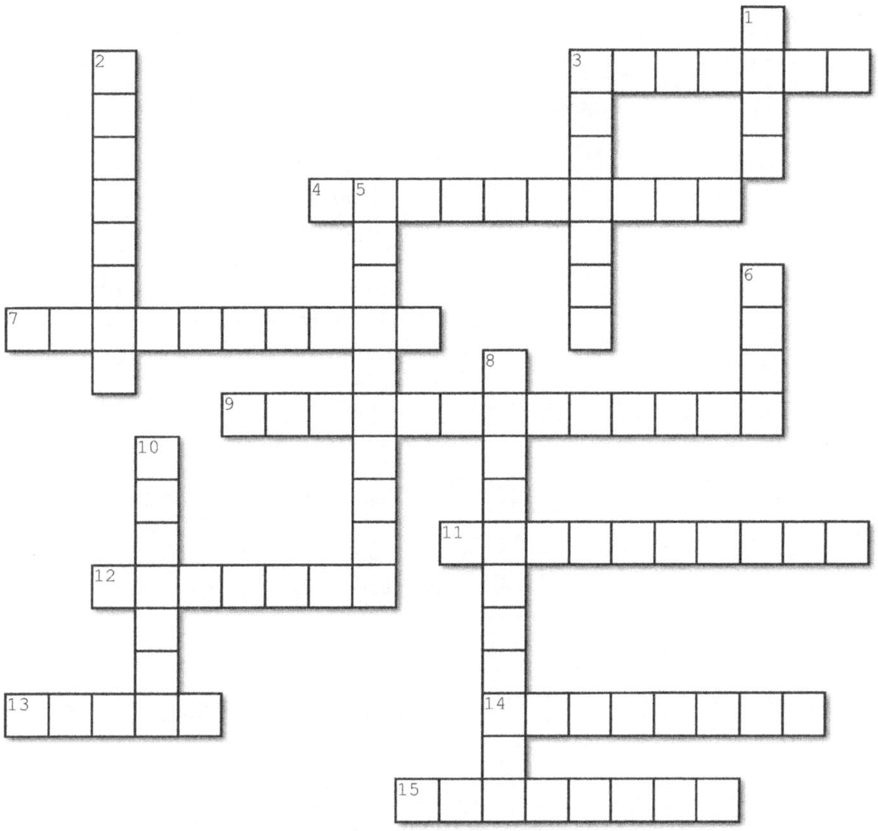

**Across**

**3.** Tissue responsible for transmitting and interpreting action potentials
**4.** Tissue responsible for protection, secretion, and absorption
**7.** Plane that splits the body into superior and inferior
**9.** Organelle that produces ATP
**11.** Tissue responsible for separating, connecting, and protecting structures
**12.** Study of the structure of the human body
**13.** The functional units of tissue
**14.** Plane that splits the body into left and right sides
**15.** Organelle responsible for breaking down protein inside the cell

**Down**

**1.** Type of connective tissue responsible for protecting the brain
**2.** Tissue responsible for movement, peristalsis, and creating body heat
**3.** Organelle that contains DNA
**5.** Study of the function of the human body
**6.** Part of a neuron that projects out and transmits action potentials to other neurons or muscles
**8.** Existence and maintenance of the body's internal environment
**10.** Plane that splits the body into anterior and posterior

Answer Key on Page 286

# Anatomy and Physiology Quiz

1. What aspect of the body is being studied in anatomy
A. Structure
B. Function
C. Diseases
D. Movement

2. Peristalsis is controlled by which of the following types of muscle
A. Cardiac
B. Skeletal
C. Smooth
D. Striated

3. Which of the following is not one of the four types of tissue
A. Nervous
B. Connective
C. Epithelial
D. Skeletal

4. The functional unit of tissue is called
A. Cell
B. Nerve
C. Blood
D. Muscle

5. Epithelial tissue
A. Holds tissue together and separates tissues
B. Provides protection, secretes substances, and absorbs substances
C. Is found inside joints and helps to lubricate joints
D. Allows nerve impulses to be transmitted from the brain to muscles

6. Function of serous membranes
A. Secreting sebum
B. Connect organs
C. Creating blood
D. Separate organs

7. Maintaining a relatively constant environment inside the body
A. Homeostasis
B. pH regulation
C. Polarity
D. Somatic holding pattern

8. Bone found in the region of the forearm
A. Radius
B. Humerus
C. Fibula
D. Hamate

9. Tissue specializing in protection, absorption, and secretion
A. Muscular
B. Connective
C. Nervous
D. Epithelial

10. Movement of the limbs is controlled by which type of muscle tissue
A. Cardiac
B. Skeletal
C. Smooth
D. Hyaline

11. The most abundant form of connective tissue found in the body
A. Fascia
B. Bone
C. Cartilage
D. Blood

12. Which of the following is a function of connective tissue
A. Absorb nutrients
B. Hold structures together
C. Sensory input
D. Regulation of hormones

13. The thoracic body cavity
A. Contains the liver, stomach, small intestine, large intestine, pancreas, spleen, and gallbladder
B. Is separated from the dorsal body cavity via the diaphragm
C. Contains the lungs, heart, and major blood vessels
D. Holds the spleen against the stomach to prevent rupture of the spleen

14. Processes branching off the cell body of a neuron responsible for bringing action potentials into the neuron for processing
A. Nucleus
B. Dendrite
C. Axon
D. Schwann Cell

15. Which of the following is not a function of connective tissue
A. Insulating the body
B. Protection
C. Separating tissues
D. Hormone release

Answer Key on Page 289

# Disease, Immunity, and Medications

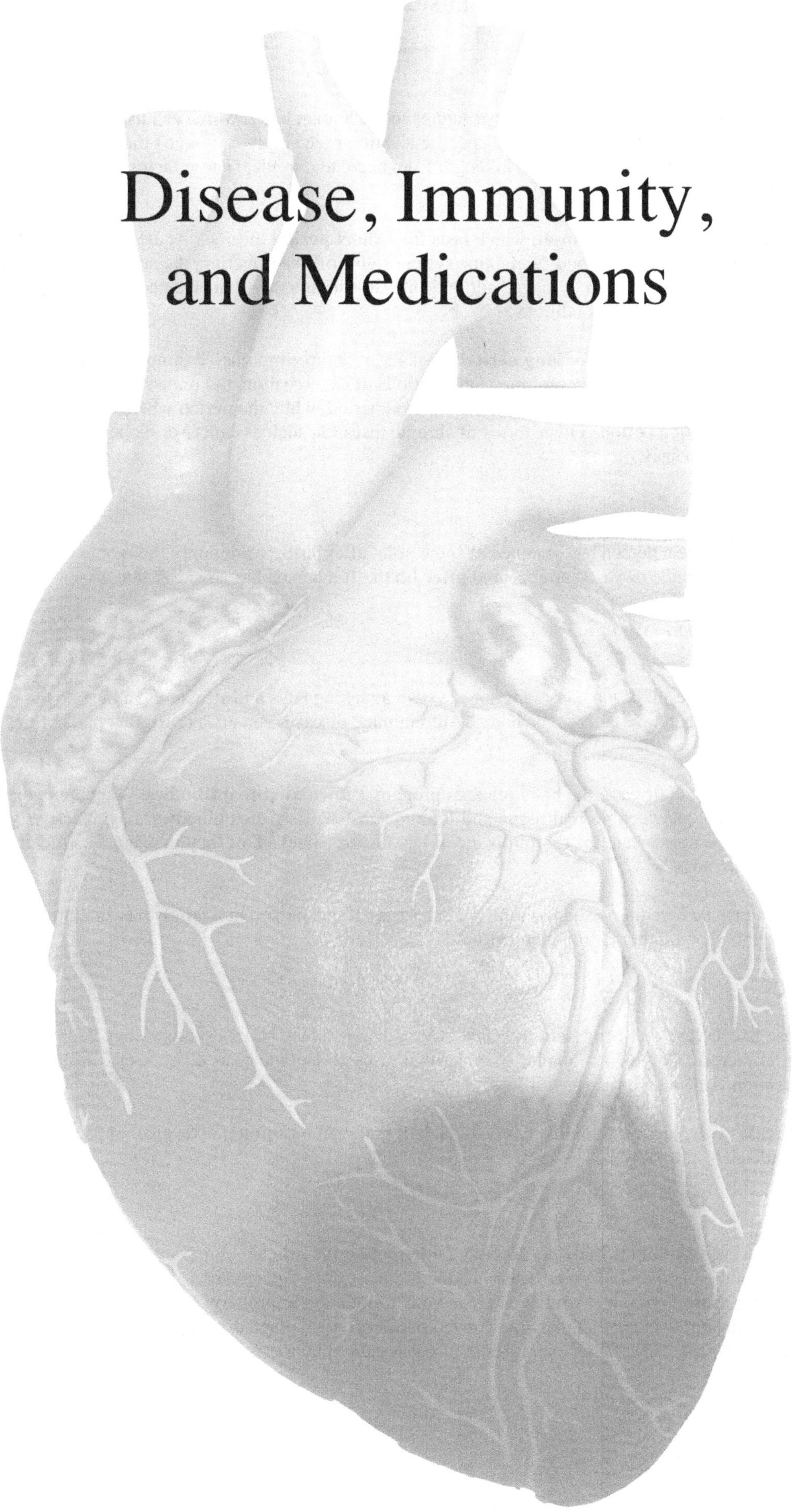

# Disease

A disease is a condition affecting certain functions or structures in the human body, which can usually be associated with signs or symptoms. Diseases most commonly affect a specific location in the body, and aren't the result of physical trauma. Diseases range in severity from mild to severe, and in length from acute to chronic. These factors are determined by the type of disease, and the ability to treat the disease.

An **acute** disease or disorder has a **sudden onset**, which lasts for a **short period** of time. Acute conditions can be seen often with infections or trauma, and as the body's immune system fights off the infection, the acute condition dissipates. However, if the condition is severe enough, it may result in death. It is in this way that acute conditions are typically more dangerous in the short term than chronic conditions.

**Chronic** diseases or disorders are present for **long periods**, usually over three months. Examples of chronic diseases include asthma and hepatitis C. Chronic diseases may have periods of exacerbation and remission. The period where the disease is not actively showing signs or symptoms is the remission period, while the period where the disease is affecting a person's health is the exacerbation period. Other forms of chronic diseases, such as cancer or diabetes, are always present, and can make a person continuously ill.

### Acquired Diseases

An acquired disease is a disease a person has obtained at some point after birth. Commonly thought of as some sort of infection, it actually just means the disease has appeared **after birth**. If a person has a disease that was not congenital, then it is referred to as an acquired disease.

### Autoimmune Diseases

Autoimmune diseases are the result of the body's immune system attacking cells and structures in the body that it cannot differentiate from pathogens that have entered the body. Autoimmune diseases can attack different parts of the body with differing levels of severity.

In a person with an autoimmune disease, the body releases proteins known as **autoantibodies**. Autoantibodies are the cells that cannot tell the difference between normal tissue and foreign substances. Autoantibodies may attack only one specific structure, such as Graves' disease where the thyroid is the only structure attacked, or they may attack structures throughout the entire body, such as in lupus.

Autoimmune diseases may be hereditary, such as multiple sclerosis. If one person in a family has an autoimmune disorder, it may increase the likelihood of another family member having it as well.

### Congenital Diseases

A congenital disease is a disease that is **present at birth**. These diseases may be inherited, or may be the result of certain environmental factors. Common examples of congenital diseases include heart defects, cleft lip, Down syndrome, HIV infection, and spina bifida(page 176).

Causes for these diseases vary, but many are likely due to lack of maternal nutrition intake, alcohol use, drug use, and the fetus not receiving adequate nutrients.

### Deficiency Diseases

Deficiency diseases are the result of the body not receiving **adequate nutrients**, vitamins, and/or minerals in the diet. Examples of these include iron, vitamin C, zinc, calcium, and iodine. When a person does not receive these nutrients in adequate amounts, it can cause organs and structures in the body to function improperly, or not at all. For example, if a person lacks sufficient vitamin C in the diet, they may develop scurvy. If a person does not consume enough calcium, they may develop osteoporosis(page 237). Other examples of diseases caused by a nutrient deficiency include anemia(page 53), goiter(page 100), and rickets.

**Hereditary Diseases**

A hereditary disease, also known as a genetic disease, is the result of some sort of abnormality in a person's **genome**. These abnormalities vary in severity, and in turn, may cause differing levels of difficulty in normal function.

Genetic disorders are commonly passed down from the parents, but some genetic disorders may be the result of mutations in the genes due to environmental factors. Other times, the mutation in the gene may be completely random.

There are differing types of gene inheritance that contribute to the development of hereditary diseases.

**Single gene inheritances** are the result of mutations occurring in one single gene. This leaves the majority of the body operating normally, but can change one specific aspect of the body. An example is cystic fibrosis(page 200), where the mutated gene causes the respiratory passages to produce an extremely excessive amount of mucous.

**Multifactorial gene inheritances** are the result of a mutation in multiple genes, in association with environmental factors. The gene may be present that can cause the disease, but it may lie dormant unless it is activated by environmental factors. Examples include cancers, hypertension, and cardiovascular disease. If the person avoids the environmental factors, they see less of a chance of developing the disease associated with the mutated gene.

Abnormal chromosomes are often caused by problems during cell division, known as **nondisjunction**, which can damage the chromosomes in the cell's DNA. An example of an abnormal chromosome disease is Down syndrome. This is caused by having an extra copy of chromosome 21. This gives the person 47 total chromosomes, instead of the standard 46.

**Idiopathic Diseases**

An idiopathic disease is a disease that has an **unknown origin or cause**. These diseases show no obvious sign of origin, and spontaneously appear. There may be theories about why a disease occurs, but the exact reason is unknown. Examples of idiopathic diseases include ankylosing spondylitis(page 225), chronic fatigue syndrome, and fibromyalgia(page 149).

**Infectious Diseases**

An infection is an **invasion** of a **microorganism** inside the body in some way, which can be localized and less serious, to systemic and life-threatening. These microorganisms are usually not inside the body, and therefore, the body does not have a knowledge of how to exactly combat the infection when first exposed. When there is an infection, the body develops antibodies, and these are used to destroy the invading microorganism.

There are four primary types of infections: bacterial, viral, fungal, and parasitic.

**Bacterial Infections**

Bacteria are single-celled organisms that can only be seen under a microscope. They have a membrane surrounding the cell, and are able to freely reproduce via cell mitosis.

Bacterial infections are caused by an invasion of certain types of bacteria, such as H. pylori, staphylococcus, streptococcus, and salmonella. Bacteria come different shapes and sizes, some looking like rods(bacillus), and others looking like balls(borrelia) or spirals(spirilla). Bacterial infections make a person sick by releasing toxic substances in their waste. An overabundance of these toxins cause a person to become ill, depending on the severity. Bacteria are known to reproduce quickly, and treatment should be sought for serious bacterial infections such as pneumonia and strep throat. Treatment for bacterial infections involves taking a course of antibiotics, such as penicillin, which destroy the bacteria. Any course of antibiotics should be completed fully, as ceasing taking the prescribed dosage could result in any remaining bacteria becoming resistant to the antibiotics. It's in these cases where infections such as MRSA(methicillin-resistant staphylococcus aureus) may appear and become extremely difficult to treat, which may be life-threatening.

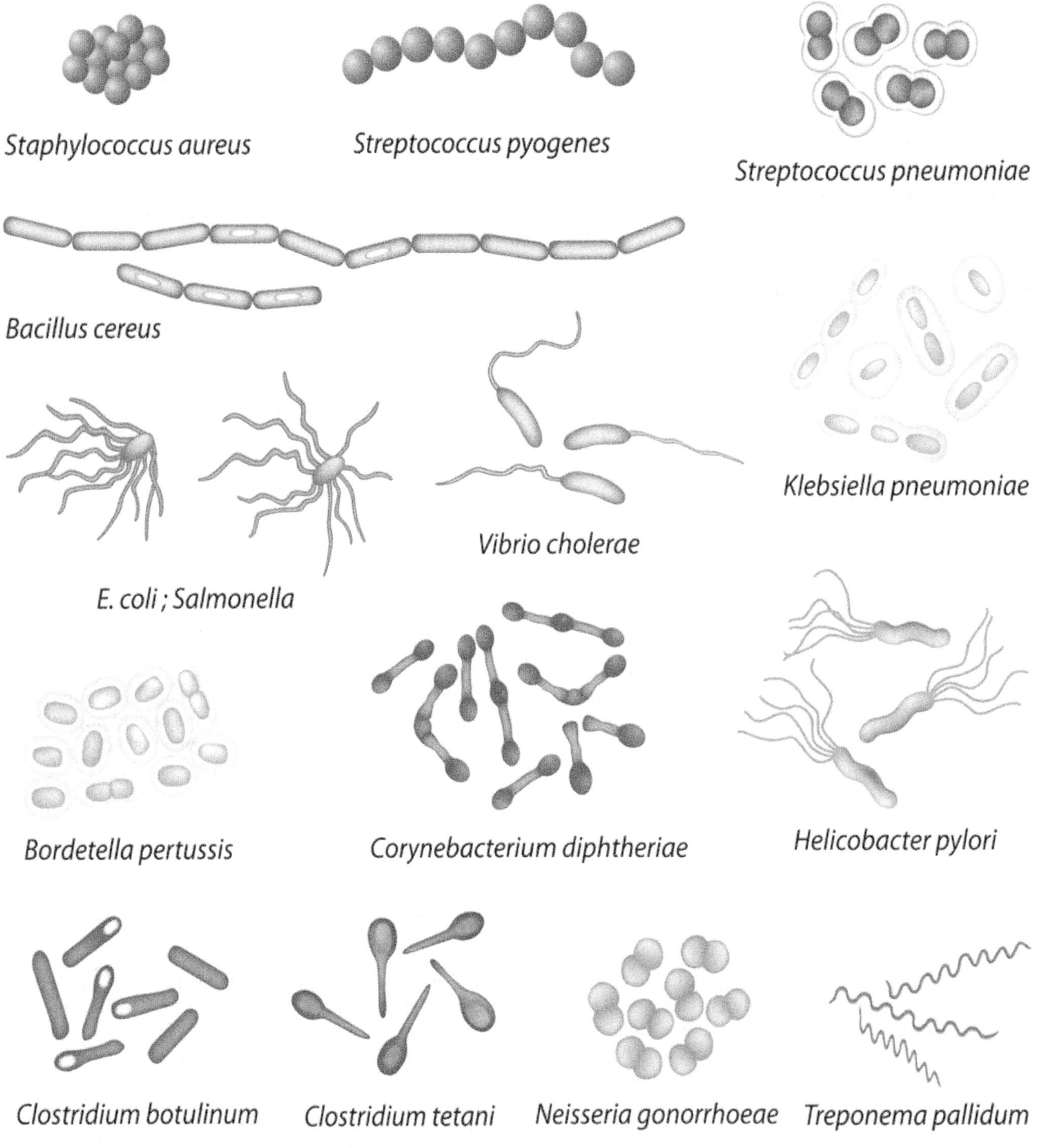
Staphylococcus aureus
Streptococcus pyogenes
Streptococcus pneumoniae
Bacillus cereus
Klebsiella pneumoniae
Vibrio cholerae
E. coli ; Salmonella
Bordetella pertussis
Corynebacterium diphtheriae
Helicobacter pylori
Clostridium botulinum
Clostridium tetani
Neisseria gonorrhoeae
Treponema pallidum

**Viral Infections**

Viral infections are caused by viruses, structures smaller than bacteria, that contain RNA or DNA in their core. They attach to healthy cells and insert code into the cell that changes the behavior in the cell and causes the infected cell to create more virus particles. These particles come together in the cell, creating new viruses. When too many of these viruses have formed, they break through the host cell and enter the body, infecting more healthy cells. This process is known as the **lytic cycle**.

When the body detects a viral infection, it releases chemicals known as **pyrogens** into the body, which elevate body temperature. This increased body temperature, known as a fever, does not give the viruses an environment to thrive in, and ultimately the viruses die or fail to reproduce due to the extreme temperature change. Treatments for viral infections typically are used to treat the symptoms, as there is no way to destroy the virus itself. Vaccines can be used to introduce dead or weakened viruses into the body, which allow the body's immune system to develop antibodies for them, preventing future infections. Antiviral medications can be used to prevent a virus from reproducing, but cannot kill the virus.

Some viruses never leave a person's body and become dormant, not always causing problems. Others never leave the body and actively affect the body, such as HIV. Most of the time, in instances such as influenza, the body's immune system naturally fights off the virus over the course of a week or two.

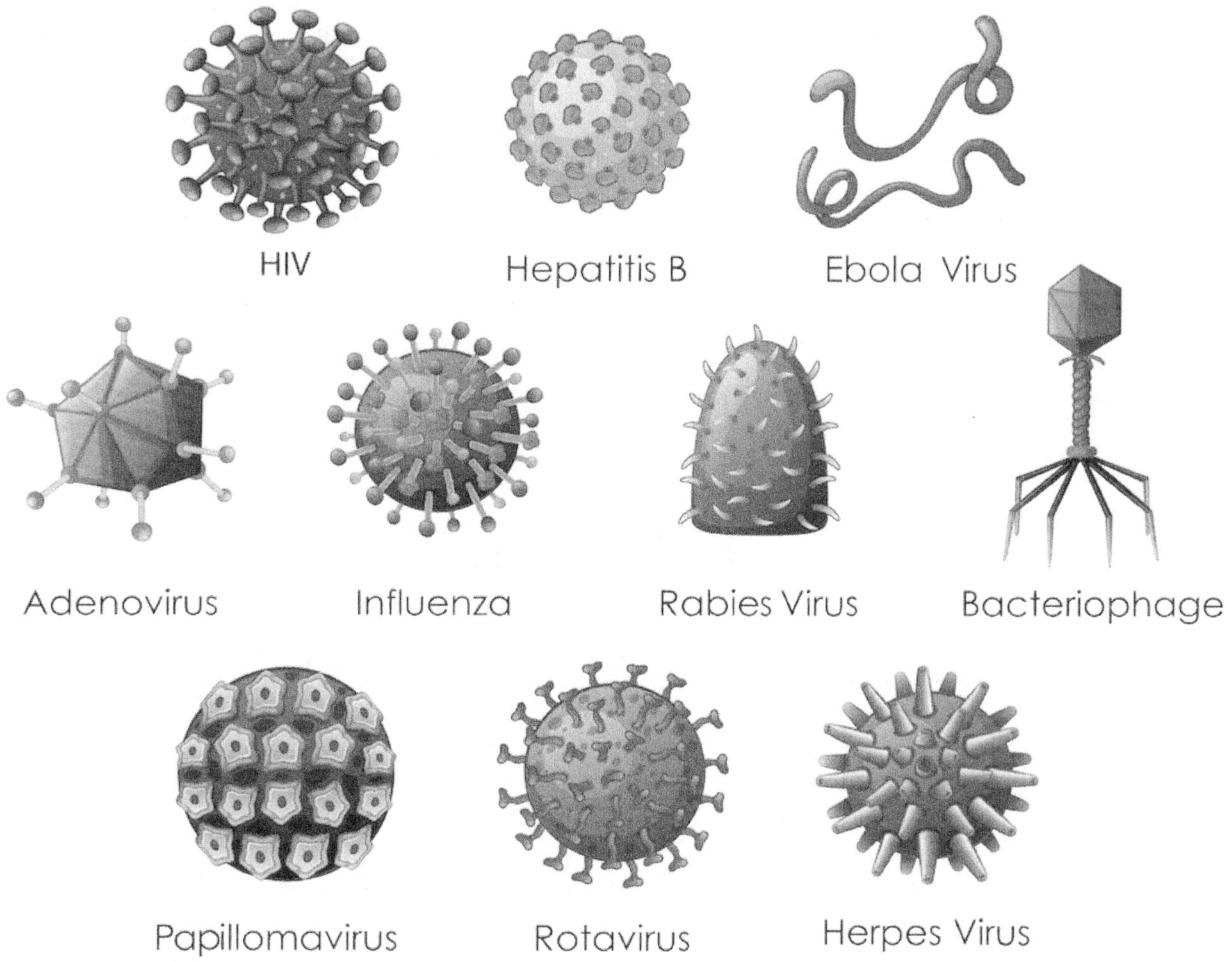

**Fungal Infections**

Fungal infections are caused by a fungus coming into contact with the skin or entering into the body via means such as inhalation. Certain fungi thrive in specific environments that are dark, warm, and humid. Examples of these include athlete's foot and jock itch. Other fungi may attach to dead tissues, such as the nails or skin. An example of these include ringworm.

Common forms of fungi that result in infection include candidiasis, aspergillosis, sporothrix, talaromyces, and histoplasma. These fungi can be found in various parts of the world, and can affect people differently depending on the strength of their immune system. Some fungi thrive in extremely moist environments, while other fungi may not need as much moisture to grow.

Fungal infections are treated with medications known as antifungals, which are designed to destroy fungus. These can be used directly on the skin as ointments or shampoos, orally in gel or liquid form, or inserted into a part of the body such as the vagina in cases such as yeast infections. Serious fungal infections may need to be treated with antifungals injected into the body.

**Parasitic Infections**

Parasitic infections are caused by small organisms that use a host in order to survive. These parasites may affect their host in some way, or they may not, depending on the type of parasite. The three types of parasites are protozoa, helminths, and ectoparasites.

**Protozoa** are single-celled organisms, and they live inside the host's body, multiplying beyond safe levels. A protozoa infection is considered serious, most commonly the result of drinking water that may contain the parasite.

**Helminths** are also known as **worms**, such as tapeworms, flukes, and roundworms. Worms most commonly enter the host's body through consuming a food or drink that contains the worm or worm larvae.

**Ectoparasites** are parasites that attach to the surface of the host, often feeding off the blood of the host to survive. Examples include mosquitoes, leeches, and ticks.

Some parasitic infections do not require treatment. If symptoms of infection appear, treatment should be sought. Common parasitic infection treatments include anti-parasitic medications used to destroy any parasites, and removal of the parasite if medication does not work.

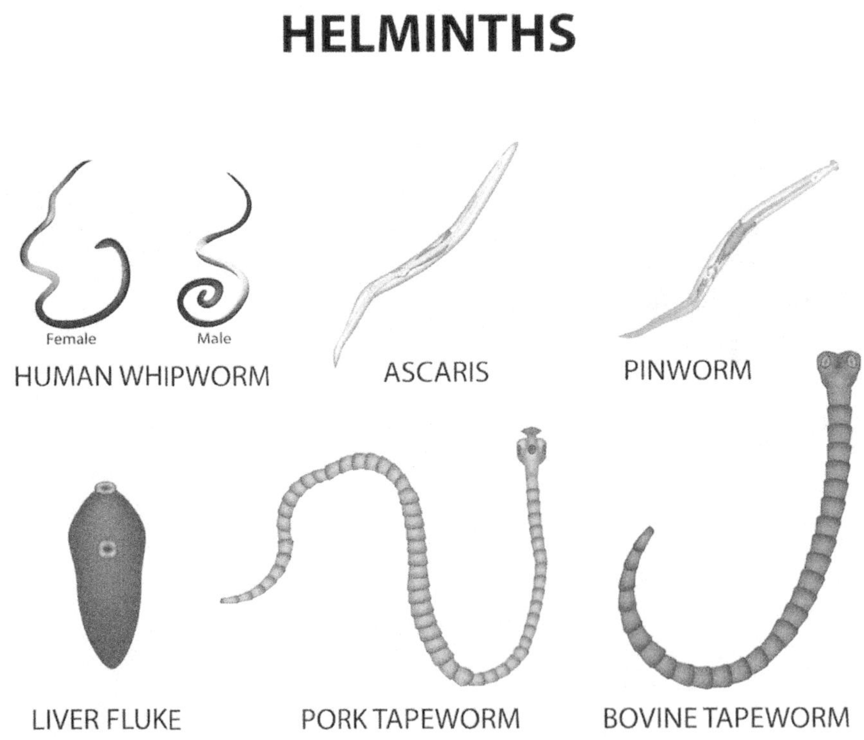

**Psychological Diseases**

Psychological diseases, often referred to as **mental disorders**, are often associated with problems a person may experience with their mood or thoughts. Causes are hard to pin-point, and may vary from person to person. These mental disorders can have an extremely adverse effect on the overall well-being of the person. Treatment via medications and psychotherapy may be available.

Mental disorders commonly seen in children include autism, ADHD(Attention Deficit/Hyperactivity Disorder), attachment disorder, and stuttering. Disorders commonly seen in adults may include addiction, depression, bipolar disorder, eating disorders, PTSD, and panic disorder.

Personality disorders are disorders that may influence how a person acts or responds to certain situations. Examples of personality disorders include Antisocial Personality Disorder, Dissociative Identity Disorder, and Obsessive-Compulsive Personality Disorder.

# Immunity

Immunity refers to the ability of the body to protect itself from disease and pathogens. Immunity is the responsibility of the **immune system**, which destroys foreign objects that enter the body that may produce infection or disease. The process through which these substances are destroyed is known as the **immune response**.

The **humoral immune system** is the part of the immune system that takes place in the body's **fluids**, known as the **humors**. This results in the production of **antibodies** when a foreign substance is observed in the body. Antibodies react by neutralizing the pathogen, or allowing the pathogen to be destroyed easier by other cells.

The **cell-mediated immune system** involves **T lymphocytes**, also known as **T cells**. These cells vary in type, depending on the kind of pathogen involved. The T lymphocytes are responsible for **destroying** the pathogen, and do not utilize antibodies. Types of T cells include effector, helper, cytotoxic, natural killer, memory, and regulatory, each responsible for a different aspect of immune support.

## T-cell activation

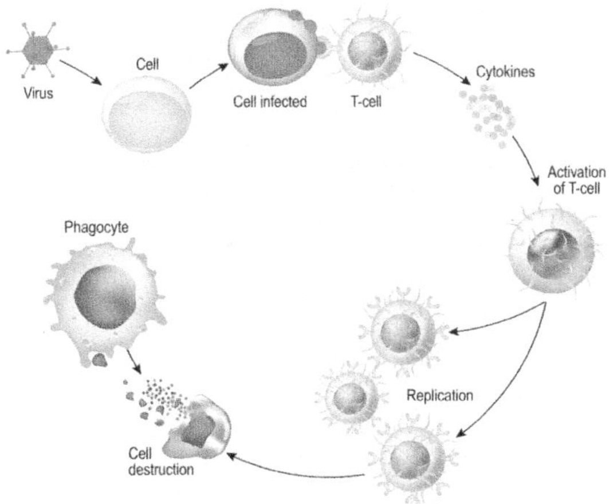


## B-cell activation

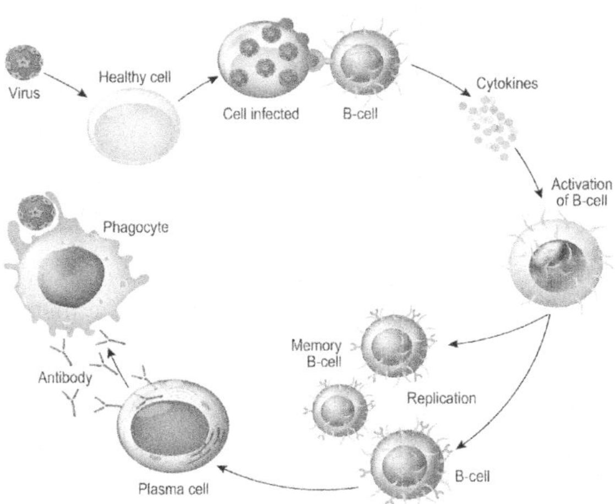


When a pathogen is detected in the body, a B cell or T cell will bind to the pathogen, and release **cytokines**. Cytokines are proteins responsible for allowing **communication between cells**. Cytokines will send a message to the immune system, which will then bring more B cells or T cells into the area to combat the pathogen.

**Phagocytes**

**Phagocytes**, which are certain types of white blood cells, are responsible for "**eating**" pathogens or debris in a process known as **phagocytosis**. Debris can include foreign objects or substances that have entered the body, or dead or dying cells that need to be removed from the body. An example is the fading of tattoos. Over time, tattoo ink is broken down by the body's phagocytes, because the body senses it is a foreign substance that should not be present. When enough ink is broken down by phagocytes, the tattoo fades. Laser tattoo removal works by breaking the ink into smaller pieces, which the phagocytes can then absorb and eliminate from the body easier.

Examples of phagocytes include neutrophils, monocytes, macrophages, and dendritic cells. Neutrophils are typically the first phagocyte into the area. **Neutrophils** release enzymes that **destroy bacteria**, and perform phagocytosis. **Monocytes** move from the blood into the area, where they are then known as **macrophages**. Much like neutrophils, they perform **phagocytosis** to eliminate the debris or infection. **Dendritic cells** are located on **surfaces** of the body such as the skin and gastrointestinal tract. Dendritic cells act by performing phagocytosis on a pathogen to retrieve its specific **antigen**. Once this information has been obtained, it is **passed on** to T cells via cytokines produced by the dendritic cells.

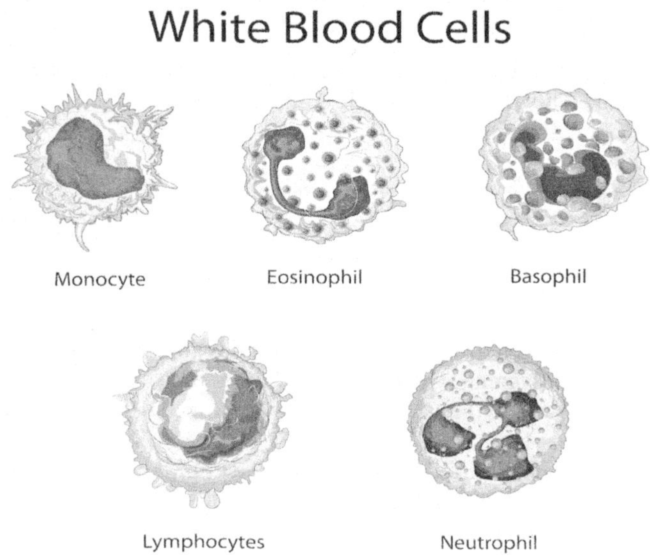


**Phagocytosis**

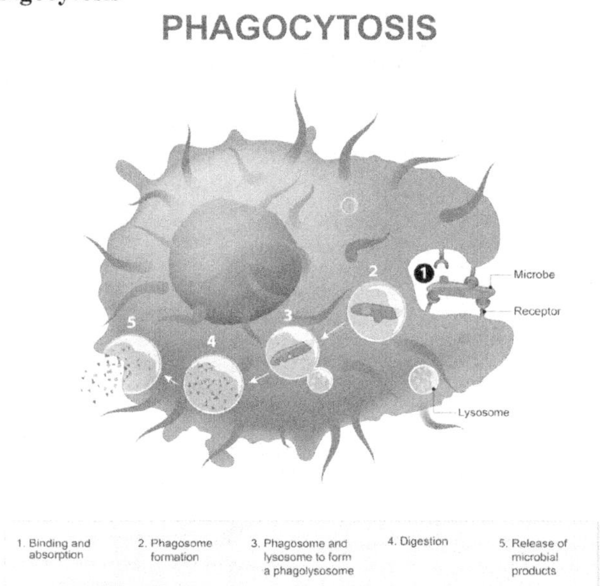


**Phagocytosis** is the process of a cell "**eating**" an object or substance, a process known as **endocytosis**. The phagocyte envelops the debris or pathogen in a vesicle known as a **phagosome**. A phagosome is produced when the cell wraps the cell membrane around the structure and the cell membrane fuses together. The phagosome is introduced into the cell, holding the substance, where the substance is broken down by granules that produce toxic or acidic matter to dissolve the substances. Once the substance has been destroyed, the waste is removed from the cell in a process that is essentially the opposite of bringing the substance into the cell. The phagosome fuses back with the cell membrane, and the waste product is expelled into the extracellular fluid. This process is known as **exocytosis**.

**Antibodies**

An **antibody**, also known as **immunoglobulin**, is a protein produced by **plasma cells** to neutralize pathogens in the body such as viruses and certain bacteria. Antibodies are **Y shaped**. The tips of the antibodies that produce the Y shape contain what's known as a **paratope**, which binds together with the **epitope**, the substance found in antigens that the body's immune system recognizes. **Antigens** are molecules the pathogen contains that the antibodies recognize and attach to, similar to a key fitting into a lock.

Antibodies are produced and secreted by **B cells**, in two different forms. The first form is **soluble** and moves freely throughout the body. These types of B cells are known as **plasma cells**. The second is a **membrane-bound form**, and it attaches to the surface of B cells. These types are known as **B cell receptors**. B cell receptors bind to the surface of B cells and are able to quickly identify pathogens seen before in the body. This allows the B cells to produce sufficient antibodies to attack the pathogen with a faster response time.

Antibodies vary depending on the type of pathogen detected. For each different pathogen, a different type of antibody is produced. The amount of pathogens exposed to the body determines the amount of different antibodies being produced. If a person has been exposed to the pathogen before, **memory cells** may be produced, which **store information** on how the immune system is to destroy the pathogen. It is when this happens that a person is considered **immune** to a certain disease.

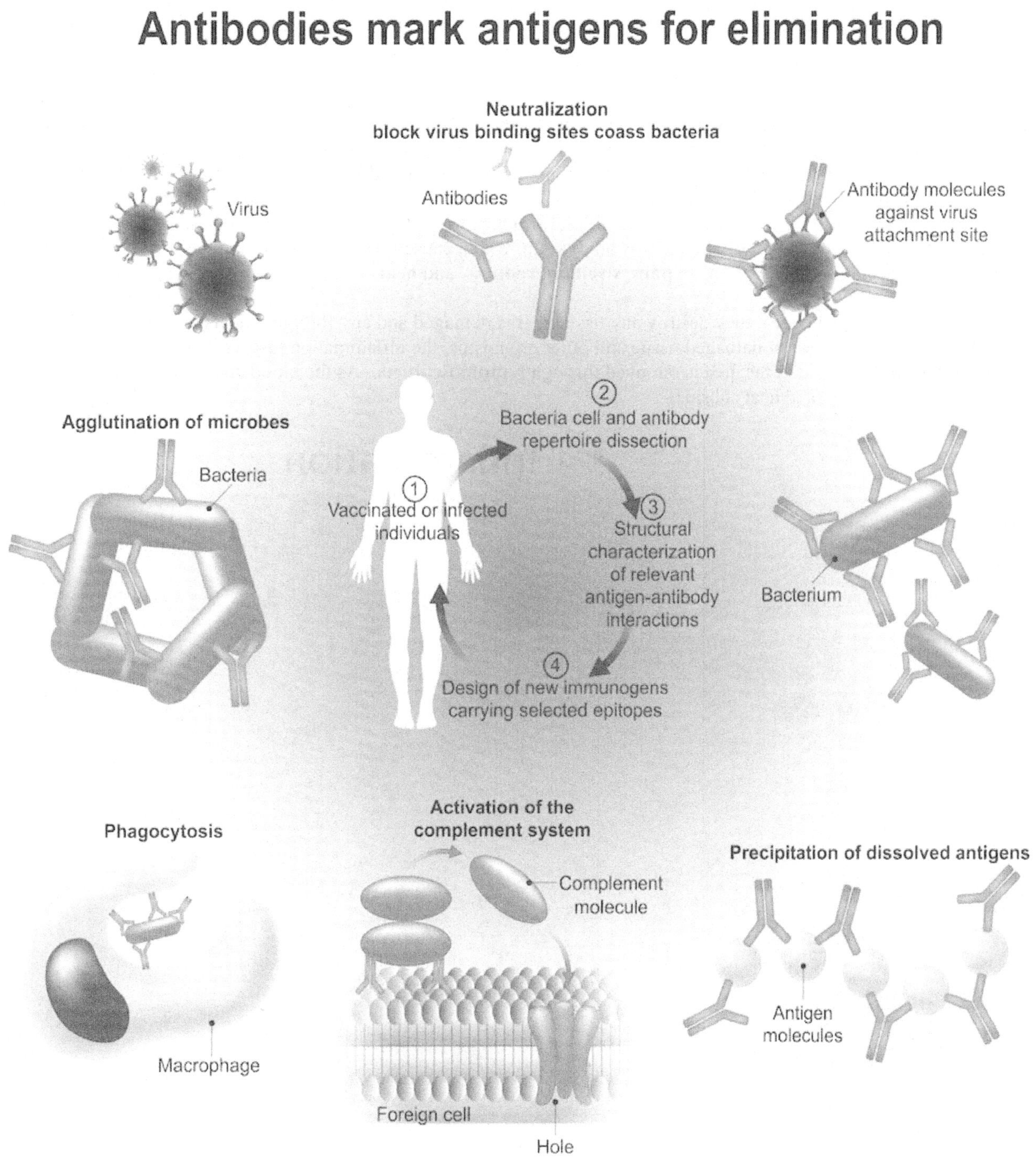

## Tissue Repair

When a part of the body is injured or damaged, the damaged tissue must go through repair to allow proper functioning of the structure once again. The amount of repair correlates to the amount of tissue damage that has occurred. Some tissue may not be able to be repaired effectively, and may require scar tissue to complete the repair.

### Inflammation

Upon damage to tissue, the tissue will experience **inflammation**. Inflammation starts with **dilation** of **capillaries** in the area of the trauma. Damaged tissues release **histamines** into the area, which stimulates the capillaries to dilate. When the capillaries dilate, the walls of the capillaries become thinner and more **permeable**. This allows **leukocytes** and **plasma** from the blood to enter the extracellular fluid in the damaged area, which is what produces inflammation. Because there is an increase in blood in the area, the inflamed area will feel **warmer** to the touch, and have a **reddish** appearance. The leukocytes release chemicals into the area, such as bradykinin, which causes **pain** by stimulating the nerve endings in the area. The four markers of inflammation are **pain**, **swelling**, **redness**, and **heat**.

As more leukocytes enter the area, they destroy any tissue that is damaged and any foreign objects or organisms that are present. Once the area is clear of damaged tissue and other organisms, the inflammation resolves. The capillary walls constrict, and the excess fluid in the area is removed through **lymphatic ducts**. As the blood and fluid is removed from the area, the swelling, redness, and heat subside.

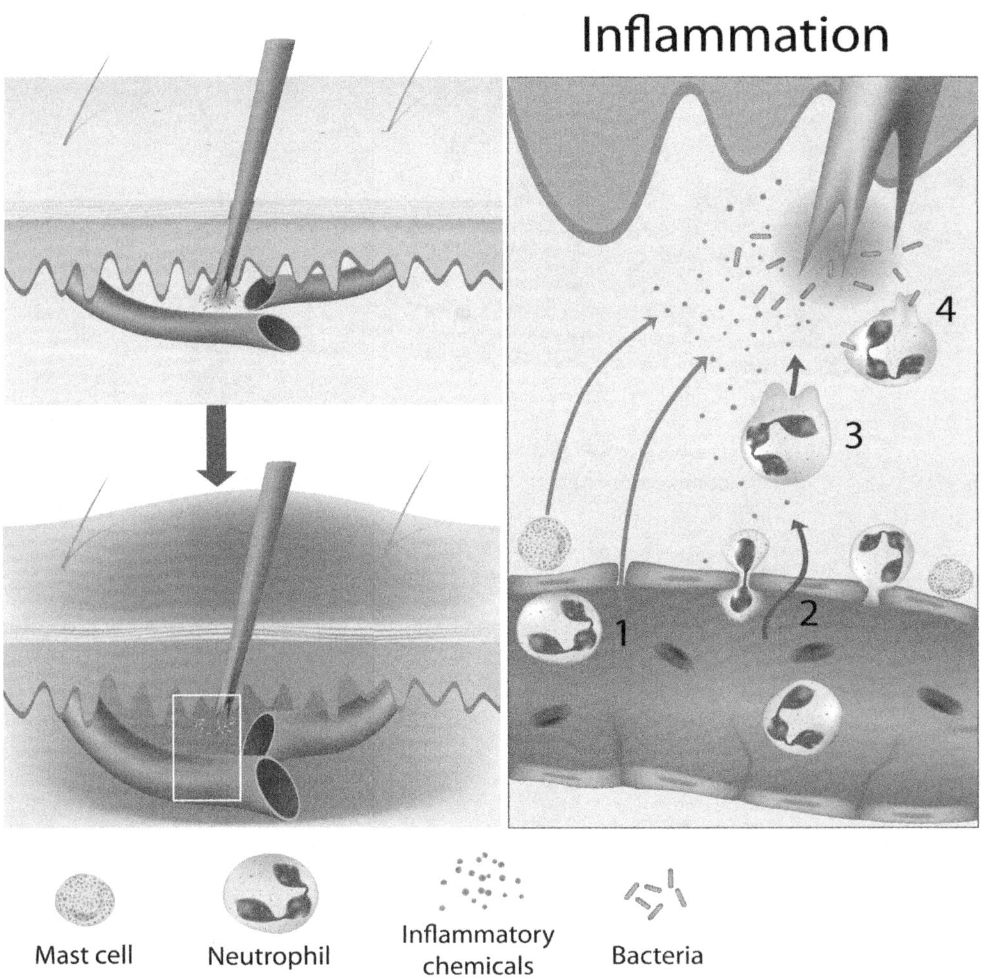


1. Histamines dilate capillaries

2. Neutrophils move from the capillaries into the area

3. Neutrophils detect foreign objects or pathogens

4. Phagocytosis is performed, pathogens and debris are destroyed

**Healing**

Most tissue in the body can regenerate and create more tissue to replace any damaged tissue. Some tissue, such as nerve tissue and brain tissue, usually cannot. If a large portion of the body has experienced damage, the tissue may need to be removed to prevent the area from becoming gangrenous.

If a person has suffered a wound(page 126), and the damaged areas are close together, the body will heal itself through a process known as **primary intention**. Examples of wounds that are healed via primary intention are small cuts, scratches, and surgical incisions. These wounds allow for **blood clots** to form that hold the tissues together and stop bleeding. Beneath the clot, which is known as a **scab**, new tissue is formed, and the two sides of the wound join together. Once the new tissue is formed, the scab sloughs off, revealing the new tissue.

If a person suffers a wound that requires healing via **secondary intention**, the edges of the wound cannot be approximated. The edges are uneven, do not properly align, and may be far apart. This type of healing requires **granulated tissue** to form at the base and sides of the wound. As the healing progresses, the granulated tissue fills in the area missing tissue. This type of healing often takes far longer than primary intention healing, and will leave the area with scar tissue to help fill the damaged area. An example of secondary intention healing is seen with decubitus ulcers(page 115).

When a person experiences a wound that requires medical intervention, delayed primary closure may be utilized. With delayed primary closure, the **wound** is **left open** to ensure it is properly cleaned and free of bacteria or other pathogens before being closed. This is also known as **tertiary intention healing**. Once it is determined that there is no infection present, the wound is then surgically closed. An example of wounds that often require tertiary intention healing is animal bites.

**Bone Healing**

Damage to bones, such as fractures(page 228), requires the use of **osteoclasts** and **osteoblasts** to help repair the structure. These cells continuously maintain the bone matrix, but if the bone is injured, they are the primary cells responsible for healing. After a bone is fractured, **osteoclasts** will begin **breaking down** the damaged bone tissue. This leaves the bone with a clean surface in which to build new bone tissue. It is similar to demolishing a building and erecting another building in its place. The rubble from the demolished building needs to be removed before another building can be constructed.

After the damaged surface has been cleared by the osteoclasts, **osteoblasts** begin forming **new bone matrix** to replace the matrix that has been lost. The material produced by osteoblasts is known as **callus**, and it binds the two sides of the fracture together, similar to scar tissue in the skin. The bone will absorb the callus, and the callus is then replaced by bone tissue. These cells are known as **osteocytes**. The bone is then remodeled into essentially its original shape, and osteoblasts stop producing osteocytes to replace the damaged bone.

**Scar**

A scar, also known as **cicatrix**, is a fibrous tissue formed to help a wound heal. Scar tissue acts as a bandage, holding the damaged tissue together when it cannot be effectively replaced on its own. Scarring depends on the size, location, and depth of the wound suffered. Other factors that may play a role in scar development is a person's age, genes, and overall health of the person and the part of the body involved.

Different types of scars include acne scars, keloid scars, contracture scars, hypertrophic scars, and striae.

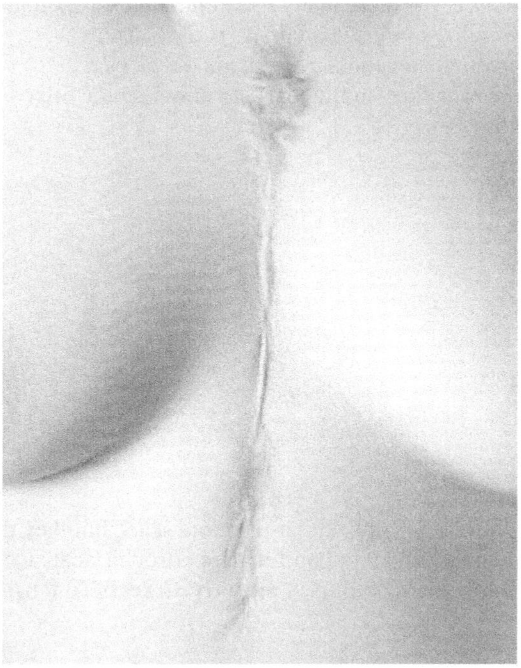

**Acne scars** may occur in a person with severe acne. These scars can leave **deep pits** in the skin, usually the result of a follicle wall being broken by an excessive accumulation of oil, bacteria, or fluid.

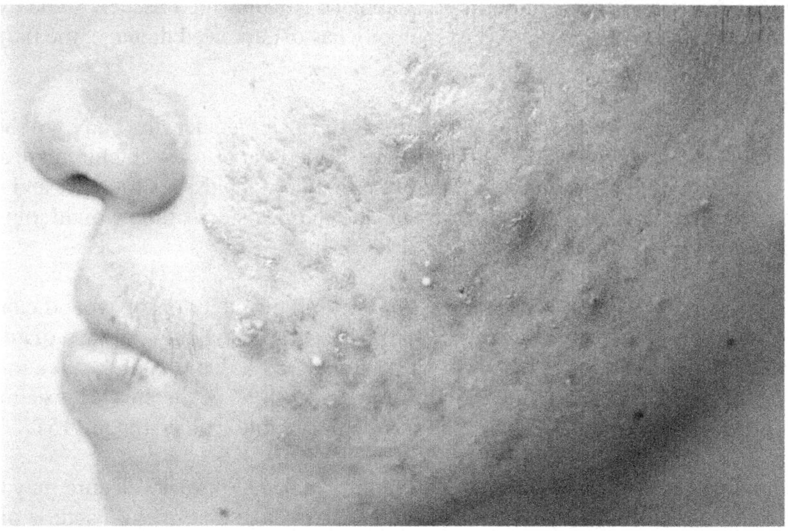

Scarring due to acne

**Keloid scars** are more commonly seen in people with darker skin tone. These scars are the result of over-healing in the area. Keloid scars are often **raised** off the skin, extending beyond the area of damage. If large enough, these may be uncomfortable, cause pain, or reduce movement.

**Contracture scars** are usually seen in people who have suffered **burns**. These scars are spread out, and may extend deeper into the skin and affect muscles and nerves. The larger the burn, the more likely it is contracture scars may affect the ability to move certain parts of the body, depending on the location. If a person develops a contracture scar early in life, the scar may become mixed with healthy tissue.

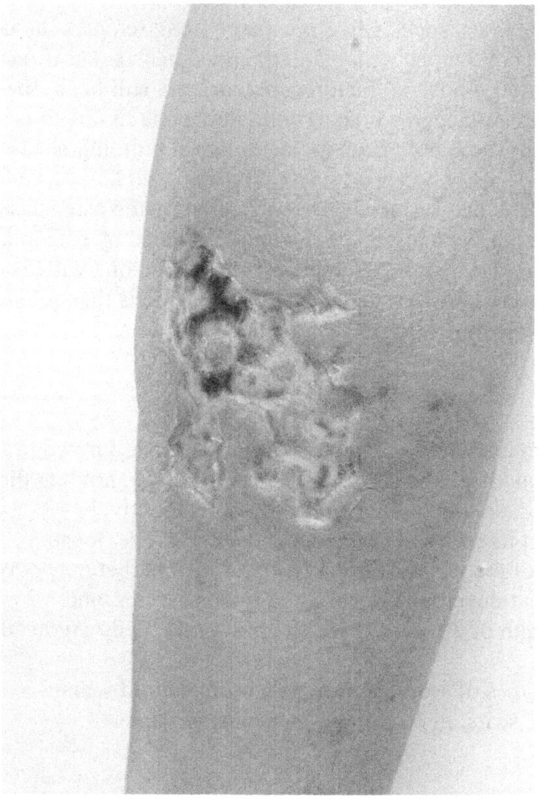

**Hypertrophic scars** are similar to keloid scars, but they do not extend past the area of damage. These scars often appear **red**, and may be tender or painful. Hypertrophic scars are the result of a **collagen imbalance** at the site of injury, which does not allow the scar to form properly. **Excessive tension** on the area may also lead to the development of hypertrophic scars.

**Striae**, also known as **stretch marks**, are scars that form in the skin when the body experiences a **rapid growth**, such as during pregnancy, puberty, or during activities such as weight lifting. These scars generally have a different color than the surrounding skin. As the area grows, the skin is stretched and pulled apart. In response, the skin develops fibrous tissue to hold the expanding area together, which produces scarring.

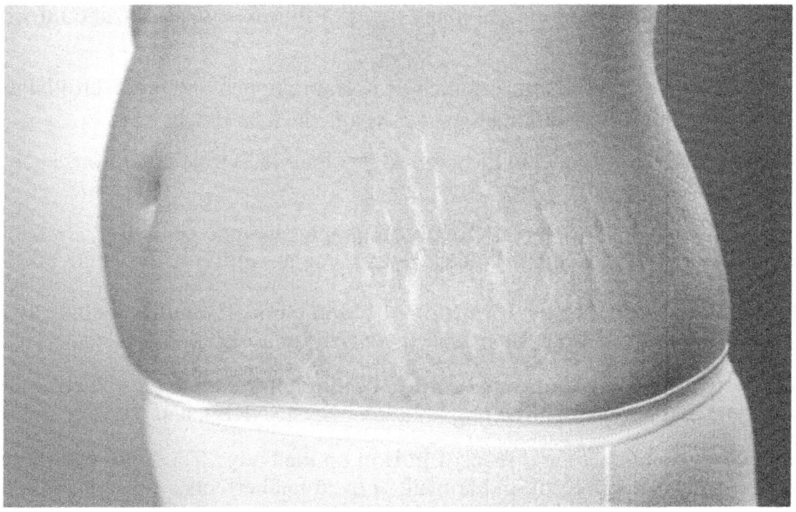

Striae commonly seen with pregnancy or weight gain

**Sutures** are used to **close wounds** produced through damage to tissues or surgery. Suturing a wound closed allows the damaged tissue to join together and produce a scar. There are many types of sutures, but all are either absorbable or non-absorbable. Absorbable sutures will be absorbed by the body and will not require surgical removal, while non-absorbable sutures require a doctor to surgically remove them.

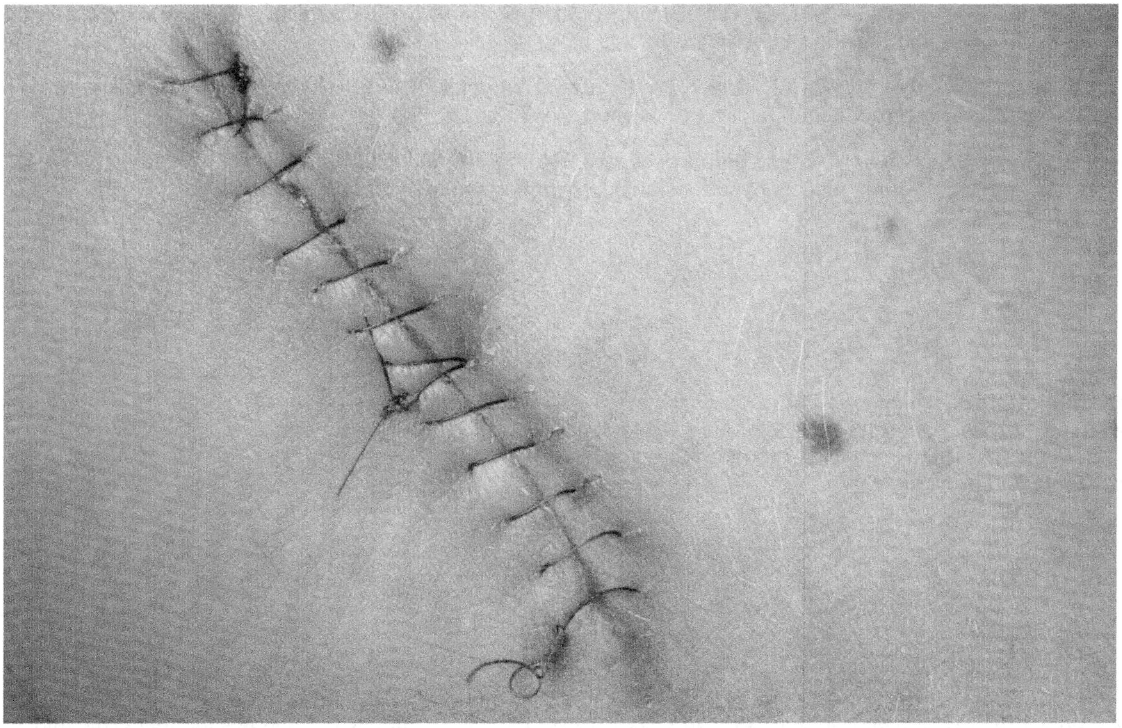

# Medications

There are many different types of medications used to treat many types of illnesses, diseases, and infections. Among the most common are:

- **Analgesics**, which help to **relieve pain**. Examples include acetaminophen and non-steroidal anti-inflammatory drugs. These help treat symptoms of conditions that cause pain, such as cancer.
- **Antacids**, which reduce the activity of **acids** in the stomach. These help treat conditions such as Gastroesophageal Reflux Disease.
- **Antibiotics**, which are used to combat **bacterial** growth. Examples include penicillin, amoxicillin, and erythromycin. These are used to treat infections in the body, such as cellulitis, impetigo, and strep throat.
- **Anticoagulants**, which are used to reduce the formation of **blood clots**. Examples include aspirin, heparin, and warfarin. These are used to treat conditions such as deep vein thrombosis and phlebitis.
- **Antidepressants**, which are used to **combat depression**. Common forms include selective serotonin reuptake inhibitors(SSRIs), serotonin and norepinephrine reuptake inhibitors(SNRIs), and tricyclic antidepressants.
- **Antidotes**, which are used to counteract the effects of **poison** on the body. These are used when too much of a substance has entered the body that can result in harmful, or even fatal effects.
- **Antifungals**, which aid in destroying **fungus**. Examples include terbinafine and fluconazole. These are used to treat any type of fungal infection, such as Tinea Pedis(Athlete's Foot) or Tinea Capitis.
- **Antihistamines**, which reduce the effects of **histamines** on the body, including runny nose and itching. These are used to treat allergic reactions.
- **Anti-inflammatory agents**, which help to reduce **inflammation**. Examples include non-steroidal anti-inflammatory drugs such as ibuprofen. These are used to help treat inflammation in conditions such as bronchitis, and potentially Alzheimer's Disease.
- **Antipyretics**, which help to reduce **fever**. Examples include ibuprofen and aspirin. These are used to treat symptoms of fever and other systemic infections.
- **Antivirals**, which aid in preventing **virus** reproduction. Examples include amantadine and rimantadine. These are used to combat virus reproduction in conditions such as encephalitis.
- **Beta blockers**, which help to reduce **blood pressure**. Examples include acebutolol, nadolol, and nebivolol. These are used to treat conditions such as hypertension, arrhythmia, and myocardial infarction.
- **Bronchodilators**, which aid in **dilation** of the **bronchial tubes**. Examples include albuterol and salmeterol. These are used to treat conditions such as asthma and bronchitis.

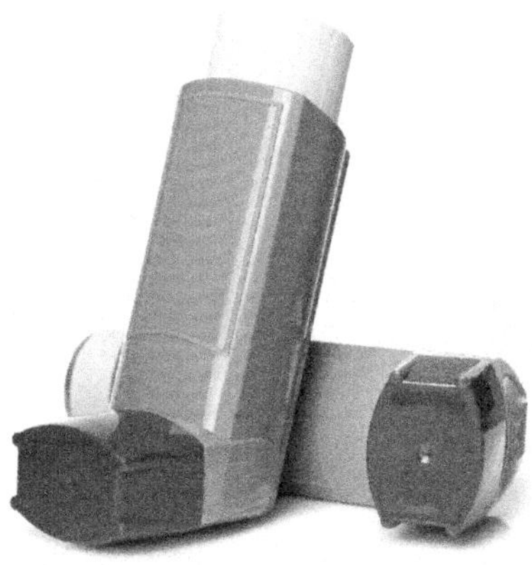

- **Decongestants**, which reduce **inflammation** in the **nasal cavity**. Examples include pseudoephedrine and phenylephrine. These are used to treat congestion caused by allergies.
- **Diuretics**, which increase the production of **urine**. Examples include bumetanide, amiloride, and mannitol. These are used to treat conditions such as edema and hypertension.

- **Expectorants**, which are used to help a person **expectorate**, or cough/spit mucous from the lungs. Common forms include over-the-counter brand names such as Mucinex and Robitussin. These are commonly used to treat chest congestion.
- **General anesthetics**, which are used to **numb** the **entire body**. Examples include propofol, ketamine, and etomidate. General anesthetics are primarily used when a person is having surgery performed that requires them to be in an unconscious state. These can be administered via needle injection or may be inhaled.
- **Insulin**, which **lowers** the amount of **sugar** in the bloodstream. Insulin is primarily used to treat diabetes.
- **Laxatives**, also known as stool softeners, which are used to help **loosen** and eliminate **feces** from the digestive tract. Common forms include mineral oil and milk of magnesia. These are used to treat constipation.

Comparison of angles of injection.

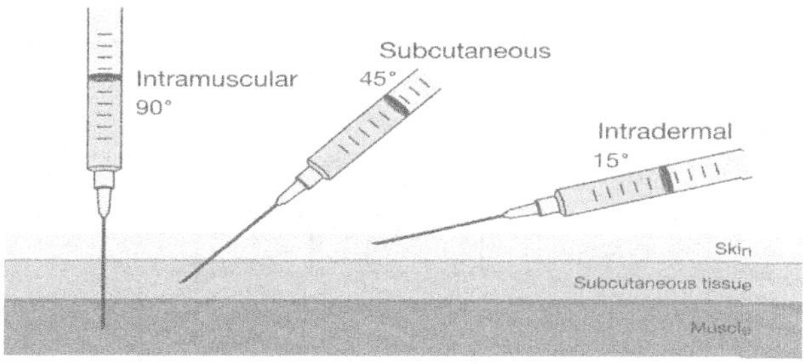


- **Local anesthetics**, which are used to **numb** an area. They are most commonly administered via **needle injection**. Examples include lidocaine and nitracaine. These are typically used before performing a surgical procedure around the area of incision.
- **Sedatives**, which are used to **calm** and **relax** the body. Examples include diazepam and clonazepam. These are typically used to calm a person before a painful or uncomfortable procedure is performed, such as a colonoscopy.
- **Statins**, which aid in lowering **cholesterol** levels in the blood stream. Examples include atorvastatin, rosuvastatin, and lovastatin. These are used to treat and/or prevent heart disease and its various symptoms, including hypertension and stroke.
- **Steroids**, which are primarily used to combat **inflammation** in specific areas. Common forms include corticosteroids and anabolic steroids. Corticosteroids are useful in treating conditions such as asthma, arthritis, and lupus.
- **Suppositories**, which are used in cases where a person may have difficulty orally consuming a medication. The most common type of suppository is a rectal suppository, but vaginal and urethral suppositories are also used. Suppositories are often used to treat constipation, hemorrhoids, fever, bacterial infections, and fungal infections.

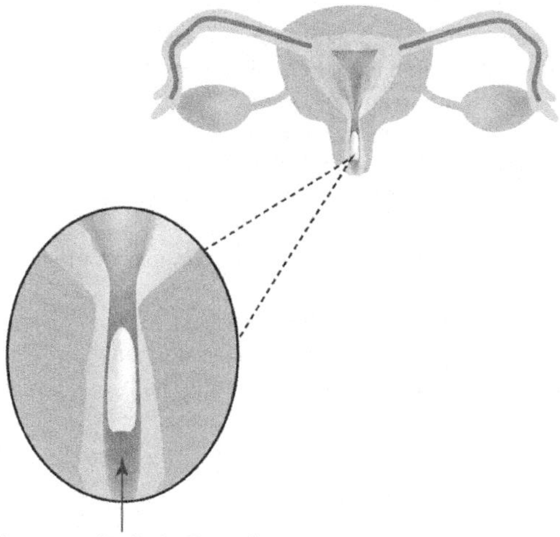

Placing suppositories in the vagina

- **Vaccines**, which are used to **prevent** a contagious disease from developing in a person. Common vaccines include MMR(Measles-Mumps-Rubella), DTaP(Diphtheria, Tetanus, and Pertussis), influenza, and human papilloma virus. Vaccines are commonly administered via intramuscular needle injection.

# Pathology

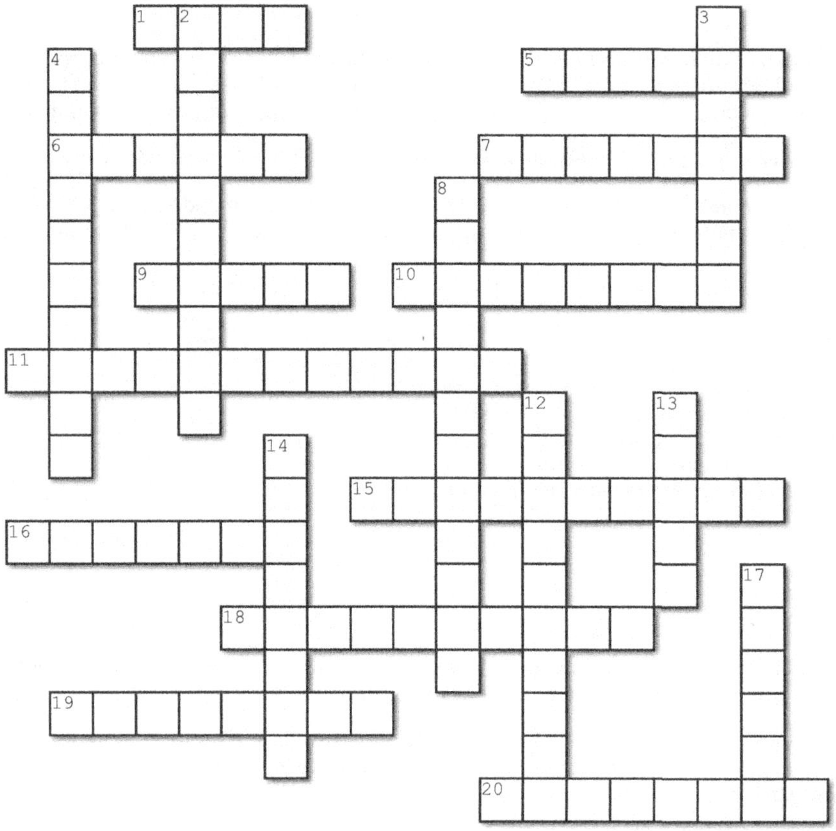

**Across**

**1.** Cicatrix is also known as this
**5.** A scar that is raised off the skin
**6.** Tinea pedis and tinea capitis are infections caused by this
**7.** Molecule pathogens contain that antibodies recognize and react to
**9.** Influenza and herpes are examples of this
**10.** Helminths are infectious agents known as this
**11.** Dilation of capillaries at the site of trauma causes this
**15.** Disorders in which the body's immune system attacks its own cells and structures
**16.** Disease that has a slow onset and persists for at least three months or longer
**18.** A disease that a person obtains through genetics
**19.** The ability of the body to protect itself from pathogens
**20.** Disease a person develops at some point after birth

**Down**

**2.** A disease that is present at birth
**3.** Condition that affects certain structures or functions of the body, typically presenting with signs and symptoms
**4.** A disease resulting from the body not receiving adequate nutrients
**8.** Process of a cell eating a pathogen or debris
**12.** A disease that has an unknown cause
**13.** Disease that has a sudden onset and lasts for a short period of time
**14.** Staphylococci and streptococci are examples of this
**17.** This is used to close a wound and bring the edges of damaged tissue together to promote proper scar formation

Answer Key on Page 286

# Disease, Immunity, and Medications Quiz

1. Signs of inflammation include
A. Heat, pain, redness, coldness
B. Pain, edema, swelling, redness
C. Swelling, heat, redness, pain
D. Redness, pain, heat, dehydration

2. Ischemia may ultimately result in
A. Phlebitis
B. Arteriosclerosis
C. Necrosis
D. Varicose veins

3. Anticoagulants are medications that prevent
A. Blood vessel dilation
B. Inflammation
C. Mucous production
D. Blood clotting

4. Medication prescribed to fight off bacterial infections
A. Anti-inflammatory Agents
B. Antivenoms
C. Antipyretics
D. Antibiotics

5. Analgesics are used to combat
A. Pain
B. Obesity
C. Inflammation
D. Gout

6. Lice, scabies, and ticks are all types of
A. Parasites
B. Bacterium
C. Fungi
D. Viruses

7. Phagocytosis is a cellular process in which
A. A cell absorbs a harmful fluid in the blood stream
B. A cell eats and destroys a harmful object or organism in the body
C. A cell begins the stages of apoptosis
D. A cell divides from one mother cell into two daughter cells

8. Cicatrix is the development of fibrous material to help a wound heal, also known as
A. Bruise
B. Hemorrhage
C. Scar
D. Chemotaxis

9. A disease a person has obtained at some point after birth
A. Acquired disease
B. Deficiency disease
C. Autoimmune disease
D. Hereditary disease

10. Parasitic worms are known as
A. Protozoa
B. Rotovirus
C. H. pylori
D. Helminths

11. Upon tissue becoming damaged, the beginning stages of inflammation begin. The first stage of inflammation is when
A. Damaged tissues release histamines to dilate blood vessels in the area
B. Scar tissue begins forming to reduce infection
C. Phagocytes enter the area and destroy pathogens
D. Lymph is emptied from the damaged area to allow blood to clot

12. Statins are prescribed when
A. A person is experiencing extreme pain in a localized area
B. A person is at risk of developing blood clots in the veins of the legs
C. A person has high levels of cholesterol in their blood
D. A person has trouble breathing due to constriction in the respiratory passages

13. Anemia, goiter, and osteoporosis are all examples of
A. Congenital diseases
B. Deficiency diseases
C. Autoimmune diseases
D. Hereditary diseases

14. E. coli, streptococcus, and Helicobacter pylori are all types of
A. Parasites
B. Viruses
C. Bacteria
D. Fungus

15. A disease or condition that has a sudden onset that typically lasts for a short period of time
A. Acute
B. Chronic
C. Acquired
D. Autoimmune

Answer Key on Page 289

# Cardiovascular System and Pathologies

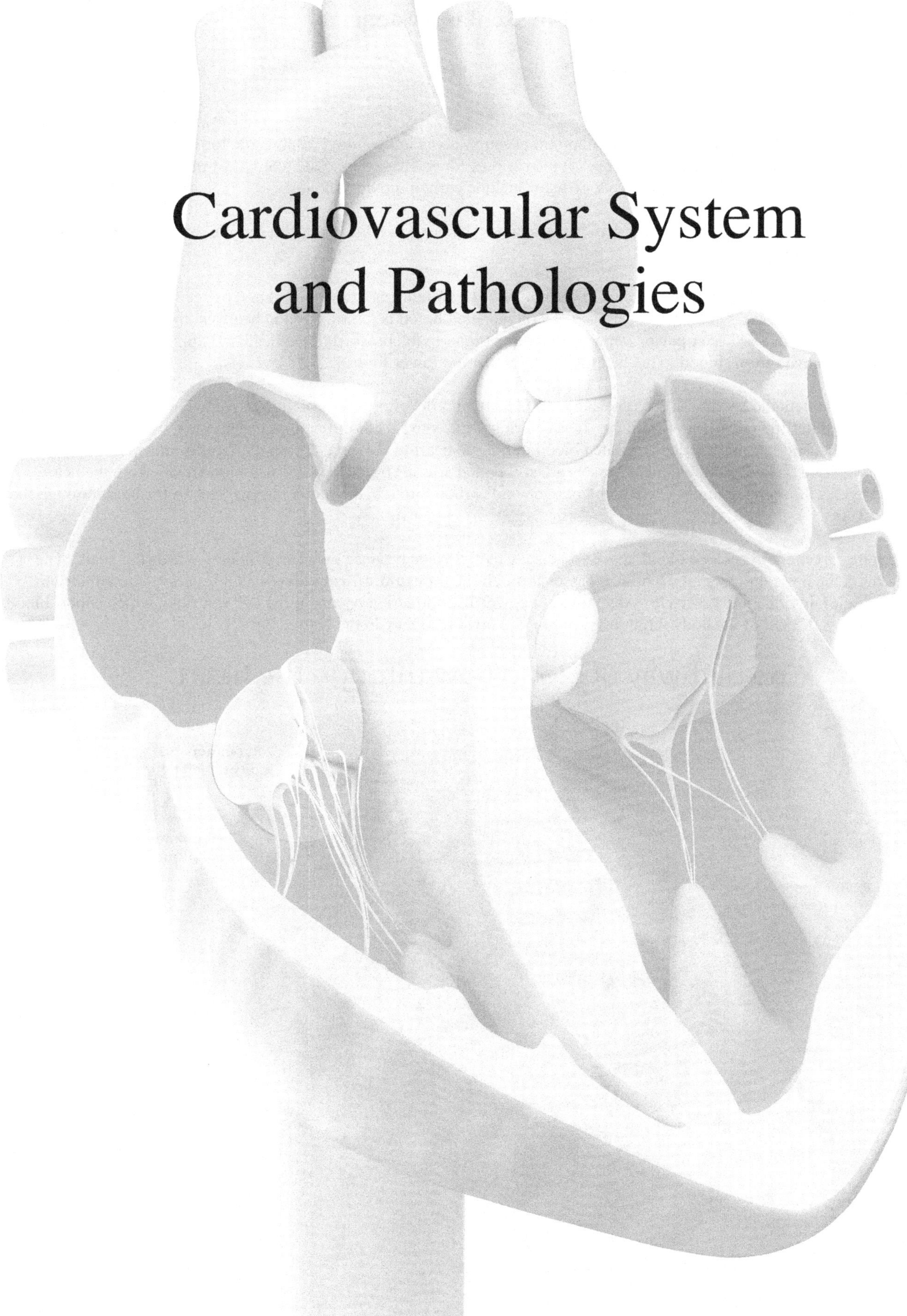

# Cardiovascular System

The Cardiovascular System is one of the most important organ systems in the body, responsible for **transportation** of nutrients such as oxygen and hormones to tissues. It also allows for waste to be moved to areas of the body where it can be eliminated, such as the lungs, liver, and kidneys. Wastes include carbon dioxide and urea.

The primary organ of the Cardiovascular System is the **heart**. The heart, a large, powerful muscle, has one function: to **pump blood** throughout the body.

Blood is sent to the body to exchange oxygen and carbon dioxide. When gas exchange occurs, oxygen detaches from the erythrocytes, and carbon dioxide takes its place. Deoxygenated blood is returned to the heart via the largest veins in the body, the vena cavae. The **superior vena cava** returns blood to the heart from the head and upper limbs, while the **inferior vena cava** returns blood to the heart from the trunk and lower limbs.

When blood first enters the heart, it is deoxygenated, and enters into the **right atrium**. It then passes through the **tricuspid valve**(which separates the right atrium from the right ventricle), into the **right ventricle**. The cardiac muscle in the right ventricle contracts, and it sends the deoxygenated blood out of the heart to the lungs through the **pulmonary arteries**. Despite carrying deoxygenated blood, these vessels are still called arteries because they carry blood away from the heart. After blood cycles through the lungs, exchanging oxygen and carbon dioxide, the blood returns back to the heart through the **pulmonary veins**.

Again, despite carrying oxygenated blood, these vessels are called veins because they carry blood towards the heart. The blood re-enters the heart into the **left atrium**. It passes through the **bicuspid/mitral valve**(which separates the left atrium and left ventricle), into the **left ventricle**. An extremely powerful contraction occurs in the left ventricle, which shoots blood out of the heart to the rest of the body through the **aorta**, the **largest artery** in the body.

## The pathway of blood flow through the heart

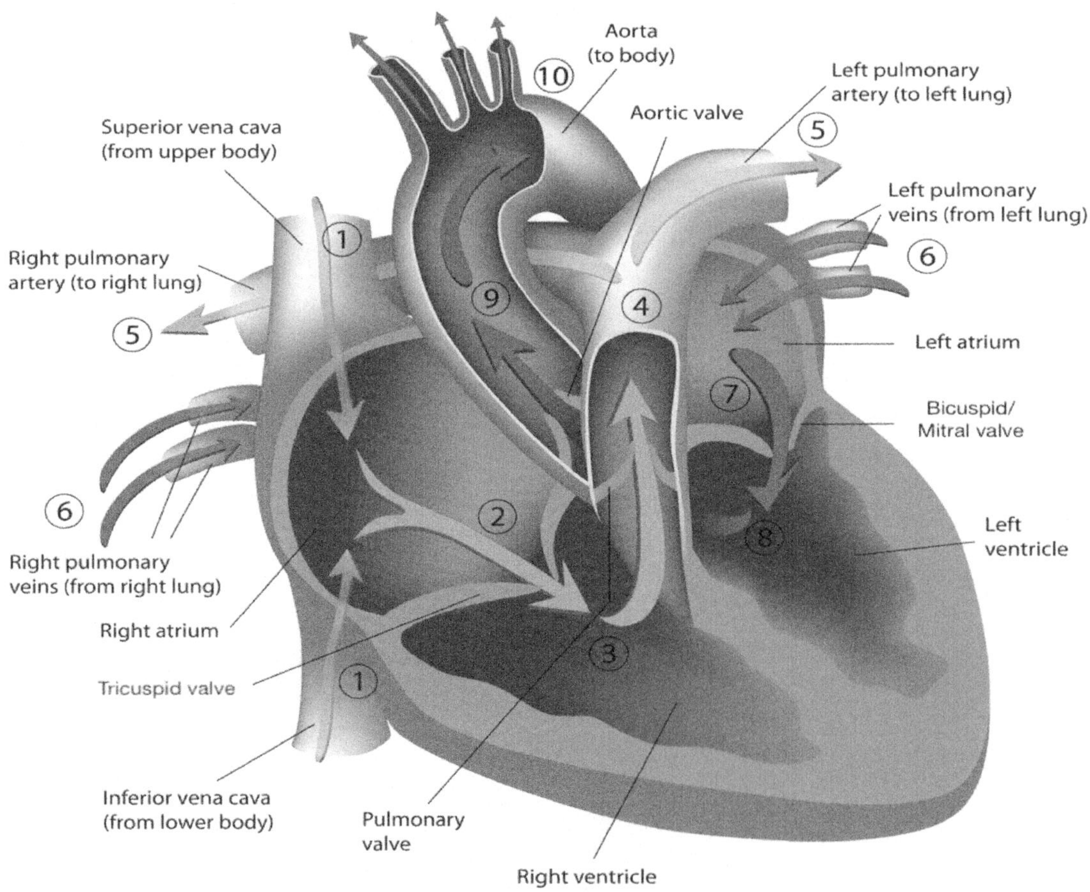

**Blood vessels** are the main route of transportation for not only blood, but other substances, such as hormones. These substances are carried throughout the body in blood vessels. The largest types of blood vessels are known as **arteries**. Arteries primarily carry oxygenated blood away from the heart, to tissues. Arteries are the deepest blood vessels due to their size and importance. Tissues surrounding the arteries help to protect them from damage, which could result in severe bleeding and loss of oxygen.

**Veins** are blood vessels that primarily carry deoxygenated blood towards the heart, where it can replace carbon dioxide with oxygen. Veins are much more superficial than arteries, often visible under the skin, whereas most arteries cannot be seen.

**Capillaries** are microscopic arteries, and are where gas exchange takes place between blood vessels and tissues.

Major arteries and veins are often named after their location in the body, such as the brachial artery/vein(in the arm), femoral artery/vein(in the thigh), abdominal aorta(in the abdomen), etc.

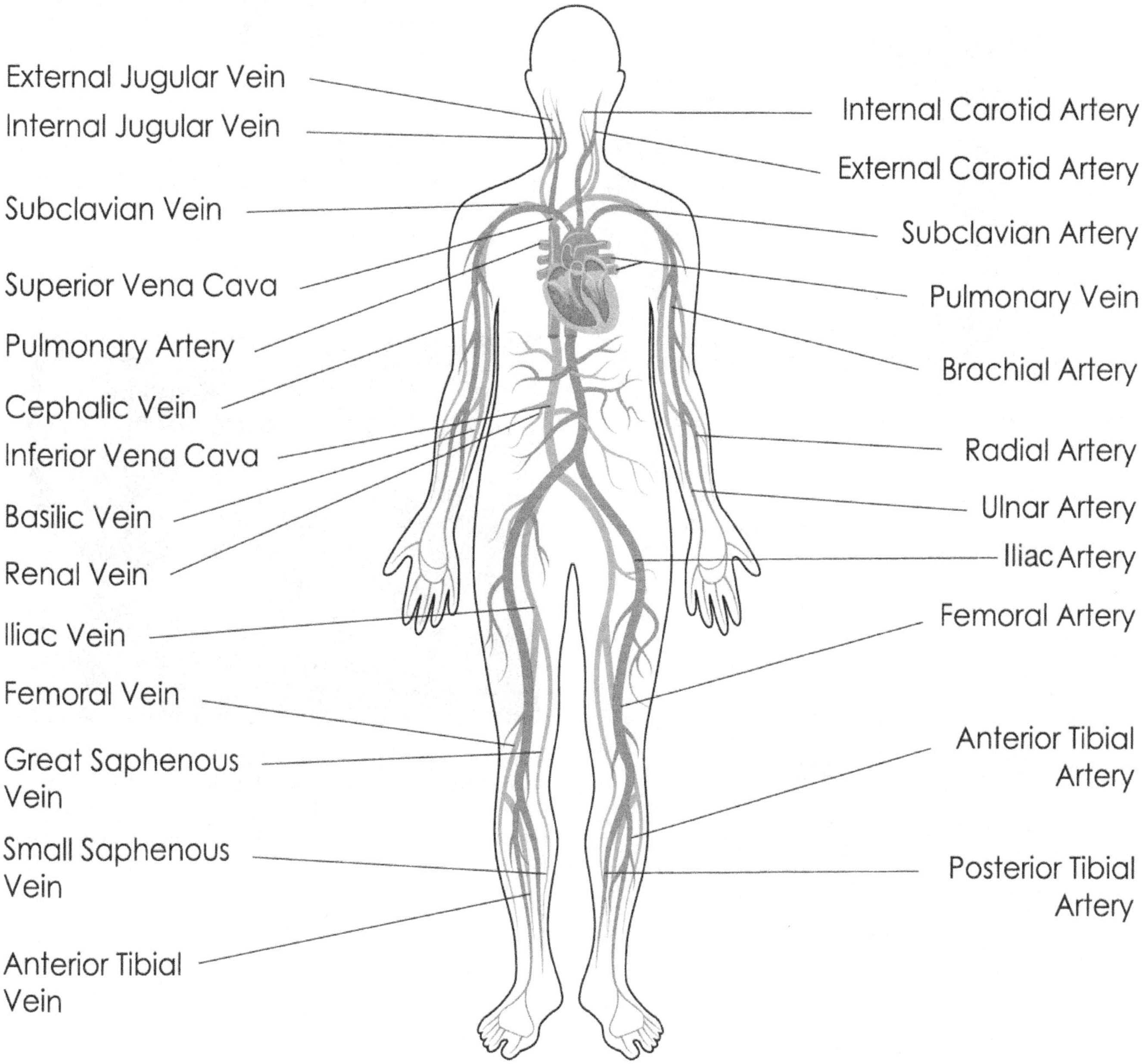

**Blood** is the most **abundant** form of connective tissue in the body. Blood is mainly a mode of **transportation** for blood cells, hormones, nutrients, and waste products. There are four parts of blood: **erythrocytes**, **leukocytes**, **thrombocytes**, and **plasma**.

**Erythrocytes**, also known as red blood cells, are responsible for **transporting oxygen** and **carbon dioxide** throughout the body. The cytoplasm of erythrocytes is made of a protein known as **hemoglobin**, which is primarily made of iron. Hemoglobin is what oxygen and carbon dioxide attach to. In the lungs, when the erythrocytes are exposed to the alveoli, carbon dioxide detaches from the erythrocytes, and oxygen then attaches in its place. This is how gas exchange occurs in erythrocytes.

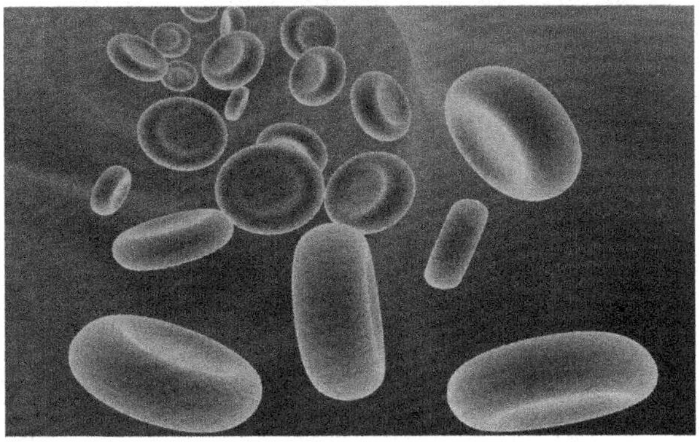

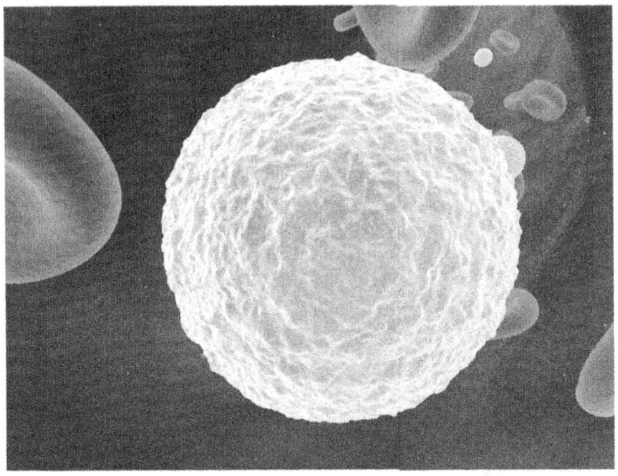

**Leukocytes**, also known as white blood cells, are the body's primary **defense** against **pathogens**. There are several different types of leukocytes, ranging from T-cells to basophils. These cells eat pathogens(such as bacteria), dead cells, and debris floating in the blood stream. When there is an infection inside the body, leukocytes move into the area of infection and destroy bacteria. The waste produced during this process becomes pus.

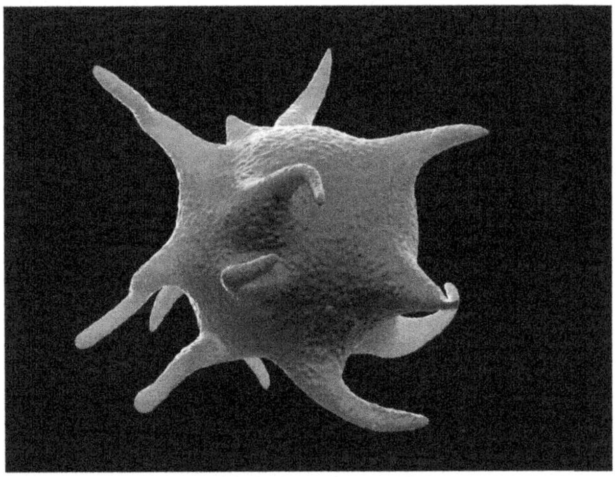

**Thrombocytes**, also known as **platelets**, have one function: to **clot the blood**. This is vitally important when a person is bleeding. If the blood does not clot, the person could continue bleeding until they lose too much blood. Thrombocytes contain proteins that allow them to adhere to a mesh of fibrin, creating a kind of natural bandage that can prevent bleeding.

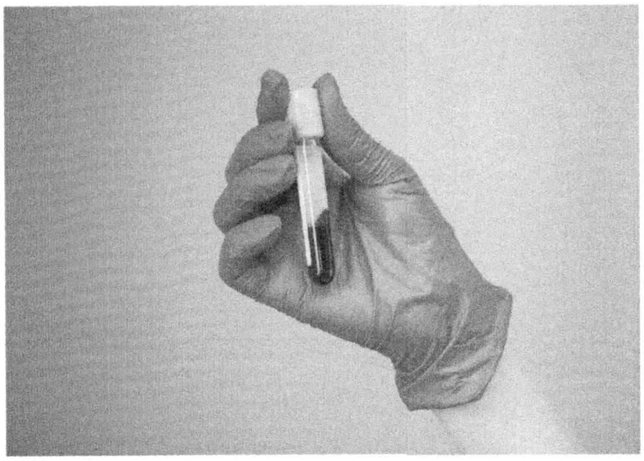

**Plasma** is the **fluid** portion of blood. The majority of blood, around 56%, is made of plasma. Plasma is what allows all of the blood cells, hormones, nutrients, and waste to move throughout the body. Without plasma, these substances would go nowhere!

## Medical Tests and Equipment

**AED(Automated External Defibrillator)**: An AED is a portable defibrillator, used to send electric shocks to the heart in a person who is suffering from sudden cardiac arrest. The person will have two sticky pads attached to their skin that connect to the AED, one pad placed on the chest and one on the left side of the trunk. The AED sends a shock to the person through the pads, directly into the heart, which can help return the heart to its normal rhythm.

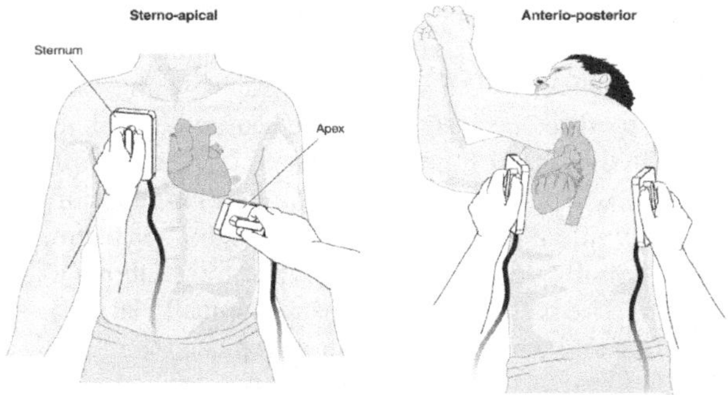


**Echocardiogram:** An echocardiogram is a type of ultrasound performed on the heart in order to view all the structures and chambers of the heart. This can be used to determine if there are any issues with the heart, such as valve defects, how strong the heart muscle is, or if there are any abnormal holes in the heart.

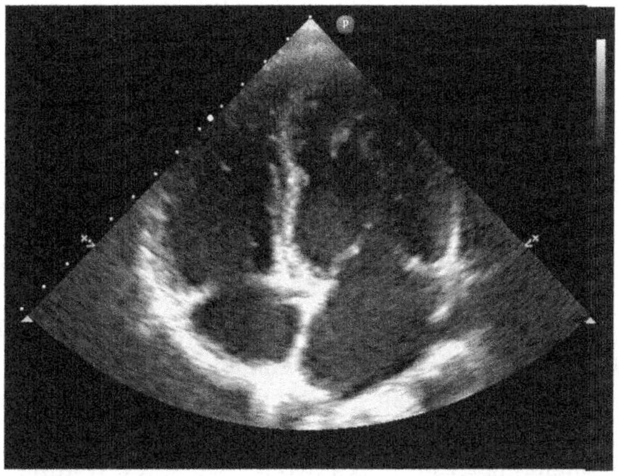

**ECG/EKG(Electrocardiogram):** If a doctor feels as if a patient needs to have their heart rhythm monitored, they may administer an ECG/EKG. During this procedure, ten pads attached to electrodes are attached to the patient's bare skin in specific points around the trunk. The ECG/EKG picks up the electrical activity of the heart, and produces a visualization that shows each wave of electrical activity. The first wave seen is known as the P wave, and shows the contraction of the atria. Next is the QRS wave, which shows the depolarization and contraction of the ventricles. Following that is the T wave, which represents re-polarization of the ventricles.

In some cases, a person may need to have heart activity recorded over 24-48 hours. In these cases, a Holter Monitor is used. These are portable machines that remain attached to a patient, continuously recording heart activity. These can be used if a person has irregular heart rhythms that come and go, and aren't present during an initial ECG reading.

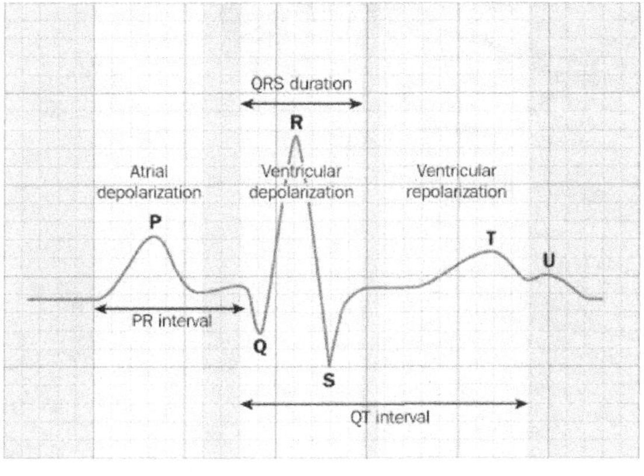


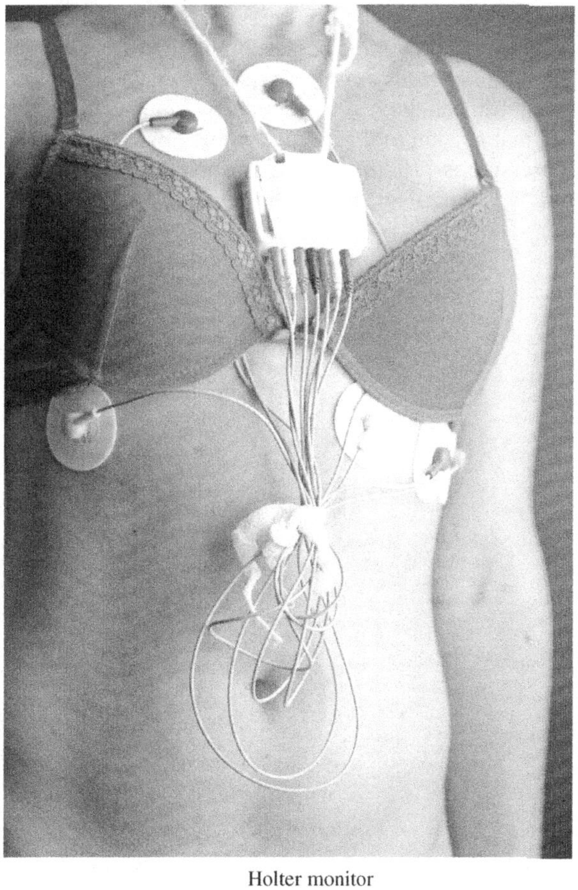

Holter monitor

**Pacemaker**: If a patient suffers from severe arrhythmia, a pacemaker may be implanted into the body to help regulate heart rhythm. The pacemaker is usually placed under the skin on the upper left side of the chest, just inferior to the clavicle. A pacemaker is a small metal device with a battery inside that sends electric shocks to the heart when it detects the heart rhythm is not functioning properly. It accomplishes this with the use of leads that travel through the superior vena cava directly into the heart. The leads go into the atrium, ventricle, or both, depending on the type of arrhythmia a person has. The battery in a pacemaker typically lasts between five and ten years, and can be replaced.

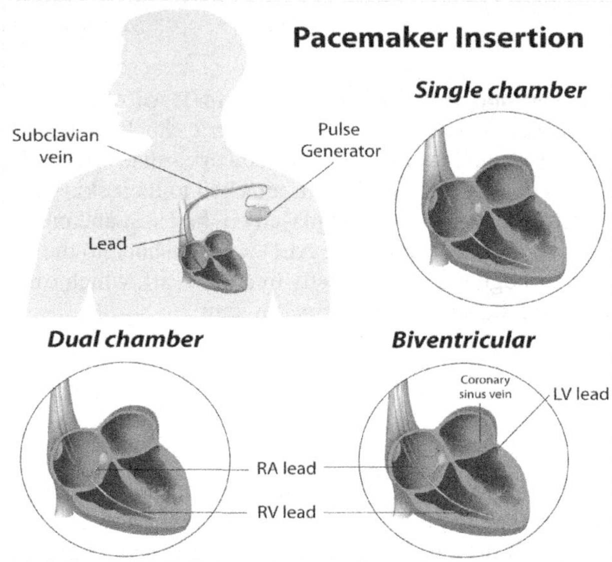


**Sphygmomanometer**: When measuring blood pressure, a sphygmomanometer is wrapped around a person's arm. The cuff around the arm inflates, and the pressure of the blood passing through the arteries can be felt. The sphygmomanometer produces two numbers: the systolic number and diastolic number. The systolic number reads systolic pressure, which is the pressure felt as blood is pumped from the heart and passes through the arteries. The diastolic number reads diastolic pressure, which is the pressure felt when the heart is at rest and blood is not passing through that portion of the arteries at that time. A normal blood pressure is 120/80 mmHg, in which the systolic pressure is 120 mmHg, and the diastolic pressure is 80 mmHg.

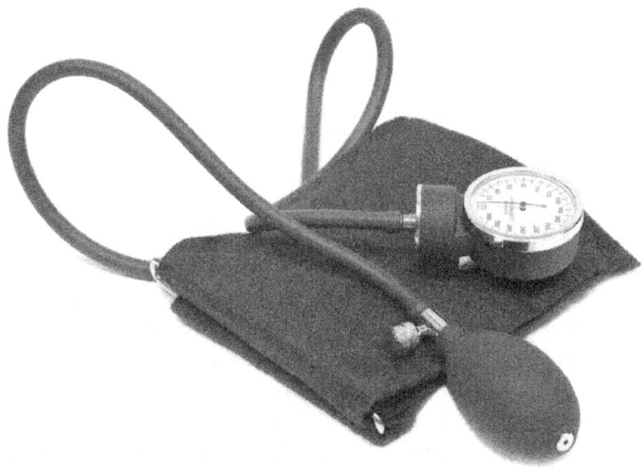

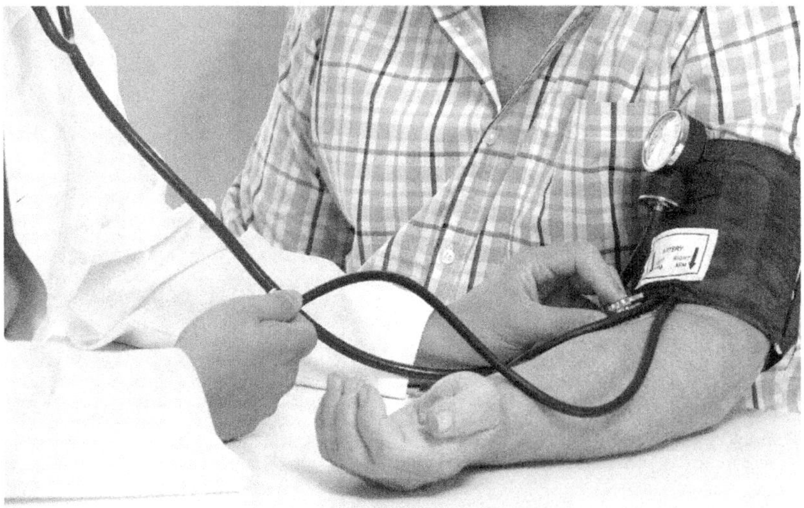

# Cardiovascular System Pathologies

## Anemia

*(an-: without; -emia: blood)*

Anemia is a disease of the blood, resulting in a **lack of oxygen** and an over-abundance of carbon dioxide in the blood. There are many different types of anemia, ranging from **iron-deficient anemia** to **sickle cell anemia**. Anemia is the most common blood condition in the United States, with an estimated 3.5-4 million people afflicted with it.

Iron-deficient anemia is the most common form of anemia. The cells in the blood that are responsible for carrying oxygen and carbon dioxide throughout the body are the erythrocytes, or red blood cells. In the cytoplasm of erythrocytes, there is a protein present known as hemoglobin, which is made of iron. The hemoglobin attracts oxygen and carbon dioxide, allowing these molecules to attach to the erythrocytes.

### *Causes*

In iron-deficient anemia, the primary cause is a lack of iron being consumed. Less iron being consumed results in less **hemoglobin** in the erythrocytes, which in turn causes a lack of oxygen and carbon dioxide attaching to the red blood cells.

Sickle cell anemia is an inherited form of anemia, in which the erythrocytes have a sickle shape, as opposed to a normal erythrocyte, which is circular. This shape can cause the erythrocytes to become stuck in blood vessels, and reduce adequate blood flow to tissues.

### *Symptoms*

People with anemia may feel sluggish, tired, have an increased heart rate, may show paleness in the skin, shortness of breath, and experience dizziness, all due to a lack of sufficient oxygen reaching tissues.

Sickle cell anemia may also result in the further development of infections due to damage caused to the spleen, pain in the thorax and abdomen(known as crises) due to blockage of blood vessels in these locations, and a lack of nutrients to the body, which can stunt growth.

People whose diet lacks proper amounts of iron or vitamin B-12 may develop anemia. Pregnancy, and a lack of folic acid, may result in anemia in pregnant women. Sickle cell anemia is primarily seen in African-Americans, resulting from a genetic defect.

### *Treatments*

Treatments for anemia vary depending on the type, but may include increasing iron intake, bone marrow transplants, or blood transfusions. Pregnant women may require an increased intake of folic acid. People with sickle cell anemia face less treatment options. The only potential cure is through a bone marrow transplant. Oftentimes, the only treatment is trying to minimize the number of crises a person may experience. Antibiotics and pain relievers may help in preventing infections in younger patients and reducing pain experienced during crises.

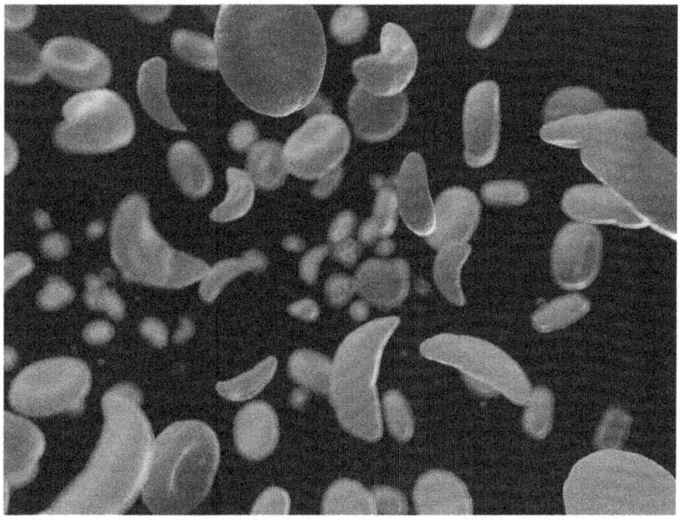

### *Contraindications*

Massage is indicated for a client with anemia. Massage helps increase circulation and oxygen intake, which provides the body with needed nutrients.

## Aneurysm

*(Greek "aneurysma": a widening)*

An aneurysm is a condition of the arteries, resulting in a **bulge** in the **wall of an artery**. There are several different forms and causes of aneurysms. Different types of aneurysms include Aortic(bulge in the wall of the aorta), Cerebral(bulge in an artery supplying blood to the brain), and Ventricular(bulge in the wall of the heart).

***Causes***

Aneurysms are the result of a part of an arterial wall becoming weakened. When the wall of the artery becomes weakened, it forces the wall out, creating a pouch or bubble. Most commonly, aneurysms are the result of hypertension putting too much pressure or strain on the artery. Ventricular aneurysms are most commonly caused by myocardial infarction, which can weaken the heart muscle.

When the arterial wall stretches due to weakness, it makes it much easier for the artery to rupture. Because the artery carries oxygen-rich blood, this makes aneurysms very dangerous, as any rupture will severely cut off blood flow to the structure supplied with blood by the artery.

***Symptoms***

Unfortunately, aneurysms that have not ruptured are asymptomatic. In fact, aneurysms themselves, unless very large, cause no symptoms at all. When an aneurysm ruptures, however, a person may experience severe chest or back pain, low blood pressure, severe headache, tachycardia, and lightheadedness.

Many different people may develop aneurysms for many different reasons, including obesity, hypertension, diabetes, advanced age, and alcoholism. Some people develop aneurysms for no apparent reason at all.

***Treatments***

Common locations for aneurysms include the abdominal aorta and the brain. Aneurysms may be treated surgically before rupture to prevent major medical emergencies in the future. Beta blockers are commonly used as medications before surgery is required.

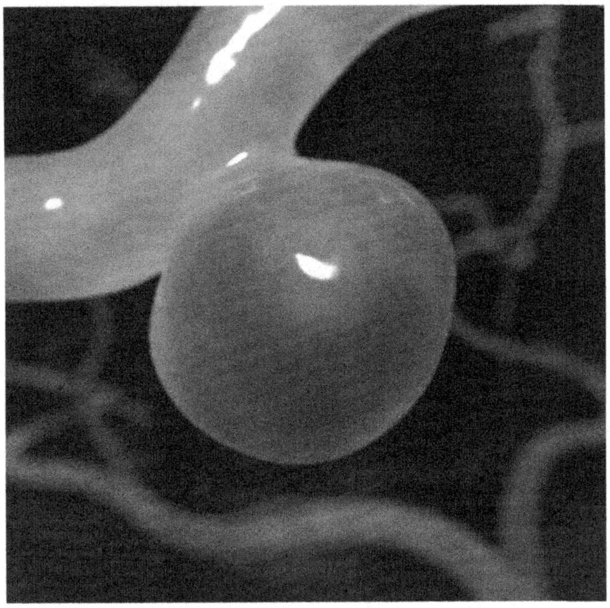

Berry aneurysm

***Contraindications***

Massage is indicated with a doctor's note. Any massage that increases blood pressure should be avoided, such as deep tissue, because it can put pressure on arteries, which may lead to bursting of an aneurysm.

## Angina Pectoris

*(Latin "angere": to strangle; pectoris: chest)*

Angina Pectoris is **pain in the chest**, which results from **ischemia in heart tissue**.

***Causes***

The primary cause of angina pectoris is **blockages** in arteries that provide the myocardium with blood. When these arteries become restricted, the heart muscle is unable to get enough oxygen-rich blood. Lack of oxygen in tissue results in ischemia. During times of physical exertion, chest pain may develop as a result of the lack of oxygen entering the heart tissue. During times of rest, however, the heart does not have to work as hard, and the pain is non-existent. People who develop angina pectoris usually have increased emotional stress, and are chronic cigarette smokers. Because the arteries are narrowed, atherosclerosis may also be a contributing factor in the development of chest pain.

***Symptoms***

Symptoms of angina pectoris include acute instances of pain(less than five minutes), pain that dissipates with medication and/or rest, and pain that only appears when the heart is required to work harder, such as during physical activity.

***Treatments***

Treatment includes rest and medication, such as nitroglycerin, which relaxes the coronary arteries and increases the volume of blood entering the myocardium.

***Contraindications***

Angina pectoris is generally indicated for massage. During acute pain, massage should be postponed until the client is comfortable enough to continue with massage.

## Arrhythmia

*(a-: without; rhythm: rhythm)*

Arrhythmia is a condition of the heart, which results in the heart's natural **rhythm** being **altered**. There are several different forms of arrhythmia. Some of the most common forms of arrhythmia are Atrial Fibrillation, Bradycardia, and Tachycardia.

***Causes***

Atrial fibrillation, the most common form of arrhythmia, results when the atria, the heart's upper chambers, contract irregularly, which sends blood into the ventricles at uncoordinated times. This is caused by an electrical signal from the SA Node not firing correctly, which disrupts the timing of the atria contracting. This can affect the ability of the heart to consistently deliver oxygenated blood to the body.

Bradycardia*(brady-: slow; -cardia: heart)* results in the heart rate being reduced to a rate of contraction that is considered too slow to deliver substantial oxygen to the body.

Tachycardia*(tachy-: rapid; -cardia: heart)* results in the heart rate being increased to a rate of contraction that is considered too rapid. In tachycardia, the ventricles of the heart are contracting too rapidly, which may cause a lack of oxygen-rich blood from reaching the body, as the quick contractions do not allow the ventricles to properly fill with blood before being pumped out to the rest of the body. Older adults, those over age 60, are more likely to develop arrhythmia than younger adults and children. Heart diseases are a main contributing factor towards older adults developing arrhythmia. Other diseases may also play a role in the development of arrhythmia, so people who have had myocardial infarction may be more prone to developing the disease. Diabetes, sleep apnea, and hypertension all have contributed to the development of arrhythmia.

***Symptoms***

There are many different symptoms seen with arrhythmia. Symptoms include dizziness, fatigue, shortness of breath, pain in the chest, lightheadedness, and fainting. Arrhythmia may also result in cardiac arrest in severe cases.

***Treatments***

Treatments vary, depending on the type of arrhythmia a person suffers from. Medical devices such as pacemakers may be implanted into the body to help regulate and control heart rhythm(IE, if a person's heart rate drops too low, the pacemaker will stimulate the heart muscle and cause it to contract, increasing heart rate back to safe levels). Alternative methods to controlling arrhythmia, such as massage therapy and yoga, may be applied in some cases.

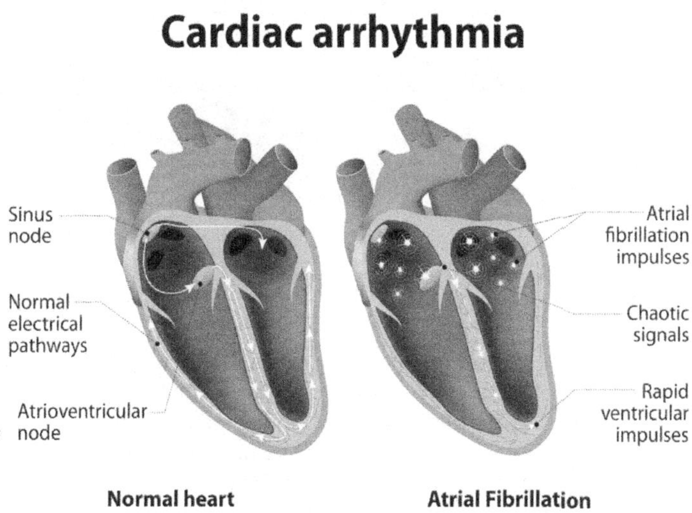

***Contraindications***

Untreated arrhythmia is an absolute contraindication for massage therapy. If a client has a pacemaker, massage may be performed. A client may have discomfort while lying prone due to pressure on the pacemaker, which may call for side-lying massage to be performed, or pillows to be used to take pressure off the area. Avoid massaging the site of the pacemaker(upper left chest just below clavicle).

## Arteriosclerosis/Atherosclerosis

*(arterio: artery; scler-: hard; -osis: condition);*
*(athero: fatty plaque; scler-: hard; -osis: condition)*

Arteriosclerosis is a **hardening** of the **walls of arteries**, a condition that progresses slowly over time. Atherosclerosis is a **build-up** of **fatty plaque** inside the arteries. These two conditions are often caused by one another, and are often interchangeable.

***Causes***

Arteriosclerosis has many different contributing factors, including hypertension, high cholesterol, and smoking. Each of these can damage an artery. The body's response to this damage is to increase the thickness of the artery to prevent further damage. When this occurs, the artery becomes much harder and unable to move and stretch normally. This may also lead to increased deposits of plaque in the arteries, a condition known as atherosclerosis. This increased plaque, along with the hardening of the artery, may restrict blood flow and lead to conditions such as angina pectoris and myocardial infarction.

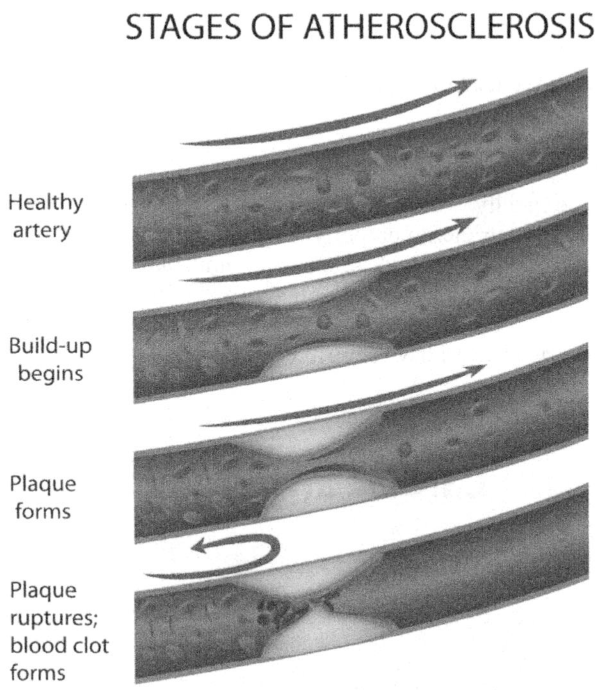


***Symptoms***

Symptoms include angina pectoris, shortness of breath, fatigue, and pain in any area of the body that may have any sort of restriction in the arteries.

***Treatments***

Medications are effective treatments for arteriosclerosis/atherosclerosis, including beta-blockers, statins, calcium channel blockers, and diuretics. If an increased plaque buildup is severe, an angioplasty may be performed, or a stent may be placed inside the artery to increase blood flow. Plaque may be surgically removed, or a bypass surgery may be performed to increase circulation into areas that may be experiencing ischemia.

***Contraindications***

Massage for atherosclerosis/arteriosclerosis may be performed. Certain medications may require a lighter massage to be performed, because they may thin the blood and damage to a blood vessel can lead to increased bleeding internally.

## Congestive Heart Failure

Congestive Heart Failure is the **gradual failure** of the **heart** to adequately **pump blood** throughout the body. There are many causes of Congestive Heart Failure. There are two types of heart failure: Systolic heart failure and Diastolic heart failure. In systolic heart failure, the heart muscle can no longer pump with enough force, and blow flow is reduced throughout the body as a result. In diastolic heart failure, the ventricles of the heart weaken, reducing the effectiveness of the heart pumping blood. To compensate, the heart pumps blood much harder than normal, increasing blood pressure. Despite the increased pressure, the walls of the heart chambers further weaken, which may lead to eventual death as a result. The condition is known as Congestive Heart Failure due to the body's inability to remove waste, such as urea, from the body as a result of the decreased ability to pump blood. The **increased amount of waste** in the body is known as **congestion**.

***Causes***

Causes of Congestive Heart Failure include coronary artery disease, such as atherosclerosis, which reduces blood flow into the myocardium and damages heart tissue, hypertension, myocardial infarction, and more. Typically, Congestive Heart Failure is the result of damage to heart tissue in some way. Commonly, people who have suffered from a heart attack are much more likely to develop Congestive Heart Failure than those who have not. Hypertension, arrhythmia, obesity, and diabetes are all contributing factors towards the development of Congestive Heart Failure. According to the American Heart Association, roughly 5.7 million people in the Unites States have been diagnosed with Congestive Heart Failure, and it is one of the leading causes of hospital visits for people over the age of 65.

***Symptoms***

People with Congestive Heart Failure may have pitting edema(page 138) due to the kidney's inability to properly filter waste, fatigue, dizziness, arrhythmia, and difficulty breathing.

***Treatments***

Treatments for Congestive Heart Failure are numerous, and many depend on the cause of the heart failure itself. Many times, treating the cause of heart failure can remedy the heart failure itself.

Medications prescribed include ACE inhibitors to dilate blood vessels, diuretics to reduce waste and fluid buildup in the body, and beta blockers to lower blood pressure and possibly reverse the damage caused by systolic heart failure.

Surgery may be an option if medication isn't effective on its own. Types of surgery include bypass surgery to return blood flow into areas of the heart that may be damaged from blockages in arteries, replacement or repair of heart valves, and in extreme cases, heart transplant.

***Contraindications***

Massage is indicated for a client with congestive heart failure, as massage may help lower blood pressure and increase oxygen intake, both vital in the treatment of congestive heart failure.

## Deep Vein Thrombosis

*(thromb/o: clot; -osis; condition)*

Deep Vein Thrombosis(DVT) is a condition in which **blood clots**(thrombi) form in the **veins** deep in the body, typically the legs. These blood clots can **block blood flow** in the veins, which can lead to several serious issues.

***Causes***

There are various causes for DVT. Primary causes are injury to a vein, surgery, impaired or limited mobility, and certain medications. An injury to a vein can result in blood clots, especially if there is significant damage to the vein. Surgery, which can result in cutting through veins, can also lead to blood clots. Post-surgery, if a patient is immobilized for extended periods, circulation starts to decrease in efficiency, which can lead to blood pooling in the veins of the legs. This pooling of blood can result in clots. It is this same reason people who have paralysis may develop blood clots as well.

***Symptoms***

Although symptoms may not be present in someone with DVT, others do show symptoms, which include a warm sensation in the affected area, pain in the affected area that can increase in intensity, and discoloration in the affected area. Most commonly, DVT affects the lower limb, so this is where a person will most likely experience these symptoms.

***Treatments***

The primary treatment for DVT is medication. Certain medications can help reduce the chance of developing DVT in the future, or even remove the blood clot from the body. Intravenous anticoagulants such as heparin help to thin the blood. Other anticoagulants, such as warfarin, work extremely well in conjunction with injectable anticoagulants.

If the blood clot is severe, the patient might be given a thrombolytic, a type of medication that destroys blood clots. These are typically only given in serious cases of blood clots, such as those that result in pulmonary embolism.

Compression socks, which compress the leg up to the knee, can help reduce the amount of swelling a patient might experience with DVT.

***Contraindications***

Deep vein thrombosis is typically a local contraindication. Avoid the site of the thrombus, as dislodging the clot may lead to circulation being cut off in organs such as the lungs, brain, or heart. Massage that increases blood pressure may be contraindicated, and deeper massages may be contraindicated due to the use of anticoagulants and thrombolytics.

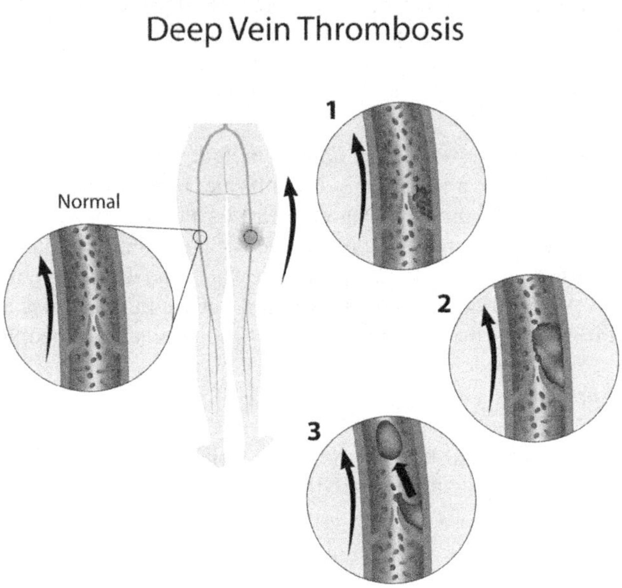


## Endocarditis

*(endo-: inside; card-: heart; -itis: inflammation)*

Endocarditis is **inflammation** of the **inner lining of the heart chambers and heart valves**, caused by some type of **infection**. Endocarditis typically affects people who have some sort of weakness in the heart valves. Because the heart valves don't have a direct blood supply, an infection of these valves can cause a lot of damage, with no effective way for the body to fight off this infection.

***Causes***

Infection that results in endocarditis is usually bacterial, but may also be caused by a fungus. These microorganisms can enter the body through poor dental hygiene, gum disease, and other infections or open sores on the body.

***Symptoms***

Common symptoms include fatigue, edema in the abdomen or lower limbs, chest pain upon inhalation, fever, and pain in muscles and joints. Symptoms vary from person to person and depend on the severity of the infection, which can range from mild to serious, based on the type of infection.

***Treatments***

Because endocarditis is the result of a bacterial or fungal infection, a patient would most likely be prescribed a course of intravenous antibiotics or antifungals to destroy the infection.

***Contraindications***

Endocarditis is a serious medical condition, and is considered an absolute contraindication to massage. A person with endocarditis should seek medical attention as soon as possible.

## Heart Murmur

*(murmur: to mutter)*

A heart murmur is a condition of the heart, which results in blood flowing **backwards** in the heart. A "murmur" refers to the sound of blood flowing through the heart. There are two types of heart murmurs: Innocent and Abnormal. Innocent heart murmurs are seen in children and infants, usually the result of congenital heart disease. Abnormal heart murmurs are much more serious, most likely due to the development of heart disease or valve malfunction.

### *Causes*

Heart murmurs may not require any medical attention, depending on the cause. Other times, medical attention may be needed. Most commonly, heart murmurs are the result of a **bicuspid/mitral valve** prolapse, where the valve is pulled backwards into the left atrium. This allows blood to flow backwards in the heart, which may reduce the ability of the heart to pump enough oxygen-rich blood to the body.

People who have developed endocarditis or Rheumatic fever often develop heart murmurs due to damage to the valves in the heart.

### *Symptoms*

While most heart murmurs aren't serious, abnormal heart murmurs may present with symptoms such as cyanosis on the fingers, chest pain, dizziness, shortness of breath, and fainting.

### *Treatments*

Heart murmurs may require the person to take anticoagulants to prevent the formation of blood clots, may be treated for hypertension if it is resulting in heart murmurs, or may need surgery to repair or replace the malfunctioning valve.

### *Contraindications*

Massage may be performed on a client with a heart murmur.

## Hematoma

*(hemat/o: blood; -oma: tumor)*

A hematoma is a **collection of blood** outside of its normal location internally, usually the result of a **breakage in a blood vessel wall**. A hematoma may be small or large, depending on the size of the rupture. The blood pools into an area, then clots, giving it a solid feel upon palpation.

### *Causes*

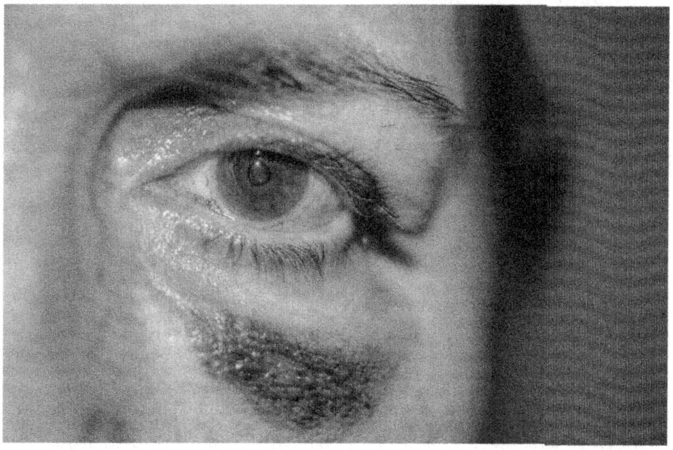

The cause of a hematoma is damage to a blood vessel. The damage does not have to be significant to cause rupture, and subsequent hematoma. As stated previously, hematomas range from tiny to large, and everywhere in between. The larger the blood vessel that is damaged, such as an artery, the more likely a larger hematoma would form.

Certain medical conditions and medications can contribute to the development of a hematoma, including aneurysms(page 54), anticoagulants such as aspirin and warfarin, and severe trauma to other structures such as fractures, which can cause extreme damage to associated and surrounding blood vessels.

When trauma occurs to the head, such as concussion(page 169), it may lead to the development of a subdural or epidural hematoma. These can be serious and lead to possible brain damage due to the pressure they can place on the brain. A subdural hematoma is a collection of blood beneath the dura mater, and an epidural hematoma is a collection of blood above the dura mater.

Another common form of hematoma is located in the ear, appropriately known as an ear hematoma. These are the result of bleeding on the cartilage of the ear, caused by trauma to the ear itself. If the hematoma is not drained, it can break down the cartilage of the ear, leaving it with a deformed, swollen appearance. Another common name for an ear hematoma is "cauliflower ear", seen most commonly in boxers, wrestlers, and mixed martial artists.

***Symptoms***

Symptoms of a general hematoma include pain, redness, swelling, possible inflammation, and warmth in the area. Depending on where it is located, it may also cause damage to other tissues, such as the brain. This can lead to painful headaches, amongst other symptoms.

***Treatments***

Treatments for hematomas vary depending on size and location. A hematoma in the skin would often require nothing but rest, ice, compression, and elevation. A hematoma in the brain or abdomen, however, may need to be fixed surgically.

***Contraindications***

Hematomas are considered local contraindications. Depending on the cause and location, the type of massage being performed may also be altered. If a client is taking blood thinners, lighter massages are indicated.

## Hemorrhage

*(hem/o: blood; -rrhage: bursting forth)*

A hemorrhage, simply put, is **bleeding**. Hemorrhages can be extremely minor, or extremely severe, depending on the amount of blood being lost while bleeding is occurring.

***Causes***

A hemorrhage is caused by trauma to a blood vessel. Trauma to the blood vessel causes blood to escape(or burst forth) from the vessel, which is bleeding. There are different types of hemorrhages, the most serious being hemorrhages that occur in the brain(cerebral hemorrhage) or hemorrhages caused by damage to major blood vessels, such as the abdominal aorta, superior vena cava, or inferior vena cava.

***Symptoms***

Symptoms vary depending on the severity. A minor hemorrhage may result in contusion, hematoma, inflammation, redness, and heat in the area. Severe hemorrhages, such as cerebral hemorrhages, can cause stroke, transient ischemic attack, brain damage, and even death.

A cerebral hemorrhage may exhibit some of the following symptoms: severe headache with sudden onset, seizure, nausea, loss of coordination and balance, weakness in limbs, possible loss of consciousness, and difficulty speaking.

***Treatments***

Treatment for hemorrhage varies, again dependent on the severity. Standard hemorrhages benefit from application of pressure at the site of bleeding to promote clot formation and reduce blood flow into the specific area. If damage is more extensive, stitches may be required to suture the wound closed. Cauterization may also help stop hemorrhage. In the case of cerebral hemorrhage, treatment can range from surgery to drain blood from the brain, to medications to help reduce fluid buildup such as diuretics, analgesics to control pain, and anticonvulsants to help control any seizures.

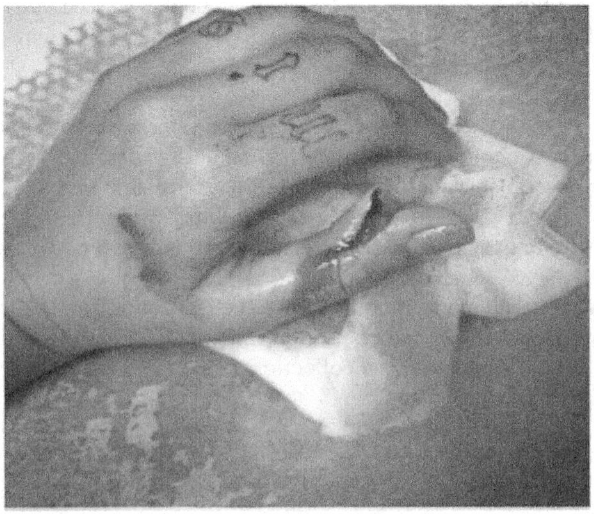

***Contraindications***

Massage is locally contraindicated for a hemorrhage. Personal protective equipment should always be utilized in the presence of a hemorrhage.

## Hypertension

*(hyper-: above; -tension: tension)*

Hypertension is a condition of the Cardiovascular System, resulting in **elevated blood pressure**. There are numerous factors that may contribute to the development of hypertension. For an average healthy adult, systolic blood pressure(pressure felt in arteries when the heart beats) is around 120 mmHg, and diastolic pressure(pressure felt in arteries when the heart is at rest) is around 80 mmHg. To be diagnosed with hypertension, a person's systolic pressure would be 140 mmHg and diastolic pressure would be 90 mmHg.

***Causes***

Hypertension may have no underlying cause, or may be the result of factors such as dysfunction of the adrenal glands or thyroid, dietary issues such as obesity or high sodium intake, kidney disease, and alcohol consumption.

Hypertension is most commonly associated with people who smoke, drink excessive amounts of alcohol, are overweight, are older in age, consume excessive salt, and more.

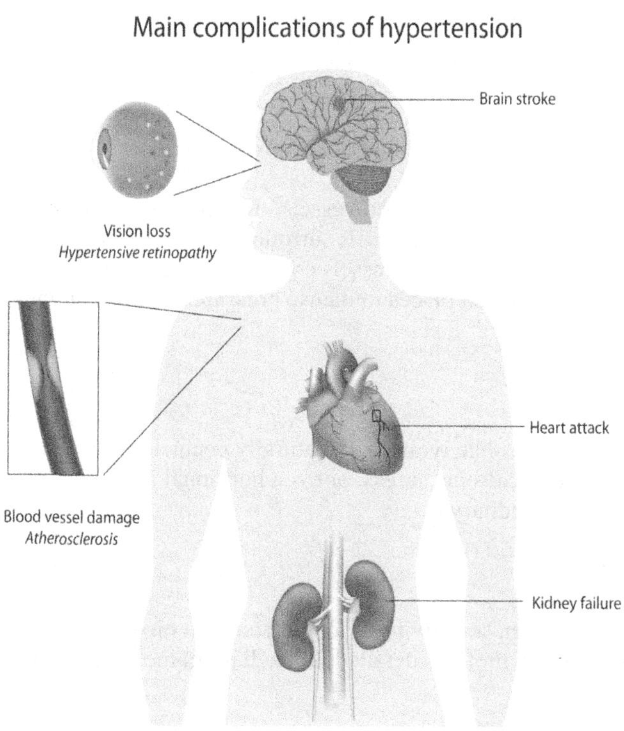


***Symptoms***

Unfortunately, hypertension is largely asymptomatic. Only in extreme cases, where the heart's blood pressure spikes extremely high, will someone experience symptoms, such as dizziness and headaches. Most symptoms people associate with hypertension are actually side effects of medications.

***Treatments***

Untreated, hypertension may lead to numerous serious medical conditions, such as myocardial infarction, stroke, atherosclerosis, and aneurysm. Luckily, hypertension is very easy to detect, and very treatable. Oftentimes, treatment is as simple as making lifestyle or dietary changes, such as consuming less sodium and increasing exercise. Other times, hypertension may require the use of medications such as beta blockers, statins, and diuretics.

***Contraindications***

Hypertension is generally not contraindicated for massage. Massage that increases blood pressure, such as deep tissue or hot stone, may be contraindicated if the client is not taking medication to control hypertension. Light massage, which promotes lowering blood pressure, should be performed.

## Hypotension

*(hypo-: below; -tension: tension)*

Hypotension is a condition of the cardiovascular system, resulting in **decreased blood pressure**. There are numerous factors that may contribute to the development of hypotension. For an average healthy adult, systolic blood pressure(pressure felt in arteries when the heart beats) is around 120 mmHg, and diastolic pressure(pressure felt in arteries when the heart is at rest) is around 80 mmHg. To be diagnosed with hypotension, a person's systolic pressure would be 90 mmHg and diastolic pressure would be 60 mmHg.

***Causes***

Causes of hypotension vary. Hypotension may even be completely normal for some people, and is only considered a problem when it leads to symptoms. Causes may include pregnancy, dehydration, serious infections, heart conditions, and severe loss of blood.

Some medications may lead to hypotension, including diuretics, beta blockers, and antidepressants.

***Symptoms***

Symptoms often do not appear in someone with non-serious hypotension. When symptoms appear, a serious problem may exist. Symptoms of hypotension include fatigue, fainting, dizziness, and nausea.

***Treatments***

The primary goal of treatment for hypotension is to increase blood pressure. Therefore, some things not recommended for hypertension are actually recommended for treating hypotension, such as increasing sodium intake. Increasing water intake is also a suitable treatment. Medications may help as well in a specific type of hypotension, known as orthostatic hypotension(lightheadedness and dizziness or fainting upon standing).

***Contraindications***

Generally, hypotension is not contraindicated for massage therapy. An invigorating massage may help increase blood pressure.

## Migraine Headaches

Migraine Headaches are a type of headache that affect the brain, which results in most side effects experienced.

Migraines have been referred to as "**vascular** headaches", due to the involvement of blood vessels. In migraines, when the brain is stimulated by a trigger, neurons rapidly send impulses which affect the blood vessels surrounding the meninges, three layers of connective tissue that surround and protect the brain. At first, the blood vessels constrict, which does not result in pain. A short time after constricting, the blood vessels will dilate, which places immense pressure on the meninges, which results in severe pain.

***Causes***

Migraines have numerous causes, which may be from exposure to substances like tyramine(a naturally occurring chemical found in foods such as aged cheese, alcoholic beverages, and cured meats), caffeine, stress, or even hormonal imbalance during stages such as menstruation. Migraines may even be considered hereditary.

***Symptoms***

Symptoms include nausea, fatigue, extreme pain, loss of sight, blurred vision, sensitivity to sound, and pain on one side of the head. Not everyone that experiences a migraine experiences all of the symptoms detailed, as each migraine is different.

***Treatments***

If a migraine is in the beginning stages, taking pain medication such as aspirin or ibuprofen can help reduce the symptoms of mild migraines. Other medications, called triptans, can help to constrict blood vessels, which can help reduce the effects of migraines.

Preventative drugs may be taken to reduce the chances of developing a migraine in the future. These medications include beta blockers, non-steroidal anti-inflammatory drugs, and even antidepressants.

***Contraindications***

Migraine headaches are generally not contraindicated for massage.

## Myocardial Infarction

*(myo-: muscle; -cardia: heart; infarct: obstruction of blood flow)*

A Myocardial Infarction, or **heart attack**, is a condition that affects the heart muscle, reducing blood flow throughout the body.

An infarction is an obstruction of blood flow to a specific part of the body. In this case, blood flow to the heart is obstructed. The two arteries that supply blood to the heart muscle are known as the coronary arteries. When an abundance of substances such as plaque build up inside these arteries, it restricts blood flow to the heart muscle. When blood flow is restricted, the tissue does not receive adequate oxygen, which results in **necrosis** of the affected tissue. When too much cardiac muscle dies, the body experiences a myocardial infarction, or heart attack.

***Causes***

Myocardial infarctions may be the result of atherosclerosis, a condition which causes the artery walls to harden and thicken due to a build-up of plaque in the arteries. Hypertension, smoking, and obesity may also contribute to the development of atherosclerosis.

***Symptoms***

Symptoms of myocardial infarction may be acute, or build up over a period of days leading up to the myocardial infarction. In the preceding days, a person may experience malaise, fatigue, and discomfort in the chest. Acute stages of myocardial infarction include intense chest pain, pain in the neck and left arm, and increased heart rate.

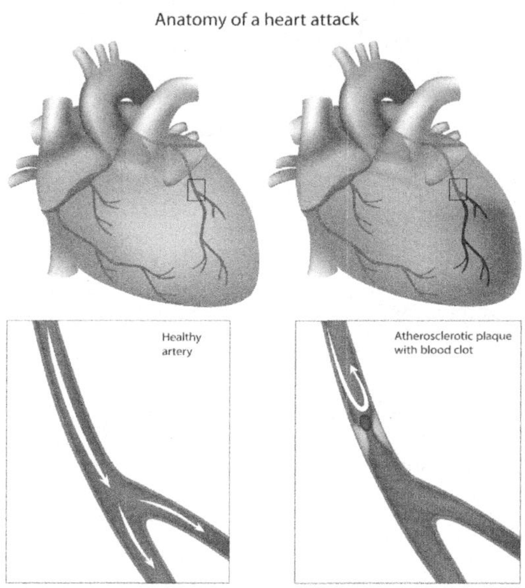


***Treatments***

A person who has suffered from a myocardial infarction may have a coronary bypass surgery performed, an angioplasty or stent placed in the affected artery, or may not need any surgery and only require medications such as aspirin, beta blockers, and statins.

***Contraindications***

Massage is an absolute contraindication during a myocardial infarction. After a myocardial infarction has occurred and a client has been treated, it is a good idea to get a note from a doctor before proceeding. Depending on the severity of the infarct and treatment, certain massages should not be performed due to strain they may place on the heart when increasing blood pressure.

## Myocarditis

*(my/o: muscle; card-: heart; -itis: inflammation)*

Myocarditis is **inflammation** of the **heart muscle**. Myocarditis may reduce the effectiveness of the heart's pumping action, leading to **arrhythmia**.

***Causes***

Myocarditis is typically caused by a **viral infection**, such as hepatitis B, hepatitis C, and adenovirus. Bacteria, parasites, and fungus have also been known to cause myocarditis, but less often than a virus. Myocarditis may also be caused by a reaction to certain drugs, such as antibiotics.

***Symptoms***

Symptoms of myocarditis include pain in the chest, arrhythmia, fatigue, edema, and dyspnea.

***Treatments***

Myocarditis often improves without treatment. Rest may be prescribed, while avoiding heavy physical exertion. Medications such as beta blockers and diuretics may be prescribed to help the heart function properly and reduce fluid retention in the limbs. Severe cases of myocarditis may require IV medications, and possibly the use of ventricular assist devices(VADs), which help pump blood from the ventricles to the rest of the body. The use of VADs is often confined to those experiencing heart failure.

***Contraindications***

Massage should be avoided until myocarditis has cleared.

## Pericarditis

*(peri-: around; card-: heart; -itis: inflammation)*

Surrounding the heart is a membrane known as the pericardium. Pericarditis is **inflammation** of the **pericardium**.

***Causes***

The cause of pericarditis is usually unknown. Viral infection may be suspected, but the exact cause has yet to be determined.

***Symptoms***

There are different types of pericarditis, each presenting with different symptoms. Acute pericarditis, which typically lasts only a matter of weeks, presents with sharp chest pain, usually felt behind the sternum or on the left side of the chest.

Chronic pericarditis, which also presents with chest pain, may result in fluid buildup around the heart.

General symptoms of pericarditis include sharp chest pain, cough, malaise, and fever.

***Treatments***

Mild pericarditis often improves without treatment. More severe cases of pericarditis, however, require treatment such as medication(pain relievers and corticosteroids are often used).

If fluid has built up around the heart(known as cardiac tamponade), hospitalization may be required, and treatments to reduce the amount of fluid around the heart may be administered, such as a pericardiocentesis. During a pericardiocentesis, the doctor will use a needle or catheter to remove fluid from the pericardial cavity.

***Contraindications***

Massage should be avoided until pericarditis has cleared.

## Phlebitis

*(phleb-: vein; -itis: inflammation)*

Phlebitis is a condition of the Cardiovascular System, affecting the **veins**, causing them to become **inflamed**. Blood clots may form in these veins.

***Causes***

Phlebitis may have numerous causes, including trauma to a vein, and immobility. Trauma to a vein results in what is known as superficial phlebitis, usually the result of IV catheters being placed into a vein via needles.

Deep vein thrombosis is another type of phlebitis, taking place deeper in the body. Deep vein thrombosis(DVT) is most commonly caused by immobility of a limb. The body's veins move and stretch with the rest of the body during movement. If the veins are immobilized, they will become irritated, due to blood pooling in the veins. The blood pooling may result in blood clot formation. If a blood clot dislodges from its location and flows freely in the blood stream, it is known as an embolus, which could become lodged in other blood vessels throughout the body, cutting off blood flow and resulting in ischemia. Depending on the part of the body this takes place, it could even lead to possible death.

***Symptoms***

Symptoms of superficial phlebitis include tenderness and swelling around the injured vein, often with the affected vein presenting with a red line in the skin following the vein. The vein may feel hard to the touch due to inflammation.

Deep vein thrombosis may present with pain in the entire affected limb(usually the leg), along with swelling. If infection results, people may have fever.

***Treatments***

Treatments of phlebitis include anticoagulants for deep vein thrombosis such as heparin, ibuprofen, and antibiotics for superficial phlebitis.

Deep vein thrombosis requires immediate medical attention, as it may result in embolism, which could potentially be fatal.

***Contraindications***

Phlebitis should be treated as a local contraindication. Because medications may be prescribed that thin the blood, lighter massage should be performed to prevent internal bleeding from damaged blood vessels. Massaging the site of phlebitis may dislodge a clot, which can result in an embolism.

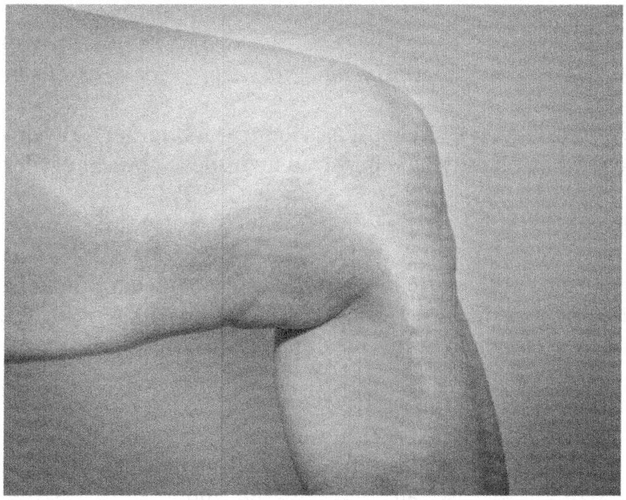

Area of the leg affected by phlebitis, presenting with redness in the location

## Raynaud's Syndrome

Raynaud's Syndrome is a condition that results in **constriction** of the **blood vessels** in the **fingers** and **toes**, reducing **circulation** to these areas. This constriction is known as "vasospasm". Primary Raynaud's Syndrome occurs independently, while Secondary Raynaud's Syndrome is typically associated with other conditions.

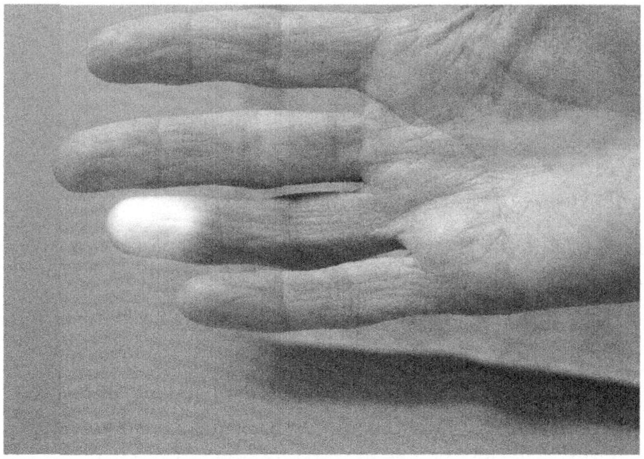

Constriction of blood vessels at the distal end of the fourth digit

***Causes***

The primary contributors to Raynaud's Syndrome are cold temperatures, stress, and cigarette smoking. Raynaud's Syndrome is typically not a debilitating disease. During a flare-up, the skin typically turns white, the person may experience numbness or pain, and the affected areas become very cold.

Secondary Raynaud's Syndrome may be associated with conditions such as lupus or scleroderma, and develops later in life than Primary Raynaud's Syndrome.

***Symptoms***

Symptoms of Raynaud's Syndrome include discoloration of the skin in affected areas, cold fingers and/or toes, numbness, and stinging pain upon warming of the area.

***Treatments***

Treatments for Raynaud's Syndrome include exercise, reducing stress, not smoking, and avoiding cold temperatures whenever possible. Secondary Raynaud's Syndrome may require medications such as statins to help regulate blood pressure and cholesterol.

***Contraindications***

Raynaud's Syndrome is indicated for massage. Using heat should be avoided, as sensation in the affected area may be decreased and tissue damage may result. Massaging the area can help dilate blood vessels and bring blood back into the fingers and toes. Increasing the temperature of the massage room may also help dilate blood vessels.

## Thromboangiitis Obliterans

*(thrombo-: clot; angi-: blood vessel; -itis: inflammation; obliterans: obstruction)*

Thromboangiitis Obliterans, also known as **Buerger's disease**, is a condition that causes **inflammation** of **blood vessels** in the arms and legs, which may lead to the development of **blood clots** and **ulcers**.

***Causes***

There is no clear cause of thromboangiitis obliterans, but **cigarette smoking** plays a very large role. Practically everyone who has been diagnosed with thromboangiitis obliterans is a chronic cigarette smoker. Why cigarette smoking plays a role in the development of this condition is unknown.

***Symptoms***

Symptoms of thromboangiitis obliterans include pain in the upper and lower limbs that comes and goes as activity using these limbs increases and decreases, ulceration of fingers and toes, phlebitis just below the surface of the skin, and Raynaud's Syndrome. A person may also experience numbness in the affected area due to lack of sufficient blood flow.

***Treatments***

Because smoking is a huge contributing factor in the development of thromboangiitis obliterans, stopping smoking is the best treatment available. This does not cure the disease, but may prevent it from advancing further. Other treatments may include medications used to dilate blood vessels in the hands and feet, surgery to remove nerves in affected areas, compression in affected areas to increase circulation, and possible amputation of fingers or toes if ulcers result in gangrene.

***Contraindications***

The area affected by thromboangiitis obliterans is generally considered a local contraindication and should be avoided during massage due to pain and possible tissue damage that has occurred.

## Varicose Veins

*(varicose: abnormally swollen)*

Varicose veins are the abnormal **swelling of veins** in the body, most commonly seen in the **legs**, but may be present in any vein. There are many different types, ranging from regular varicose veins, to spider veins, and even hemorrhoids.

***Causes***

Inside the veins, there are valves that push deoxygenated blood back up to the heart. Typically, as a person ages, the valves stop working as efficiently, which allows blood to pool **backwards** in the veins. This added pressure causes irritation and swelling of the veins. Blood pooling in the veins may also lead to complications such as the development of blood clots.

Because veins are much more superficial than arteries, when a vein becomes swollen, it is often visible. Varicose veins often present with a purple color, may look cord-like, and may even cause pain and discomfort. Causes of varicose veins include sitting or standing for prolonged periods, age, and even pregnancy.

***Symptoms***

Oftentimes, varicose veins occur with no symptoms other than visual symptoms, such as discoloration of veins. If a varicose vein becomes painful, a person may experience burning, itching, edema, and cramping in the legs around the site of the varicose vein.

***Treatments***

Treatment is often unnecessary, outside of self-care. Self-care may include wearing compression socks, exercise, diet, and elevating the legs to help circulation. If treatment is required, there are a number of different things that can be done, all the way up to removing the varicose vein from the body.

***Contraindications***

Varicose veins are a type of phlebitis, and are considered a local contraindication. Massaging a swollen vein may dislodge a clot, which could become an embolism.

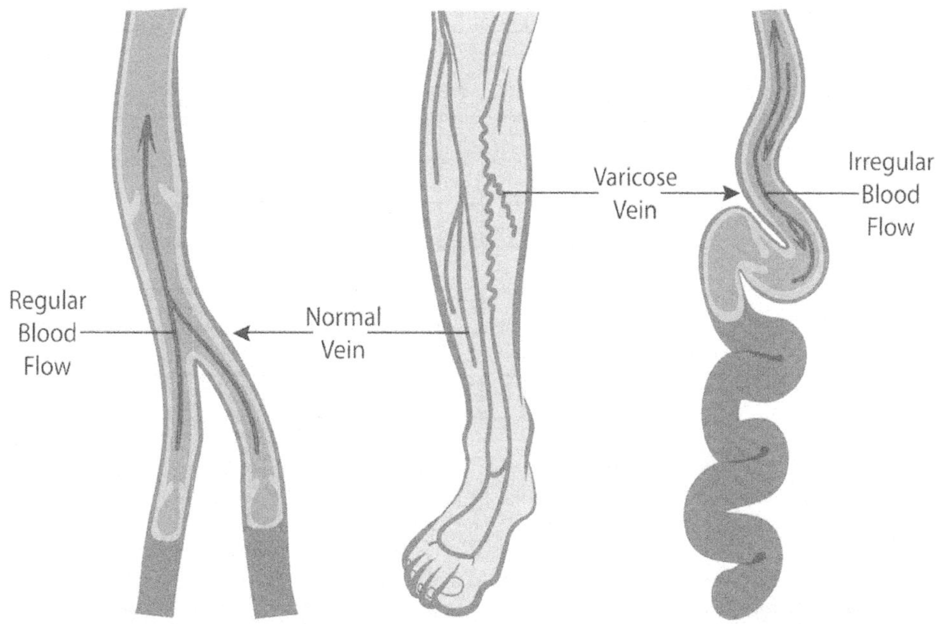


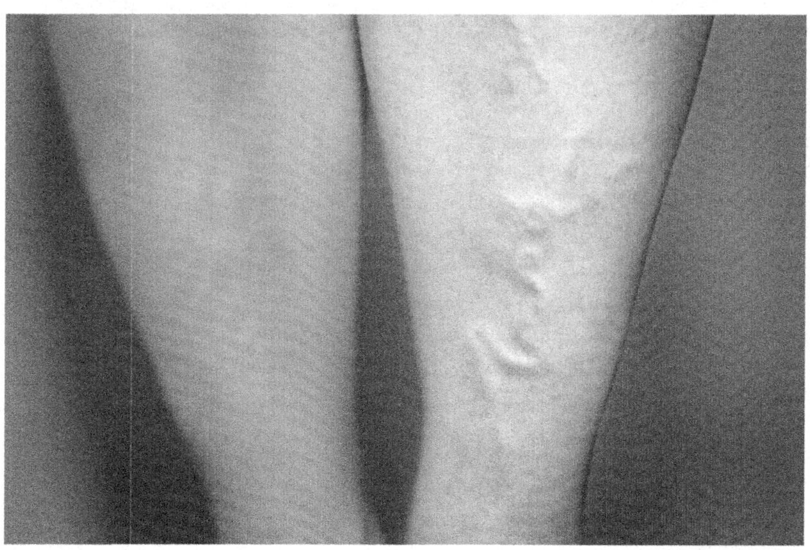

# Cardiovascular Pathologies

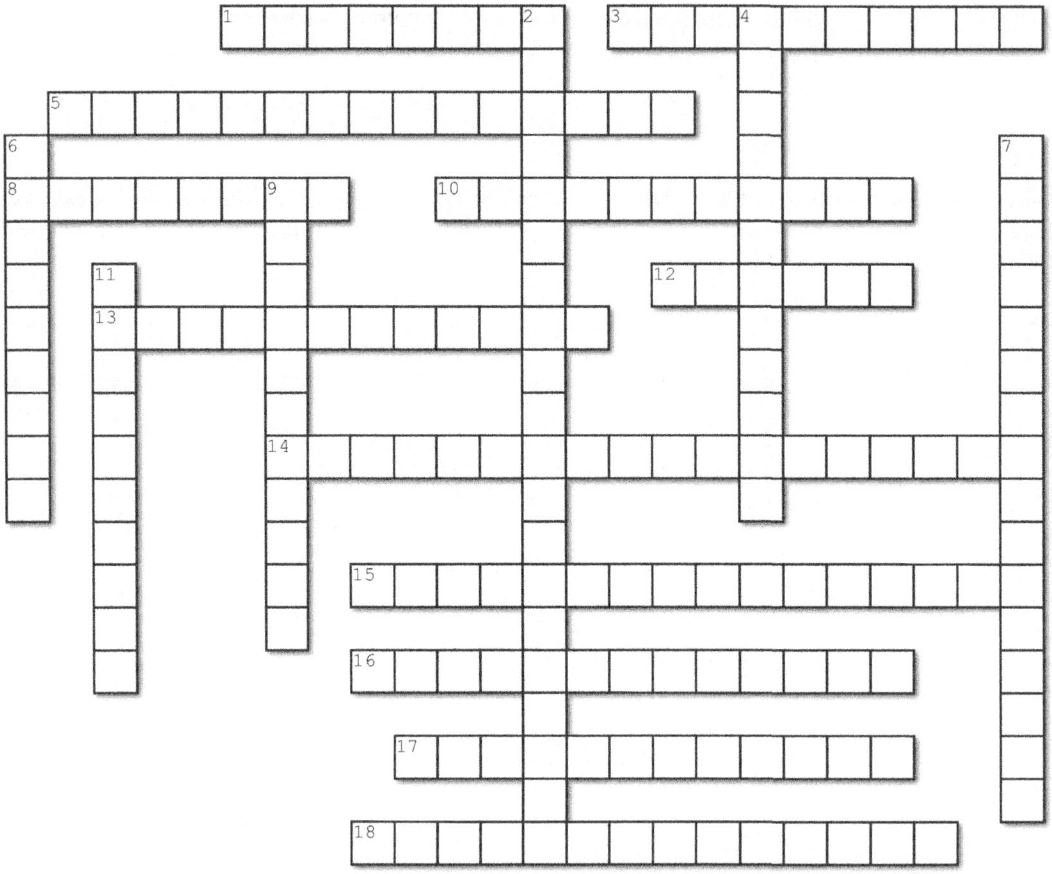

**Across**

**1.** A bulge in the wall of an artery, caused by excessive pressure on and weakening of the artery wall
**3.** Irregular heart beat
**5.** Excessive build-up of fatty plaque on an artery wall
**8.** Breakage of a blood vessel that causes blood to pool in an area and clot
**10.** Blood flowing backwards in the heart due to malfunctioning heart valves
**12.** Lack of oxygen circulating through the body due to insufficient iron in erythrocytes
**13.** Inflammation of the inner linings of the heart due to an infection
**14.** Formation of blood clots in the veins, most commonly in the legs
**15.** Constriction of blood vessels in fingers and toes, reducing circulation in these areas
**16.** Swelling of veins in the legs, caused by valves not functioning effectively
**17.** Inflammation of the membrane surrounding the heart
**18.** Pain in the chest caused by necrosis of heart tissue

**Down**

**2.** Necrosis of cardiac tissue causing insufficient circulation throughout the body
**4.** Excessive blood pressure
**6.** Inflammation of a vein, commonly caused by trauma or immobility
**7.** Hardening of the wall of an artery
**9.** Inflammation of heart muscle, typically caused by a viral infection
**11.** Bleeding, caused by damage to a blood vessel

Answer Key on Page 286

# Cardiovascular Quiz

1. Erythrocytes
A. Carry oxygen and carbon dioxide throughout the body
B. Are also called neutrophils and perform phagocytosis
C. Produce thrombi at an area of trauma
D. Allow transport of blood cells throughout the body

2. Phlebitis
A. Swelling of veins as a result of valve incompetence, causing blood to flow backwards
B. Inflammation of a vein due to excessive fat accumulation in the vein
C. Swelling of a vein due to excessive lymph fluid in a limb
D. Inflammation of an artery due to immobility as a result of surgery

3. A patient with severe bradycardia would most likely need a pacemaker implanted into their body to regulate
A. Embolism formation
B. Lipid accumulation
C. Heart rhythm
D. Phlebitis

4. All of the following carry blood away from the heart except
A. Capillaries
B. Arteries
C. Arterioles
D. Veins

5. Blood passes from the right atrium through the tricuspid valve into the
A. Left ventricle
B. Left atrium
C. Right ventricle
D. Pulmonary artery

6. If systolic pressure measures 140 or higher, a person may be diagnosed with
A. Hypotension
B. Hypertension
C. Hyperemia
D. Myocardial infarction

7. Ulceration may occur in the fingers and toes in severe cases of
A. Emphysema
B. Cyanosis
C. Raynaud's syndrome
D. Paraplegia

8. Hypotension is also referred to as
A. Low blood pressure
B. High blood pressure
C. Arrhythmia
D. Varicose veins

9. Protein found inside of red blood cells, responsible for transporting oxygen and carbon dioxide throughout the body
A. Mitochondria
B. Hemoglobin
C. Hemophilia
D. Leukocyte

10. Another term for a blood clot within a blood vessel
A. Thrombus
B. Embolus
C. Aneurysm
D. Fibrin

11. Dilation of a small portion of an artery, caused by a weakened arterial wall
A. Embolism
B. Aneurysm
C. Thrombus
D. Murmur

12. Chris, who has recently suffered from a heart attack, has requested a massage. The proper course a massage therapist should take is
A. Reschedule the massage until medical clearance has been provided from the client's physician
B. Perform the massage to promote circulation
C. Perform the massage and use a cold compress to lower blood pressure
D. Perform the massage while avoiding shaking or trembling actions

13. A blockage of a blood vessel may result in
A. Arrhythmia
B. Phlebitis
C. Ischemia
D. Hypotension

14. A lack of erythrocytes in the body results in
A. Myocardial infarction
B. Raynaud's syndrome
C. Anemia
D. Decreased immune response

15. Arteriosclerosis
A. Hardening of the walls of the arteries
B. Fatty plaque buildup in the arteries
C. Bulging of an arterial wall
D. Inflammation of a vein

Answer Key on Page 289

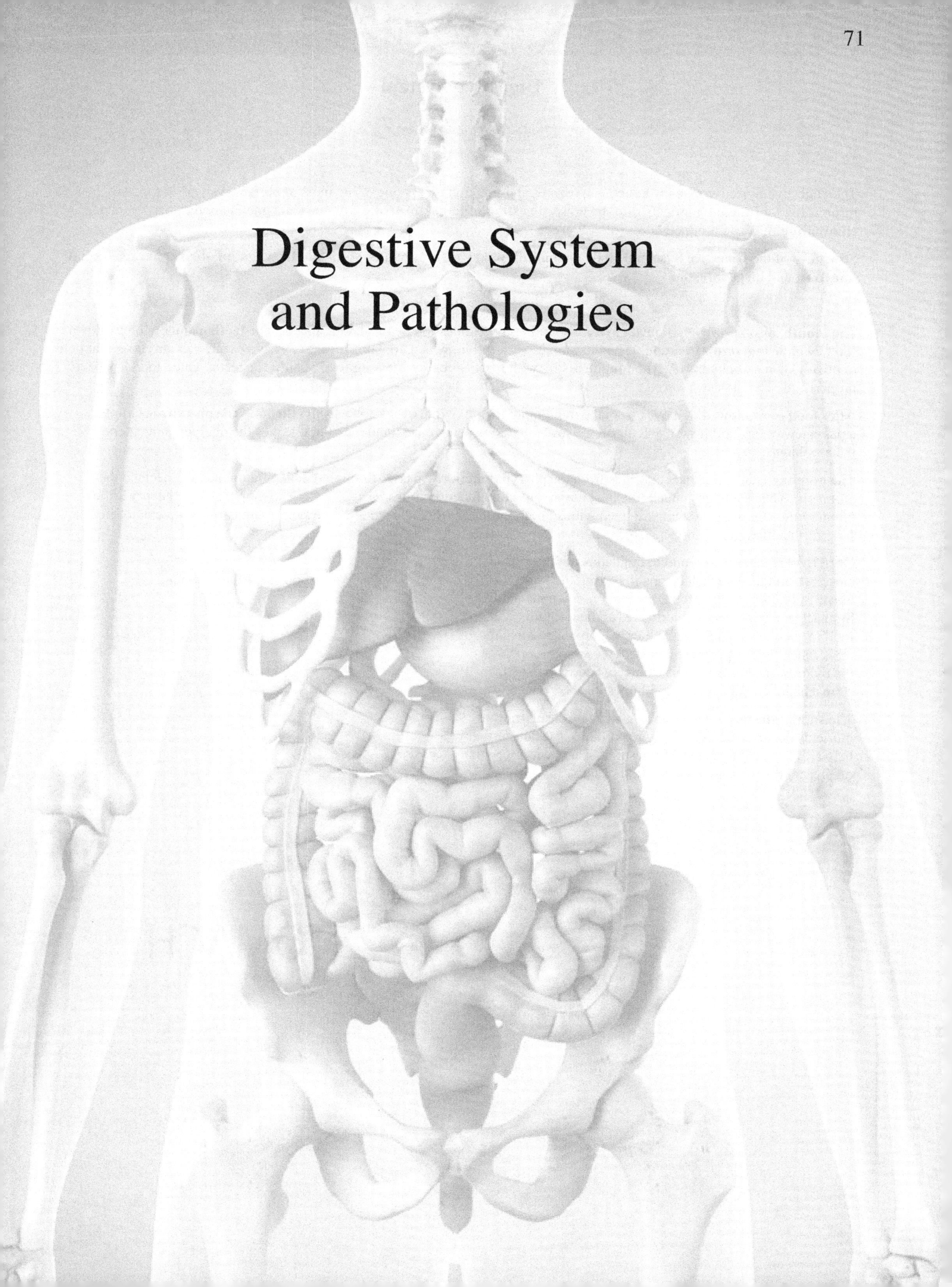

# Digestive System and Pathologies

# Digestive System

The Digestive System has many structures, organs, and functions. It is one of the most important systems in the body, responsible for bringing nutrients **into** the body, **digestion** of food, **absorption** of nutrients into the body's tissues, and **elimination** of waste products.

Structures of the Digestive System include the **mouth, pharynx, esophagus, stomach, liver, gallbladder, pancreas, small intestine**, and **large intestine**.

## Digestion

The **mouth**, also known as the **oral cavity**, is the first place digestion begins taking place. The **teeth** manually break down food by **chewing,** or **mastication**. The food mixes with **saliva**, which contains digestive enzymes such as **amylase**, that help to break down carbohydrates. The **tongue** assists with mastication by pressing food against the teeth. Once food has been properly chewed, it is swallowed.

After food is swallowed, it moves from the mouth into the **pharynx**, also known as the **throat**. The pharynx is simply a passageway for food, water, and air on the way to their respective destinations. Food leaves the pharynx and enters the esophagus.

The **esophagus** is a long tube that runs from the pharynx inferiorly, passes through the diaphragm, and connects to the **stomach**. The esophagus, much like the pharynx, has one function: transporting food. The esophagus, and every hollow organ of the Digestive System, are lined with smooth muscle. When the smooth muscle rhythmically contracts, it forces food further along in the organ. This is known as **peristalsis**.

Once food reaches the **stomach**, both ends of the stomach close off, and the stomach begins **digesting** the food. Powerfully, it churns the food, breaking it down manually. Stomach acids like hydrochloric acid and pepsin mix with the food inside the stomach and further help to break down the food. Once food is properly digested, the stomach opens at the pylorus, the bottom of the stomach, and food exits the stomach and enters into the small intestine.

The **small intestine** is where the majority of **absorption** of nutrients occurs. **Accessory organs** produce substances that help aid the small intestine in digestion. These accessory organs are the liver, gallbladder, and pancreas.

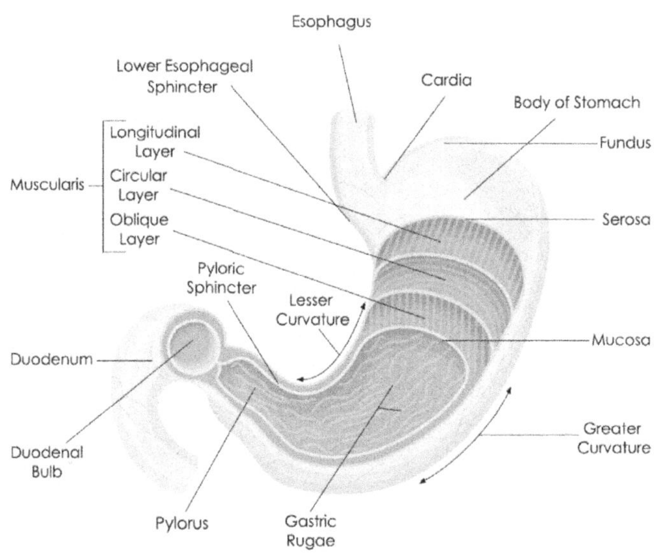


STOMACH

## Liver, Gallbladder, Pancreas and Bile Passage

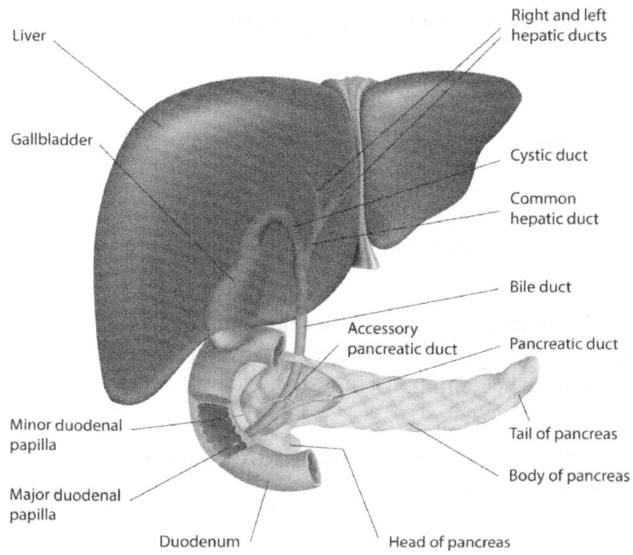


The **liver**, the heaviest internal organ, mainly acts as a **blood detoxifier**. It filters harmful substances from the blood. However, it aids in digestion by producing **bile**, a yellowish substance that aids in the emulsification of fats. Connecting to the liver is the gallbladder. Once the liver produces bile, it empties the bile into the gallbladder, where it is stored until it is needed.

The **gallbladder** simply has one function: to **store bile** and empty bile into the small intestine through the bile duct, which connects to the duodenum, the first section of the small intestine.

The **pancreas** is an extremely important organ, and is vital in the processing and breaking down of glucose in the body. The pancreas produces **glucagon**(created by alpha cells), which aids in increasing glucose concentration in the blood. It also produces **insulin**(created by beta cells), which aids in lowering glucose concentration in the blood. These substances enter the blood stream directly. The pancreas also produces **pancreatic juices**, which empty into the small intestine through the bile duct, which further aid in digestion.

Food moves from the stomach into the **small intestine**. The first section of the small intestine is known as the **duodenum**. The duodenum is the last section of the Digestive System where digestion of food takes place. Bile and pancreatic juices mix with food in the duodenum and further break down substances. Peristalsis forces the food from the duodenum further into the small intestine, into the middle portion, known as the **jejunum**. The jejunum is where the majority of nutrient absorption takes place in the small intestine. As the food is forced through the small intestine, it moves into the final section, known as the **ileum**. Final absorption occurs in the ileum. Food moves through the ileum and into the large intestine.

The large intestine has two primary functions: **absorption** of water, and **elimination** of waste. As feces moves through the large intestine, water is absorbed. If too much water is absorbed, constipation may result. If not enough water is absorbed, diarrhea may result. The large intestine has four sections: the ascending colon, the transverse colon, the descending colon, and the sigmoid colon. As the feces leaves the sigmoid colon, it enters the rectum, where it is ready to be eliminated from the body.

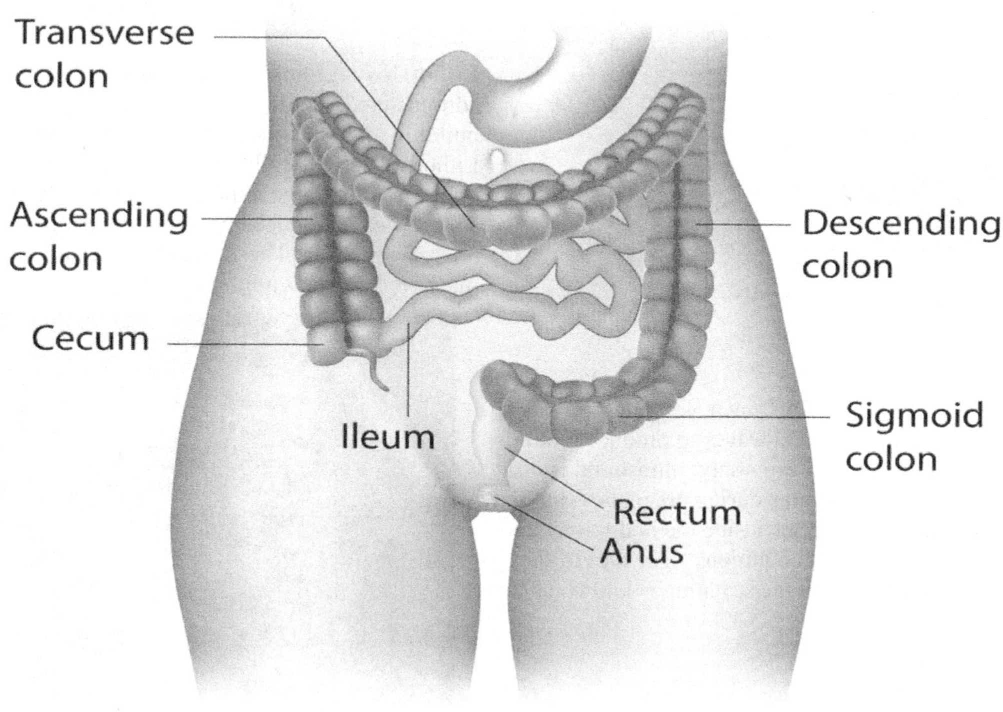

### Sphincters

In the Digestive System, there are **ring-like** bands of **muscle** between digestive organs, known as **sphincters**. Sphincters function to allow food to enter into an organ, or to keep food from moving backwards.

There are four primary sphincters in the Digestive System:

The **esophageal** sphincter is located between the **pharynx** and the **esophagus**. It opens and allows food to move down into the esophagus.

The **cardiac** sphincter is located between the **esophagus** and the **stomach**. It is named after the region of the stomach it connects to, which is known as the cardia. When food enters the stomach, the cardiac sphincter closes, preventing food and stomach acid from ascending into the esophagus.

The **pyloric** sphincter is located between the **stomach** and the **small intestine**. It is named after the region of the stomach it connects to, which is known as the pylorus. When food enters the stomach, the pyloric sphincter closes, preventing food from leaving the stomach before digestion has taken place. When food has been properly digested, the pyloric sphincter opens, and food leaves the stomach and enters the small intestine.

The **ileocecal** sphincter is located between the **small intestine** and the **large intestine**. It is named after the parts of the two organs that come together, the ileum(small intestine) and cecum(large intestine).

### Medical Tests and Equipment

**Endoscopy**: An endoscopy is a procedure in which a tube is inserted into a part of the digestive tract with a camera and light attached, allowing a doctor to see inside the organs. Commonly, this is performed to view the esophagus, stomach, and small intestine. An endoscope used to view the large intestine is known as a colonoscopy.

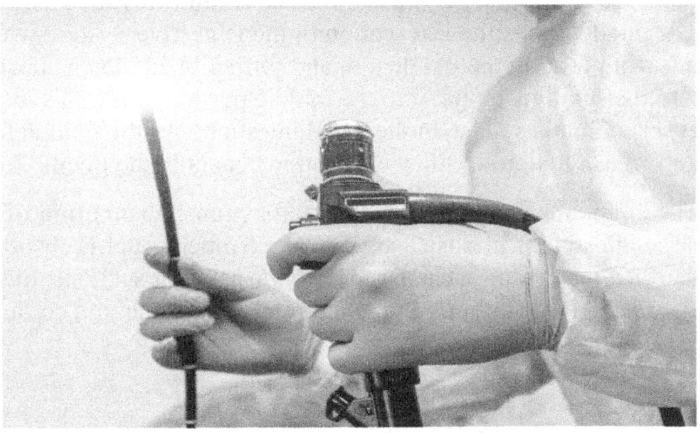

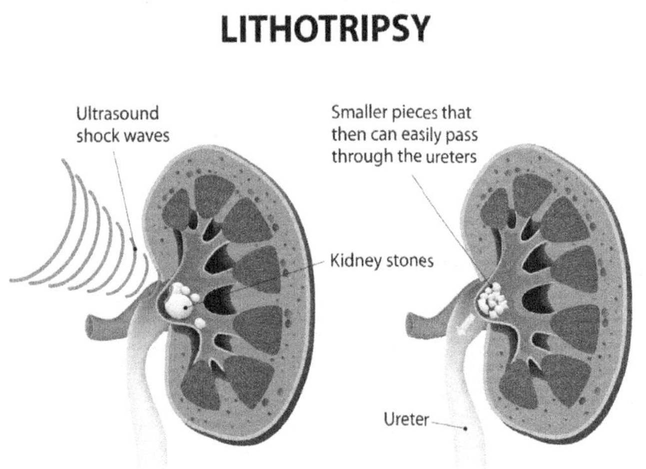


**Lithotripsy**: Lithotripsy is the use of sound waves administered via ultrasound to break up or destroy deposits building up in the body, such as kidney stones and gallstones. Lithotripsy is typically only performed if one of these deposits is too large to pass from the body on its own. The sound waves produced break up the deposit, and allow it to be passed normally. These sound waves are produced by a machine known as a lithotripter.

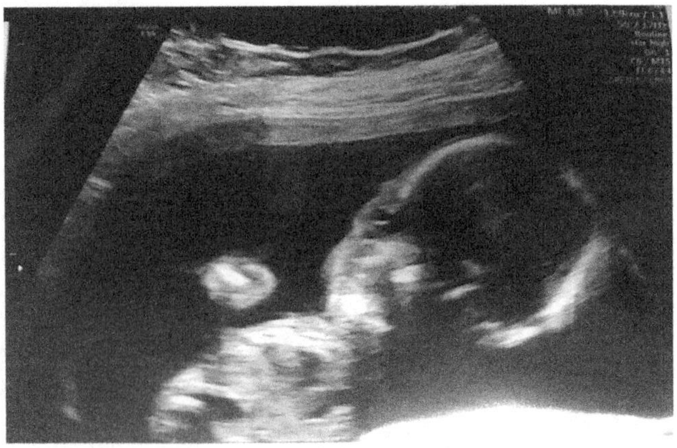

**Ultrasound**: An ultrasound, also known as sonography, is an imaging technique utilizing sound waves to produce pictures of structures inside the body. Commonly, ultrasound is used to view the development of a fetus during pregnancy, but may also be used to examine infections inside the body, liver and gallbladder function, and heart conditions. The part of the machine that is used to perform the scanning is known as the transducer.

# Digestive System Pathologies

## Appendicitis

*(append: appendix; -itis: inflammation)*

Appendicitis is **inflammation** of the **appendix**, a small tube extending off the ascending colon. The exact function of the appendix is unknown, but it is entirely possible to live without the appendix. When the appendix becomes inflamed, it risks **rupturing** and dumping infectious substances into the abdomen. This can possibly lead to peritonitis(page 88), which may be life-threatening. Appendicitis is always considered a medical emergency and must be treated immediately.

***Causes***

The most common cause of appendicitis is blockage of the appendix by fecal matter. This blockage keeps infectious material in the appendix, which may then become abscessed. A tumor may also block the appendix.

***Symptoms***

Symptoms of appendicitis include pain in the upper portion of the abdomen that moves down into the lower right abdomen which becomes extremely sharp, nausea and/or vomiting, low-grade fever, and loss of appetite. Painful urination, cramping, constipation, or diarrhea may also accompany appendicitis.

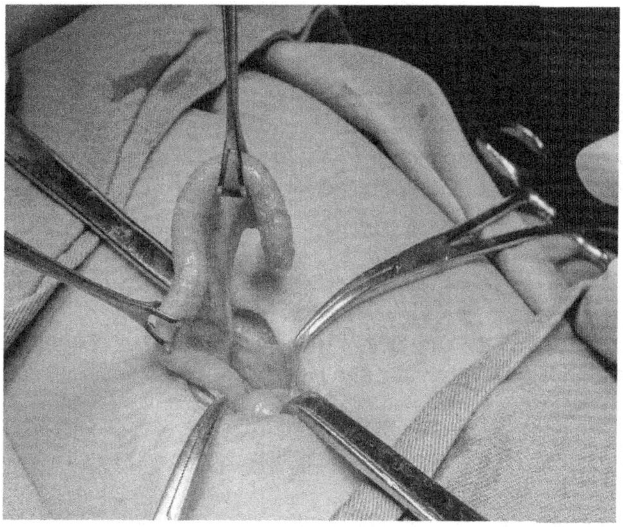

Inflamed appendix and subsequent surgical removal

***Treatments***

Most commonly, appendicitis is treated by complete removal of the appendix, known as an appendectomy(surgical removal of the appendix). This ensures the appendix will not rupture and introduce infectious substances into the abdomen.

***Contraindications***

Appendicitis is considered an absolute contraindication for massage, and is a medical emergency.

## Cholecystitis

*(chole-: bile; cyst-: bladder; -itis: inflammation)*

Cholecystitis is **inflammation** of the **gallbladder**. If untreated, cholecystitis may lead to extremely serious conditions, such as rupture of the gallbladder.

***Causes***

Most commonly, cholecystitis is the result of formation of **gallstones**. Gallstones can block the cystic duct, which connects the gallbladder to the bile duct on its way to the duodenum, causing inflammation of the gallbladder as bile backs up in the organ.

There is no consensus on what causes gallstones to form. Some theories state gallstones form because the bile contains too much cholesterol, too much bilirubin, or the gallbladder doesn't properly empty bile into the duodenum.

***Symptoms***

Symptoms of cholecystitis include severe abdominal pain in the upper right quadrant near the liver, nausea, vomiting, fever, and pain in the right shoulder/back. These symptoms often occur after ingesting large meals.

***Treatments***

A diagnosis of cholecystitis almost always results in a hospital stay. Treatments may include antibiotics to fight off any associated infection, pain medication to reduce discomfort, and fasting to let the gallbladder rest and reduce inflammation.

Cholecystitis often recurs, and therefore most people who are diagnosed with cholecystitis require surgery to completely remove the gallbladder. The liver is then connected directly to the duodenum, allowing bile to enter into the small intestine.

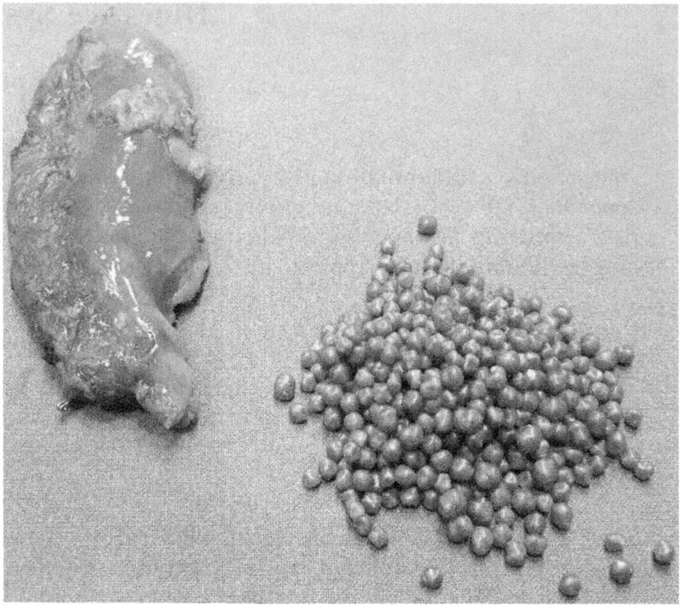

***Contraindications***

Cholecystitis is considered an absolute contraindication in the acute stage. After the underlying cause has been determined, medications may be prescribed to help deal with the formation of gallstones and infection, or the gallbladder may be removed completely. This will require a hospital stay, in which massage will not be performed.

## Cirrhosis

*(Greek "kirrhos": yellowish; -osis: condition)*

Cirrhosis is **scarring of the liver**, due to other conditions such as **hepatitis**(page 84). Each time the liver is damaged, it repairs itself. During this repair process, scar tissue is formed. As the liver is damaged over time, more scar tissue forms, which makes liver function difficult. Cirrhosis gives the liver a cobble-stone, yellow-orange appearance.

***Causes***

Most commonly, cirrhosis is the result of chronic hepatitis and alcohol abuse. Every time there is a flare-up of chronic hepatitis(HBV and HCV), it damages the liver, resulting in scar formation. Non-alcoholic fatty liver disease may also contribute to the development of cirrhosis.

***Symptoms***

Cirrhosis often does not present with symptoms until the damage caused is excessive. Symptoms may include nausea, weight loss, jaundice, bleeding and bruising easily, fatigue, edema in the legs, and an accumulation of fluid in the abdomen.

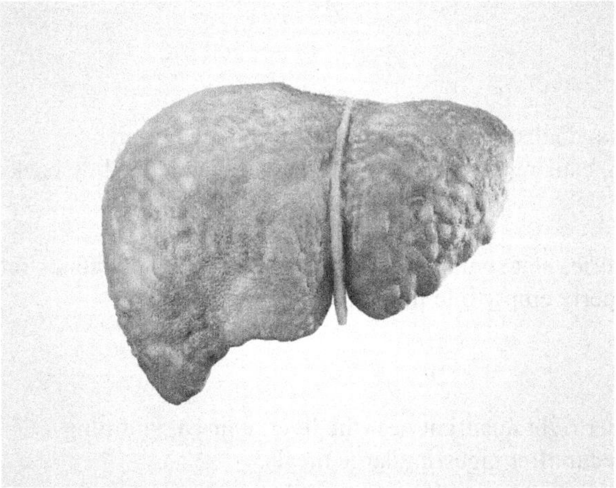

Yellowing and scarring of the liver, giving it a cobblestone appearance

***Treatments***

Early stages of cirrhosis are treated by addressing the underlying cause, not the scarring itself, as the scarring is irreversible. A patient with early stages of cirrhosis may seek treatment for alcohol dependency to reduce the intake of alcohol, look into weight loss to reduce nonalcoholic fatty liver disease, and medications to help control HBV and HCV, which can substantially damage the liver.

Advanced stages of cirrhosis may require liver transplantation to provide the body with a liver that functions properly.

***Contraindications***

Massage should be avoided in a client with cirrhosis, due to increased waste products being filtered through the liver.

## Constipation

Constipation is a **lack of bowel movement** for an extended period of time, usually longer than three days. Most people have bowel movements at differing intervals, but three days seems to be the longest amount of time for a normal bowel movement across all demographics.

Acute constipation is typically nothing to worry about. Chronic constipation could be a sign of a more serious condition, such as colon cancer.

### *Causes*

Causes of constipation vary, but may include dehydration, lack of fiber in the diet, excessive dairy consumption, antacids, stress, and even hypothyroidism(page 104).

### *Symptoms*

Symptoms of constipation include lack of bowel movements, hard stool, small stool, swollen abdomen, and difficulty defecating.

### *Treatments*

Treatment of acute constipation may include increasing water intake, increasing the amount of fiber in the diet, and the use of over-the-counter laxatives to soften the stool and make it easier to pass. Chronic constipation should be treated by a doctor, with treatments aimed towards the cause of the constipation, whether it be cancer or laxative abuse.

### *Contraindications*

Massage is indicated for constipation. Massaging the abdomen in a clockwise motion may help promote peristalsis and improve the likelihood of defecation.

## Crohn's Disease

Crohn's Disease is an **inflammatory bowel disease**, which causes **inflammation** of the **digestive tract**. Crohn's has periods of exacerbation and remission, where the disease is actively causing inflammation, then periods where it is not. Crohn's disease typically appears in younger people, people who are of East European Jewish descent, people who have relatives with the disease, and people who smoke cigarettes.

Damage to the digestive tract, including ulcerations and scarring, may result. Depending on the location of ulceration and scarring, abscesses and constipation may result.

### *Causes*

The exact cause of Crohn's disease is unknown. The leading theory is that heredity and an immune system that does not function properly are the main causes of Crohn's.

### *Symptoms*

In acute stages of Crohn's, symptoms may include diarrhea, abdominal pain, cramping, fatigue, fever, and bloody stool. Depending on the severity of these symptoms, a person may need to visit a doctor.

### *Treatments*

A variety of medications may be prescribed for a patient with Crohn's, including anti-inflammatory drugs such as corticosteroids to reduce inflammation in the digestive tract, immunosuppressants to help regulate the effects of the immune system on the digestive tract, and antibiotics to reduce any abscesses that may result. Pain relievers may also be prescribed.

In serious cases, surgery may be required. During Crohn's, scarring in the ileum or large intestine may result. In this surgery, the damaged portion of the digestive tract may be removed. This does not cure Crohn's, but can make it easier to manage.

Changes in diet, especially in acute stages, may be beneficial.

***Contraindications***

Massage in the acute stage of Crohn's disease should be avoided, as the client may be in pain and experience symptoms such as diarrhea. In the post-acute stage, massage is indicated for Crohn's disease.

**Sofia, Crohn's Disease**

What kind of symptoms were you experiencing leading up to the diagnosis?

*In the afternoon on my wedding day, I remember feeling this odd folding sensation in my upper left quadrant. It's odd to explain but I kept trying to stretch it out by doing a side bend to stretch my left side out. The reason I mention it was the afternoon on my wedding day is because leading up to my wedding, I've never been so stressed out in my life. Two months prior, I sat for my x-ray boards which was also a very intense and stressful time for me. I have this theory that I stressed myself into Crohn's because there's nothing out there that explains how or why someone would get this disease. They sometimes link it to genetics but even if someone in your family gets it, you're not certain to get it yourself.*

*The day after my wedding, I felt okay. Not the best but nothing too alarming. The following day, however, we took a flight to Cancun, Mexico and I remember sitting on the plane in so much discomfort. I was wearing leggings and thought they might be too tight around my tummy. But then again, I've always had that issue. Looking back I never liked anything pressing too tight on my stomach. During the flight, I would have to hold my hands under my belt line and on top of my tummy to relieve some of the pressure. Not fun but also nothing too alarming. Once on our honeymoon, I started feeling what I thought might be acid indigestion, as well as a lot of gas. Nate(my husband) and I thought it might be heart burn, so for 11 days straight, I took an antacid. That helped enough to relieve my discomfort for a little while, but all these symptoms(folding sensation, tender tummy, GERD) wouldn't quite go away. They were muted. It prevented me from eating as much or drinking as much as I had planned on our honeymoon, but we still had a good time.*

*When were returned to Reno, I had a ton of diarrhea(gross, I know) but when I went to the urgent care, they chalked it up to being in Mexico and having Montezuma's Revenge, and gave me antibiotics for ten days. Urgent care also mentioned to me that the antacids might have done it to me too, because I guess you're not supposed to take over-the-counter antacid for that long. So I took the antibiotics, and by day ten I was good to go. Four days later, I woke up with the worst gut pain and consistent cramping. So much green diarrhea, it was awful. There was no position I could put myself in to relieve the awful cramping that occurred every 15 seconds or so. I was on the ground in my bathroom completely helpless. Part of me will always wonder if all of that was brought on by some bad edamame. To this day, I won't touch the stuff! Anyway, I was taken to the ER where they did blood work and an ultrasound. They ended up finding a mass on my liver, which they chalked up to a parasite, so they gave me two really hard antibiotics to clear that and sent me on my way.*

*I was established at a GI Doctor and before my first exam, I remember the medication they gave me making me feel faint. I couldn't open my eyes or hardly breathe. I called a nearby girlfriend who rushed me to the doctor and my O2 levels were 74. Definitely something was up. When I finished that round of medication, I felt decent enough to move on, but not quite right. By this time, it was early October and I was on my way to Miami to take a cruise to the Bahamas for a bachelorette party. For once, it was the first time I could really eat, so I did! But halfway through the trip, it all started back up and I couldn't understand why.*

*When I got back to Reno a few days later, things progressively got worse. The cramps in my belly were unreal. I couldn't stand up straight and I couldn't eat. Every time I even put something in my mouth, the cramps would intensify. It was miserable. So, a few days before Halloween, I finally caved and submitted to a CT scan. I didn't want to because of the radiation, but I was in so much pain, I couldn't refuse. I also did some stool samples and blood work just before my CT and was waiting for the results. The radiologist at my work went over my CT with me in detail. The mass on my liver was still there, but hadn't grown. I had loose fluid in the pelvic cavity, and inflammation all over my intestines. That night around 4pm, I got a call on the results of my stool samples and blood work. It turns out I had C-Diff(clostridium difficile, a bacterial infection in the intestines). They explained I probably got it from all the antibiotics I took, but I had to go on more medication to clear the C-Diff. But this time, nothing worked. I was in so much unbearable pain at this point, I didn't know what to do. C-diff is known to cause inflammation in the gut, but only in the colon. I have inflammation in my small intestine and at the terminal ileum which is indicative of Crohn's. I was in denial, I thought there's no way I could have Crohn's. In my mind, I was dead set that it was C-Diff and stress but nothing was working to relieve my symptoms.*

*I was still coming into work throughout all of this and a few days after my CT scan, one of the radiologist reviewed my scan again and thought I could be perforated! He sent me straight to the ER from work. I was so scared. This was November 7th. The ER made me comfortable(for once) while I was there, but refused to send me home with any pain medication. I was shocked. And looking back, I always thought it was weird that I didn't receive one freaking pain pill until I was actually diagnosed. Anyway, they did an abdominal x-ray and didn't see any free fluid so they sent me home. I was kind of pissed because here I am in all this pain, with no explanation and nothing to curb my symptoms. My GI talked me into an endoscopy and colonoscopy for November 15th. I had to do it in the hospital because I was high risk and still might be perforated. After being scoped and biopsied in six places, I was awoken to my doctor telling me that my entire left side was inflamed so badly that he had to puff my intestines open just to get his scope through. He said at one point he didn't think he could complete the exam but I'm glad he did. He sent me home with steroids and medication to stop the contractions in my intestines brought on by peristalsis and segmentation. The meds really helped, not completely but enough to finally eat something. My doc said with certainty that I had Crohn's, but wanted to wait for the results of the biopsy.*

*By this time, I was on my way to NYC for my friend's wedding on November 18th. I was miserable. I spent almost the entire trip in my hotel room. I also developed an upper respiratory infection. Perfect. I just remember walking around the corner from my hotel to a ramen noodle place and wondering if I'd even be able to make it. I was in so much pain. It felt like acid was flooding my abdominal cavity. I would never wish this on my worst enemy. I was constantly calling my GI doc and they kept saying the steroid would soon kick in and help but it was all LIES. Nothing helped.*

*When I got back to Reno, it was Thanksgiving and I was still not eating. I remember just trying to slowly eat a palm sized amount of mac 'n cheese. Everyone at the table felt so awful for me. I had to leave the table to cry. It was awful. I can't believe it took as long as it did, but a few days before Christmas, I finally got my diagnosis and was cleared for some real medication. The first week of January, I started Humira, which is a biologic that needs to be stored in the refrigerator. I started with four injections in my legs and abdomen. Two weeks after that, I did two more injections and finally I felt some real relief. Every other week after that and for the rest of my life, I have to inject.*

*For 13 months now, I have been pain and symptom free, mostly! I can eat and drink any thing I want, but I don't. I'm still traumatized from that experience that I take my consumption in stride. I also refuse to do any cardio workout that involves moving my stomach around. I won't jump or run or anything like that because I can feel my intestines move. Also, I can feel a bowel movement long before it's ready. I can feel it moving through my intestines and what's weird is, I remember feeling that particular symptom while I was in x-ray school. My doc said that I had been inflamed for a long time but didn't know it until I had a flare. So I guess all the stress I went through caused my first Crohn's flare. I still get cramps intermittently and the weird folding sensation every day, but I'm not in pain hardly and I don't have diarrhea. I do have BM's more frequent than before but they are manageable.*

*The unsettling part about all this is I won't be able to have children. Sure, I can get pregnant and carry if I want, but I would have to go off my medication to do so and there's no telling how my body will respond to the biologic medication as well as it is now post-baby. It's just not a risk I'm willing to take. Lucky for me, I never really saw myself having children, but occasionally I get that maternal pull, which sucks, but I'd rather be healthy.*

*The only positive thing, in my opinion, to come for all of this is the weight loss. I lost nearly 50 pounds! It's been nice! I didn't go to the high school reunion, but occasionally I get a patient in for an x-ray from high school and they can't believe how much I've changed. Even people from the x-ray program are shocked. They say, I knew you were sick, but damn, it really took a toll on you. It's crazy. But now I'm noticing a change in the way people respond to me. Women mostly. They are way more bitchy to me because they assume I've been this skinny all my life. It's kind of funny to watch their demeanor change once they find out I have a disease and can't change it. In my head, I think, "That's right you fake judgemental bitch, suck it." Haha!*

How helpful is Humira?

*Extremely helpful. I feel like I'm normal again. No pain, hardly any symptoms. I get the occasional upset stomach which is to be expected with Crohn's, but it works so well I often think I don't have a disease. I do still have to go to the bathroom more than normal but it's manageable.*

How often do flare ups occur?

*At this point, it's too early to tell. I haven't had a flare since my first one that lasted eight months. Hopefully I'll be able to go the rest of my life without experiencing another flare.*

Do you experience any side effects from your medication?

*None so far. Humira does put me at high risk for lymphoma, and because of that, I have to do lab work every six months to check my chemistry.*

Have you had any issues with other illnesses since starting Humira?

*Yes. Chronic pink eye(I wash my hands all the time) but I still get it, and UTI's. I had my first kidney stone in September last year. That was fun. I do notice it takes twice as long for a simple paper cut to heal and minor cuts get infected easily.*

Have you received massage since being diagnosed?

*Yes.*

Have you received massage during a flare up?

*No. After thinking about it, having a massage during a flare is probably the last thing I'd be seeking. My stomach was so tender and I was in so much pain, it was difficult to let the doctor even do an exam. I wore clothes that barely hung on to me because any pressure would have sent me through the roof.*

## Diarrhea

*(dia-: through; -rrhea: discharge)*

Diarrhea is **stool** that is **runny**, **watery**, or **loose**. It is a very common condition, usually not serious. Extended bouts of diarrhea may lead to **dehydration** due to water loss, however, and may need to be treated.

### *Causes*

There are numerous causes of diarrhea, including eating foods that aren't agreeable with the stomach, alcohol consumption, infections that result in food poisoning, laxative use, diabetes, etc. The most common cause of diarrhea is some sort of bacterial infection, usually the result of eating contaminated food.

### *Symptoms*

Symptoms may include the feeling of needing to use the restroom right away, bloating, cramps, nausea, and watery stools. In severe cases, blood may appear in the stool, along with fever and weight loss. If these symptoms occur, a patient should visit a doctor.

### *Treatments*

Oftentimes, no treatment is needed, and the condition will resolve itself. Over-the-counter medications may help in easing the diarrhea. A patient suffering from diarrhea needs to drink plenty of fluids to remain hydrated, as they are losing water with every defecation.

Severe cases need to be treated by a doctor.

### *Contraindications*

Massage is indicated for a client with diarrhea. Massage of the abdomen, if performed, should be done counter-clockwise along the path of the large intestine to help the feces from moving further along in the colon.

## Diverticulitis

*(diverticula: tubular sac branching off a cavity; -itis: inflammation)*

Diverticulitis is a condition affecting the large intestine, but may also affect other structures such as the abdomen, or the entire cardiovascular system. If a person is affected by diverticulosis, they have small pouches that develop in the large intestine. In certain cases, these pouches may become **inflamed** and/or **infected**, which then becomes diverticulitis.

### *Causes*

Because diverticulitis puts strain on sections of the large intestine that are already weakened, ulcerations or open sores may result. These open sores may lead to infection, and leaking of feces into the abdomen, which results in peritonitis(inflammation of the peritoneum, a very serious condition that requires medical attention).

### *Symptoms*

Symptoms of diverticulitis include fever, nausea, vomiting, pain in the lower left abdomen, and constipation. Tenderness in the abdomen may also be present.

### *Treatments*

Diverticulitis may be treated in several different ways, depending on the severity. Pain medication may help with discomfort in less severe cases. In recurring diverticulitis, scarring may be present, which could lead to backing up of fecal content in the large intestine. Infections will require antibiotics.

If scarring is severe due to ulceration, surgery to remove the damaged part of the large intestine may be required.

### *Contraindications*

Diverticulitis is considered an absolute contraindication to massage.

## Diverticulosis

*(diverticula: tubular sac branching off a cavity; -osis: condition)*

Diverticulosis is a condition affecting the large intestine, which presents with **pouches** forming in the walls of the large intestine, typically in the descending and/or sigmoid colons. It is a common condition seen in roughly half of people over the age of 65.

### *Causes*

During peristalsis, the smooth muscle located in the walls of the large intestine contract, forcing food to move further through the organ and eventually out of the body. If the large intestine does not contain enough fecal matter, as in the case of a low-fiber diet, the contractions may result in weakening of the wall of the large intestine. As a result, small pouches may develop.

If a person develops diverticulosis, small pieces of feces, nuts, seeds, etc, may become stuck inside the pouches. If feces becomes trapped in a pouch, the large intestine will absorb all of the water from it, and it will become very solid and extremely hard to remove. This may result in pain in the abdomen.

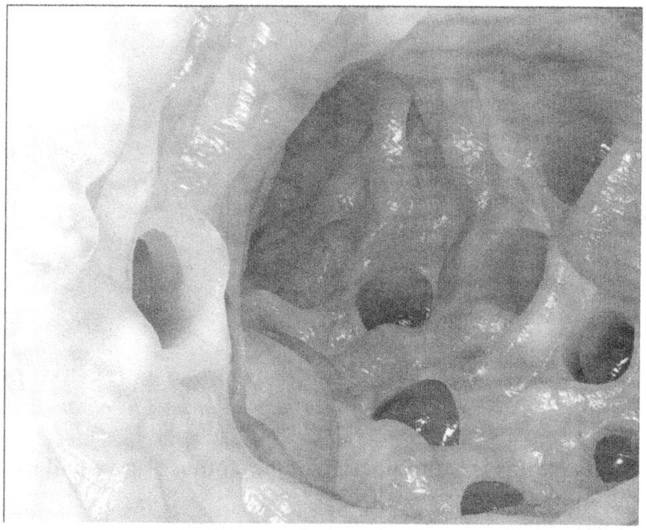

Pouches forming in the large intestine

### *Symptoms*

Typically, people with diverticulosis don't exhibit symptoms. When they do, however, symptoms may include diarrhea, abdominal cramping, or fever. These are typically the result of infection, which may lead to diverticulitis.

***Treatments***

Treatment primarily includes increasing intake of fiber via fruits and vegetables, and increasing fluid intake to make passing of stool easier to manage.

***Contraindications***

Diverticulosis is not contraindicated for massage. If pain is present, massage of the lower back and abdomen should be avoided, but may be performed elsewhere.

## Gallstones

See: Cholecystitis, page 75.

## Gastritis

*(gastr/o: stomach; -itis: inflammation)*

Gastritis is **inflammation** of the **stomach**, specifically the **lining** of the stomach. Gastritis may occur suddenly or slowly over time.

***Causes***

Some primary causes of gastritis include infection by **H. pylori bacterium**, excessive use of **alcohol**, use of anti-inflammatory drugs, vomiting, and stress. Gastritis should be treated, as it may lead to more serious conditions such as stomach cancer.

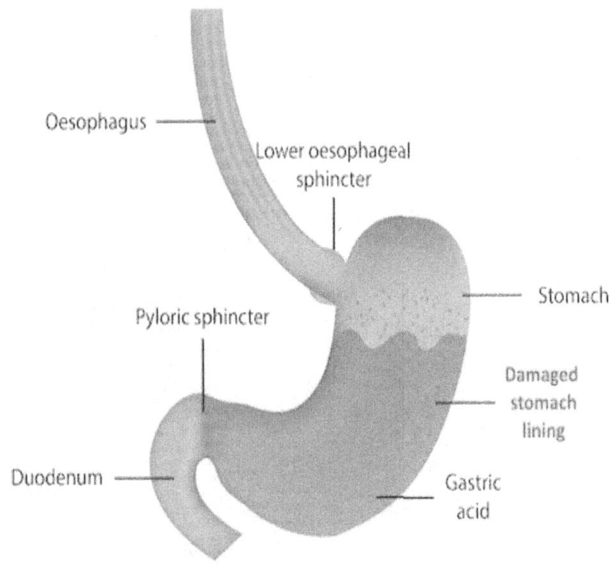


***Symptoms***

Some people with gastritis actually don't exhibit any symptoms. Those that do, however, may present with nausea, vomiting, loss of appetite, pain in the abdomen, and bloating in the abdomen.

***Treatments***

Treatment often consists of dietary changes, such as avoiding spicy food and dairy, taking antacids to reduce the amount of stomach acid present, and possibly even a round of antibiotics to combat infection by the H. pylori bacterium.

***Contraindications***

Massage on a client with gastritis is dependent on the cause and severity. If gastritis is causing nausea and vomiting, massage should not be performed.

## Gastroenteritis

*(gastr/o: stomach; enter/o: small intestine; -itis: inflammation)*

Gastroenteritis is **inflammation** of the **stomach** and **small intestine**, commonly known as the "**stomach flu**".

***Causes***

The primary cause of gastroenteritis is a **viral** or **bacterial infection**. These infections can be spread by coming into contact with someone who has it, or consuming contaminated food or water that contains the virus or bacterium. The main types of viruses that cause gastroenteritis are **rotavirus** and **norovirus**. The main types of bacteria that cause gastroenteritis are **E. coli** and **salmonella**.

***Symptoms***

Symptoms of gastroenteritis include diarrhea, vomiting, fever, abdominal pain, and body chills.

***Treatments***

Most people recover from gastroenteritis without requiring any treatment. The primary goal of treatment for gastroenteritis is to prevent dehydration. Therefore, drinking plenty of fluids is advised. Over-the-counter medications that help with nausea and vomiting may also help.

***Contraindications***

Gastroenteritis is often caused by a viral infection, and is contagious. Therefore, gastroenteritis is an absolute contraindication to massage.

## Gastroesophageal Reflux Disease

*(gastr/o: stomach; esophag/o: esophagus; reflux: flowing back)*

Gastroesophageal Reflux Disease(GERD) is a condition in which **stomach acid**, or food from the stomach, comes back up **into the esophagus**, causing **irritation and burning** in the lining of the esophagus.

***Causes***

GERD is the result of acid flowing backwards into the esophagus. This is primarily caused by the lower gastroesophageal sphincter(also known as the cardiac sphincter) relaxing when it normally is contracted and tightened. This can happen abnormally, or be caused by the sphincter weakening over time.

***Symptoms***

Symptoms include burning in the chest, pain in the chest, a dry cough, a sour taste in the mouth, and a sore throat. It is advisable to seek medical attention if chest pain is present, because symptoms are very similar to those seen in myocardial infarction.

***Treatments***

Over-the-counter medications, such as antacids, are the primary treatment for GERD. Other medications may be prescribed by a doctor if the GERD is not helped by antacids, such as H-2-receptor blockers, which reduce stomach acid production, and proton pump inhibitors, which completely block the production of stomach acid and give the lining of the esophagus time to heal.

***Contraindications***

Unless chest pain is present, massage is indicated for Gastroesophageal Reflux Disease. Semi-reclined position may help reduce acid from moving into the esophagus.

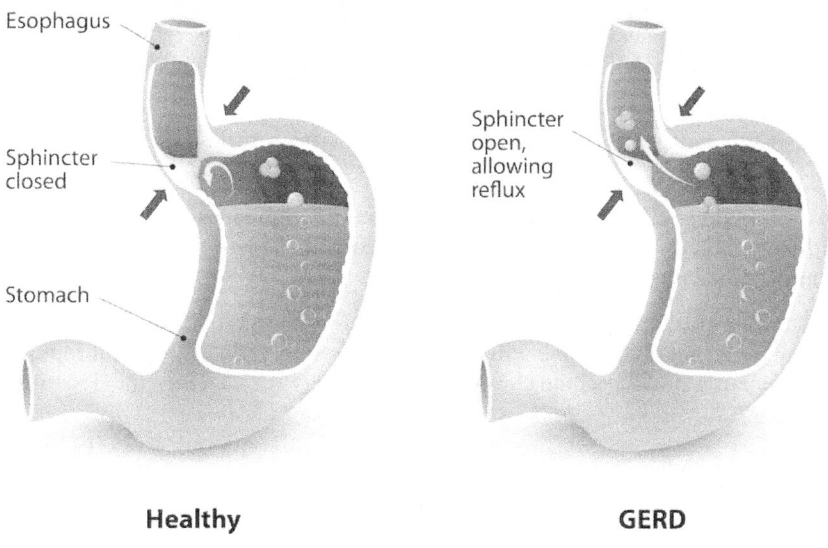

## Hemorrhoids

*(hemo-: blood; -rrhoid: protrusion)*

Hemorrhoids are swollen veins in the rectum and anus. There are two types of hemorrhoids: internal hemorrhoids and external hemorrhoids. **Internal hemorrhoids** are further inside the rectum, and are usually unable to be felt. **External hemorrhoids** are lower in the rectum and anus, and may even be seen. These can cause pain and bleeding.

***Causes***

The main cause of hemorrhoids is straining while defecating or lifting heavy objects, such as performing squats. This causes blood to rush to the area, which can put excessive pressure on the veins. This causes them to become swollen.

People who sit for long periods, people who are obese, and people who are pregnant may also be prone to developing hemorrhoids.

***Symptoms***

Hemorrhoids may be asymptomatic, or may present with itching or discomfort around the anus, or blood on toilet paper after wiping.

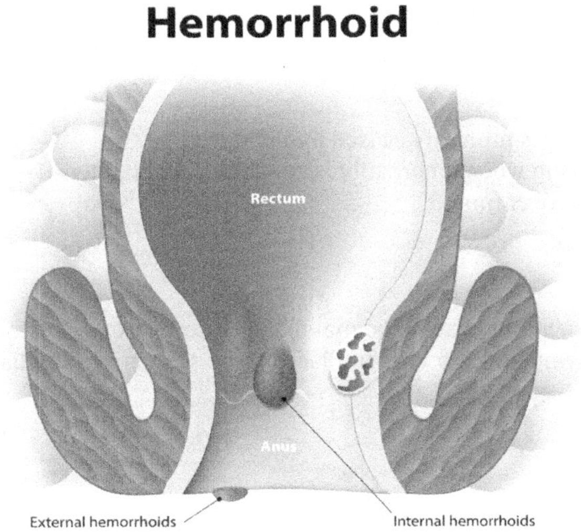


***Treatments***

Hemorrhoids typically resolve on their own without treatment. A high-fiber diet can be extremely beneficial, helping stool become easier to pass, resulting in less straining. If hemorrhoids don't clear up over the course of two to three weeks, medical attention may be needed. Surgical removal of the hemorrhoid may be an option, along with tying a rubber band around the hemorrhoid to cut off blood flow, after which it will become necrotic and fall off.

***Contraindications***

Massage is considered a local contraindication for hemorrhoids.

## Hepatitis

*(hepat-: liver; -itis: inflammation)*

Hepatitis is a condition that results in **inflammation** of the **liver**.

***Causes***

There are numerous causes of hepatitis, which affect numerous different organ systems. Most commonly, hepatitis is the result of a **viral** infection, but may also result from **toxic substances** entering into the body, such as **alcohol**. Short-term symptoms of hepatitis include jaundice(yellowing of the skin due to increased bilirubin in the blood stream), fever, and nausea. Long-term symptoms include cirrhosis(destruction of healthy liver cells), scarring of the liver, liver cancer, and liver failure.

There are five known hepatitis viruses: Hepatitis A, B, C, D, and E. Each varies in mode of contraction and severity of symptoms.

Hepatitis A is the most common form, and is typically transmitted through ingestion of fecal matter(most commonly seen in parts of the world with low sanitation standards). People infected with Hepatitis A most frequently make a full recovery, and develop an immunity to the virus.

Hepatitis B is typically transmitted through exposure to body fluids such as blood. The virus produces symptoms for a period greater than Hepatitis A, but most people will develop an immunity to it after about four weeks. A small percentage of people who contract Hepatitis B will become chronically affected by it. Vaccines for Hepatitis B are available.

Hepatitis C, much like Hepatitis B, is contracted through exposure to body fluids such as blood. Hepatitis C is a chronic condition which damages the liver even further each time the person's symptoms are in the acute stage. Hepatitis C is one of the leading causes of liver failure.

Hepatitis D is an infection that only results in symptoms if the person is also infected with the Hepatitis B virus. When this occurs, major complications may arise. Because Hepatitis D is only activated by the Hepatitis B virus, the Hepatitis B vaccine may contribute to the prevention of Hepatitis D.

Hepatitis E, like Hepatitis A, is contracted through exposure to fecal matter. It is most commonly seen in developing countries, where sanitation standards may not be high. Hepatitis E, if severe, may lead to liver failure, despite being an acute infection.

***Symptoms***

Hepatitis often results in no symptoms. More severe cases of hepatitis may result in a person presenting with nausea, fatigue, mild fever, loss of appetite, abdominal tenderness, and jaundice, among others.

***Treatments***

Treatments vary, depending on severity. Immunizations are available for Hepatitis B, and medications may help reduce the symptoms.

***Contraindications***

In the acute stage, massage is an absolute contraindication for hepatitis. In the post-acute stage, massage is indicated.

## Hernia

*(hernia: a rupture)*

A hernia is a rupture in a muscle or connective tissue, allowing an organ or other tissue to **protrude** through its normal location. There are many different types of herniae in the digestive system, including **hiatal**, **umbilical**, and **inguinal**.

***Causes***

A hernia is caused by a weakness in the affected tissue, and/or straining of the tissue. When the tissue tears, the organ, usually the small intestine, protrudes through it. This can lead to many complications, such as organ strangulation, constipation, pain, or even trauma to other structures, such as the testes.

A hiatal hernia results from part of the stomach protruding upwards through the diaphragm, into the chest. Gastroesophageal Reflux Disease may result from this type of hernia, where stomach acids leak from the stomach backwards into the esophagus.

An umbilical hernia, most commonly seen in infants, is caused by the small intestine protruding through the abdominal wall and into the umbilicus. This condition usually resolves on its own.

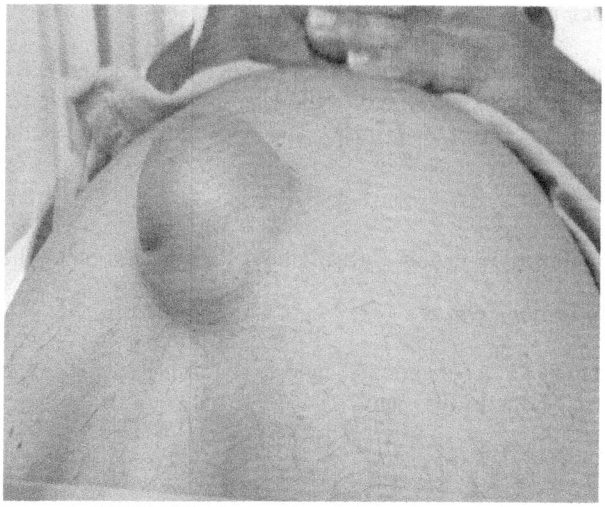

Umbilical hernia, a portion of the small intestine protruding through the peritoneum

An inguinal hernia, most commonly seen in men, is caused by the small intestine protruding through the wall of the abdomen, which typically descends into the scrotum. This may cause trauma to the testes. Sometimes, the small intestine may even drop farther down the body, into the thigh.

***Symptoms***

Symptoms vary depending on the type of hernia suffered. Examples include swelling beneath the skin in the abdomen or groin in an inguinal or umbilical hernia, and heartburn and pain in the upper abdomen in hiatal herniae.

***Treatments***

Treatments may include dietary changes in cases such as a hiatal hernia, weight loss, medication such as antacids, or even surgery to repair the hernia.

***Contraindications***

Massage of a hernia is locally contraindicated.

## Jaundice

*(jaund/o: yellow)*

Jaundice, also known as **icterus**, is a condition that causes the **skin** to turn a **yellowish** color. Jaundice is the result of an increased amount of **bilirubin** in the **blood stream**(hyperbilirubinemia). Bilirubin is a byproduct of the breakdown of heme in the body, a normal process in which the body recycles blood cells. Bilirubin is filtered through the liver and into the digestive tract, binding with bile, where it will then be eliminated from the body. Bilirubin is a yellow substance. When there is an abnormal amount of bilirubin in the blood, it can be absorbed into the skin and whites of the eyes,resulting in the yellow pigment.

***Causes***

Jaundice may result when there is damage to the liver. Examples include viral infections such as hepatitis(page 84) or alcoholism. Blockage of the gallbladder resulting from gallstones may contribute, as can certain medications taken over a prolonged period such as acetaminophen.

Neonatal jaundice occurs in infants, usually due to the breakdown of erythrocytes in the fetus at a higher level than normal. Neonatal jaundice is sometimes considered a serious condition, as excessive bilirubin is considered a neurotoxin and may damage the Nervous System. Usually, however, neonatal jaundice resolves itself within a day or two without any issues.

***Symptoms***

Jaundice is usually the result of another problem, and is considered a symptom of other conditions such as hepatitis. People with jaundice may exhibit yellowing of the skin and whites of the eyes, nausea, pale stools, dark urine, fever, chills, and diarrhea. When the primary cause of jaundice resolves, the jaundice should resolve with it.

***Treatments***

Treatment for jaundice usually revolves around treating the underlying cause, whether it be hepatitis, malaria, or gallstones.

***Contraindications***

Massage of a person with jaundice is considered an absolute contraindication, due to damage to the liver that may further result from the massage.

## Mumps

Mumps, also known as **parotitis**, is a **viral infection** resulting in **inflammation** of the **parotid salivary glands**, the largest salivary glands located near the ears. Mumps has become extremely rare due to the development of the mumps vaccine.

***Causes***

The mumps virus is contagious, so mumps is spread from one person to another. Because most people receive the mumps vaccine, contracting the virus is extremely rare, but may still occur if exposed to the virus for extended periods of time.

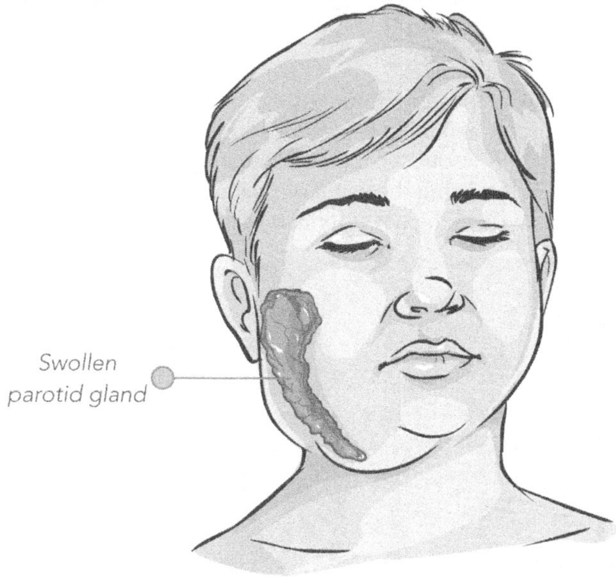


***Symptoms***

Swelling of the face and salivary glands, either on one or both sides, is the primary symptom of mumps. Fever may result, along with fatigue, body aches, and loss of appetite.

***Treatments***

Mumps is caused by a virus, and there are essentially no treatments for it aside from rest. After one week with the condition, a person is no longer considered infectious. Most healthy adults can recover from a mumps infection around two weeks after contracting the virus.

***Contraindications***

Massage is an absolute contraindication for mumps, because mumps is a contagious viral infection.

## Pancreatitis

*(pancreat/o: pancreas; -itis: inflammation)*

Pancreatitis is **inflammation** of the **pancreas**. Pancreatitis may be either acute or chronic, each presenting with differing levels of severity.

***Causes***

Pancreatitis results when **enzymes** produced by the pancreas, **insulin** and **glucagon**, **become active in the pancreas** before entering into the digestive tract or blood stream. This causes the pancreas to become irritated and inflamed. Things that may contribute to pancreatitis include blockage of the bile duct by gallstones, alcoholism, pancreatic cancer, infection, and cystic fibrosis(page 200).

***Symptoms***

Acute pancreatitis presents with fever, nausea, vomiting, pain in the upper abdomen, abdominal tenderness, and pain radiating to the back. Chronic pancreatitis may also present with the same symptoms in the acute stage, but weight loss may also occur.

Pancreatitis may lead to the development of other serious conditions such as diabetes, pancreatic cancer, and kidney failure.

***Treatments***

Upon admission to a hospital, a patient with pancreatitis will be prescribed pain medication. Fasting reduces the production of insulin and glucagon, and is therefore beneficial to decrease irritation. Other treatments that treat the underlying causes of pancreatitis can include removal of the gallbladder or gallstones, and treatment for alcohol dependency.

***Contraindications***

In the acute stage, pancreatitis is considered an absolute contraindication. In a client with chronic pancreatitis, massage may be performed in the post-acute stage.

## Peptic Ulcer

*(peptic: digestion; ulcer: open sore)*

An ulcer in the digestive tract is typically referred to as a stomach or peptic ulcer. These ulcers are **open sores** in the **inner linings** of the **stomach**, which can cause pain in the stomach.

***Causes***

Peptic ulcers are usually caused by **stomach acid** such as pepsin eating away the inner lining of the stomach and/or small intestine. Mucous lines the stomach, but when acid levels in the stomach rise and mucous production fails to match the rise in acid levels, the acid will eat through the mucous and the stomach lining. Reasons for increases in stomach acid can vary between prolonged use of things like aspirin, or a bacterial infection(H. pylori being the primary type of infection causing peptic ulcers). Excessive prolonged alcohol consumption may also contribute to the development of ulcers.

***Symptoms***

Peptic ulcers may cause painful burning sensations in the stomach, heartburn, nausea, and bloating. In less common cases, a person may also experience vomiting and have bloody stool.

***Treatments***

Treatment for peptic ulcers largely revolves around the cause of the ulcers. If H. pylori is the suspected cause, antibiotics will be prescribed to fight off the infection. Antacid medications may also be prescribed to lower the acid content of the stomach back to normal levels, giving the stomach lining a chance to heal and recover mucous.

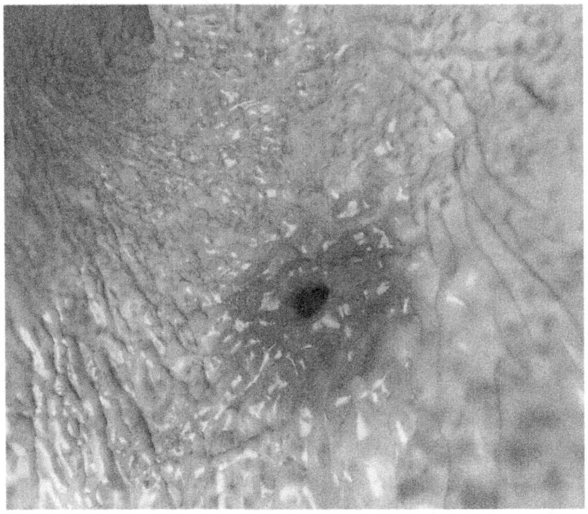

Ulceration of the stomach lining

***Contraindications***

Massage of a client with peptic ulcers often depends on the symptoms and their severity. If a client is nauseated, massage should be postponed.

## Peritonitis

*(periton/o: peritoneum; -itis: inflammation)*

Peritonitis is **inflammation** of the **peritoneum**, the serous membrane covering the abdominal and pelvic cavities.

***Causes***

Peritonitis is primarily caused by a **bacterial** or **fungal** infection. Bacteria and fungus may be introduced into the peritoneum via medical procedures such as peritoneal dialysis, and conditions that result in the formation of ulcers in the gastrointestinal tract such as diverticulitis, pancreatitis, or trauma to the peritoneum.

***Symptoms***

Peritonitis may present with tenderness in the abdomen, fever, nausea, bloating, fatigue, diarrhea, and loss of appetite.

***Treatments***

Treatment is typically a prescription of antibiotics to fight off bacterial infection, or antifungals to destroy fungus. Surgery may be required if peritonitis is the result of some sort of trauma or rupture in the peritoneum, or if inflammation is the result of something like a ruptured appendix. Surgery is also useful in fixing the underlying cause and removing any infected tissue.

***Contraindications***

Peritonitis is considered an absolute contraindication to massage.

## Pharyngitis

*(pharyng/o: pharynx; -itis: inflammation)*

Pharyngitis is **inflammation** of the **pharynx**, or the throat. A **sore throat** is considered pharyngitis.

### *Causes*

Pharyngitis is usually the result of a **viral infection** from the **common cold** or the **flu**. Bacterial infections may also result in pharyngitis, such as **strep throat**. Non-exudative pharyngitis, the kind usually caused by a virus, does not produce increased mucous, while exudative pharyngitis, the kind usually caused by bacteria, does produce mucous. Both types of pharyngitis are contagious.

### *Symptoms*

Pain in the throat is one of the main symptoms of pharyngitis. Speaking and swallowing food may be painful. A person may develop a fever, and the tonsils and lymph nodes in the neck may enlarge. Excessive mucous may be produced if it is caused by bacterial infection.

### *Treatments*

Antiviral medications may prevent the condition from worsening. If the condition is caused by bacterial infection, antibiotics can help combat the infection and improve the condition.

### *Contraindications*

Pharyngitis is commonly considered an absolute contraindication to massage during the acute stage. After the infection has cleared, massage may be performed.

## Strep Throat

Strep throat is a **bacterial infection**, resulting in **sore throat**. Typically, a throat culture is performed in order to diagnose strep throat.

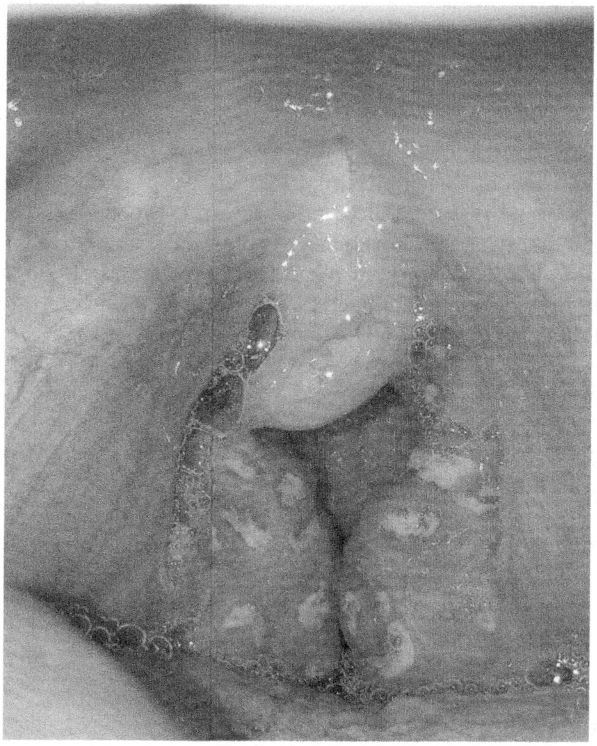

### *Causes*

Strep throat is caused by an infection of the **streptococcal** bacteria, which is contagious. Children are most at risk of contracting strep throat, but it can occur in people of all ages.

### *Symptoms*

In addition to sore throat, a person with strep throat may exhibit red spots on the roof of the mouth, white patches on the tonsils, swollen lymph nodes in the neck, pain upon swallowing, and fever, amongst others. If left untreated, strep throat may contribute to the development of Rheumatic fever, which can cause damage to heart valves.

### *Treatments*

Because strep throat is caused by bacteria, antibiotics are the primary treatment. Acetaminophen is useful in treating any pain that may be present due to the infection. After starting a course of antibiotics, a person should begin feeling better within a couple days. Taking all the medication prescribed is required to prevent the infection from returning and becoming resistant to antibiotics.

### Contraindications

Because strep throat is highly contagious, it is considered an absolute contraindication until the condition has completely cleared.

## Thrush

Thrush, also known as candidiasis, is a **fungal infection** affecting the **mouth**. This infection coats the linings of the mouth, inner cheeks, and tongue with white lesions.

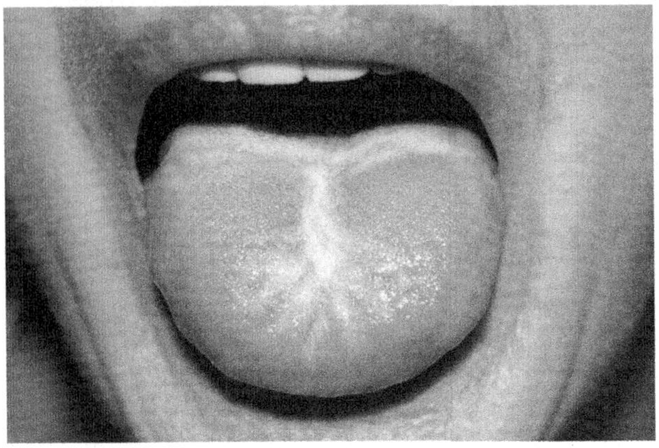

### Causes

Usually, a person's immune system will help destroy any fungus that may enter the body. If a person's immune system is weakened, the fungus may not be properly destroyed, and it could grow into thrush. Persons that take immunosuppressant medications may be more at risk than others.

### Symptoms

Thrust usually presents with white lesions on the inside of the mouth, cheeks, and tongue. It may spread further into the mouth and throat, making swallowing painful and difficult.

### Treatments

Antifungal medication is the primary treatment for thrush. These medications may be taken as topical medications, such as lozenges, or if the infection is more severe, full-body antifungals may be prescribed.

### Contraindications

Thrush is generally considered a local contraindication, and the face would be avoided. However, the massage therapist should determine if thrush is the result of another type of disorder that affects the immune system, and proceed based on those findings.

## Ulcerative Colitis

*(ulcer: open sore; col/o: large intestine; -itis: inflammation)*

Ulcerative colitis is an **inflammatory** disease of the digestive tract, specifically affecting the **inner walls** of the **large intestine** and **rectum**. Ulcerative colitis presents with chronic inflammation and ulcers, which can result in several symptoms. There are several different types of ulcerative colitis: Proctosigmoiditis(ulcers in the sigmoid colon and rectum), Ulcerative proctitis(ulcers in the rectum), Left-sided colitis(ulcers in the descending and sigmoid colons), and Pancolitis(ulcers throughout the entire large intestine). All forms of ulcerative colitis are chronic conditions, aside from acute severe ulcerative colitis, which is not common.

### Causes

Direct causes of ulcerative colitis are unclear, but heredity may play a role. There is some belief that ulcerative colitis may be caused by an autoimmune disorder of some sort.

### Symptoms

Symptoms of ulcerative colitis may include bloody diarrhea, weight loss, fever, fatigue, pain in the abdomen, difficulty defecating, and pain in the rectum. Symptoms are usually mild, and a patient may go long periods without developing symptoms.

### Treatments

There are several treatments available for ulcerative colitis, but there is no cure. Treatments include application of corticosteroids to reduce inflammation, antibiotics to combat any infections that may be present, acetaminophen to reduce pain, and possibly immunosuppressants to prevent inflammation.

***Contraindications***

Massage of a client with ulcerative colitis depends on the client's symptoms and how they are feeling that day. If a client presents with fever and body aches, massage should be postponed until the symptoms resolve. If symptoms are generally mild, massage may be performed.

Ulcerative colitis

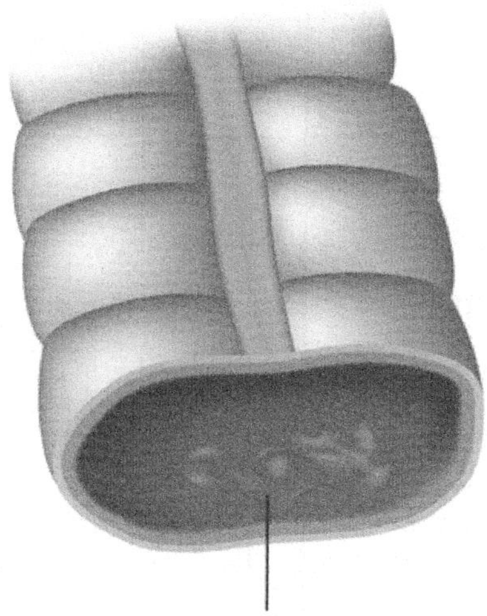

# Digestive Pathologies

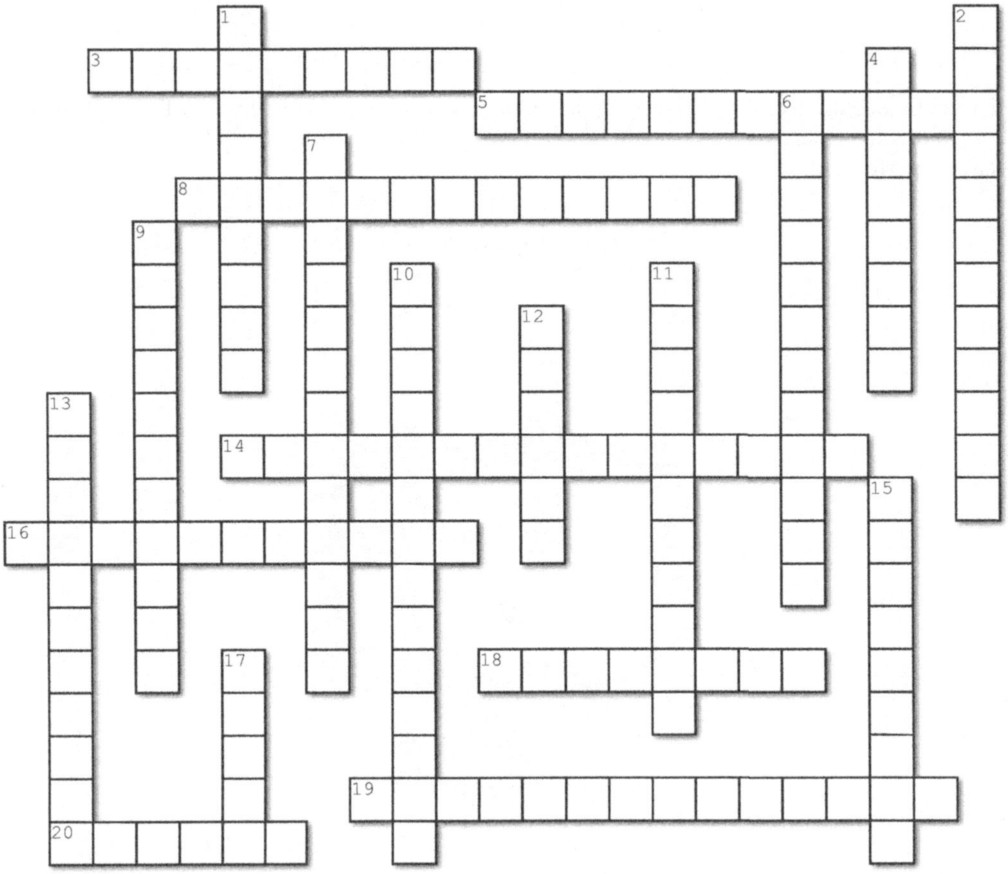

**Across**

**3.** Inflammation of the liver
**5.** Lack of regular bowel movement for an extended period
**8.** Inflammatory bowel disease that causes inflammation throughout the digestive tract
**14.** Inflammation of the stomach and small intestine, commonly referred to as the stomach flu
**16.** Inflammation of the peritoneum, usually the result of a bacterial infection
**18.** Increased levels of bilirubin, causing the skin to turn a yellowish color
**19.** The development of small pouches in the large intestine
**20.** Fungal infection affecting the inner linings of the mouth, and the tongue

**Down**

**1.** Inflammation of the stomach, commonly caused by infection from H. pylori bacteria
**2.** Inflammation of the pancreas
**4.** Loose, watery stools that may lead to dehydration over time
**6.** Inflammation of the appendix
**7.** Inflammation of the gallbladder, usually caused by the formation of gallstones
**9.** Inflammation of the pharynx, usually the result of a viral infection
**10.** Inflammation of diverticular pouches that can become infected and ulcerated
**11.** Swollen veins in the rectum or anus
**12.** Protrusion of a structure through its normal location
**13.** Streptococcal infection of the throat
**15.** Scarring of the liver, giving it a cobble-stone appearance
**17.** Viral infection causing inflammation of the parotid gland

Answer Key on Page 286

# Digestive Quiz

1. The cardiac sphincter is located in which body system
A. Urinary
B. Cardiovascular
C. Nervous
D. Digestive

2. The descending order of the small intestine is
A. Duodenum, ileum, jejunum
B. Ileum, jejunum, duodenum
C. Duodenum, jejunum, ileum
D. Jejunum, duodenum, ileum

3. The pyloric sphincter is located between which two structures
A. Stomach and small intestine
B. Stomach and esophagus
C. Pancreas and small intestine
D. Small intestine and large intestine

4. Substance produced by the liver which aids in the digestion of lipids
A. Bile
B. Vitamin A
C. Insulin
D. Glucagon

5. Nausea, vomiting, and fatigue with yellowing of the skin may be the result of
A. Hepatitis
B. Food poisoning
C. Diarrhea
D. Meningitis

6. Absorption of nutrients primarily takes place in what part of the small intestine
A. Jejunum
B. Ileum
C. Duodenum
D. Cecum

7. Autoimmune disorder in which the immune system attacks the inner linings of the digestive tract, possibly causing ulcers and scarring
A. Crohn's Disease
B. Diverticulosis
C. Pyelonephritis
D. Gastroesophageal Reflux Disease

8. Excessive alcohol consumption may result in
A. Nephritis
B. Cirrhosis
C. Gastritis
D. Diverticulitis

9. Glucagon is a digestive enzyme produced by the pancreas responsible for
A. Decreasing glucose levels in the blood
B. Increasing glucose levels in the blood
C. Increasing potassium levels in the blood
D. Decreasing potassium levels in the blood

10. Inflammation of the gallbladder, commonly caused by the development of gallstones
A. Hepatitis
B. Gastritis
C. Cholecystitis
D. GERD

11. Viral infection that causes inflammation of the parotid gland
A. Mumps
B. Measles
C. Herpes Simplex
D. Strep Throat

12. A peptic ulcer is an open sore that develops in which structure
A. Liver
B. Small intestine
C. Esophagus
D. Stomach

13. Streptococcus can result in the following condition, which causes a sore throat and white patches to appear on the tonsils
A. Pharyngitis
B. Laryngitis
C. Strep Throat
D. Tonsillitis

14. Thrush present with white lesions on the tongue, caused by what type of infection
A. Parasitic
B. Fungal
C. Bacterial
D. Viral

15. The development of small pouches that emerge from the lining of the large intestine, caused by a lack of substances for the large intestine to push against
A. Diverticulosis
B. Ulcerative colitis
C. Diverticulitis
D. Crohn's Disease

Answer Key on Page 289

# Endocrine System and Pathologies

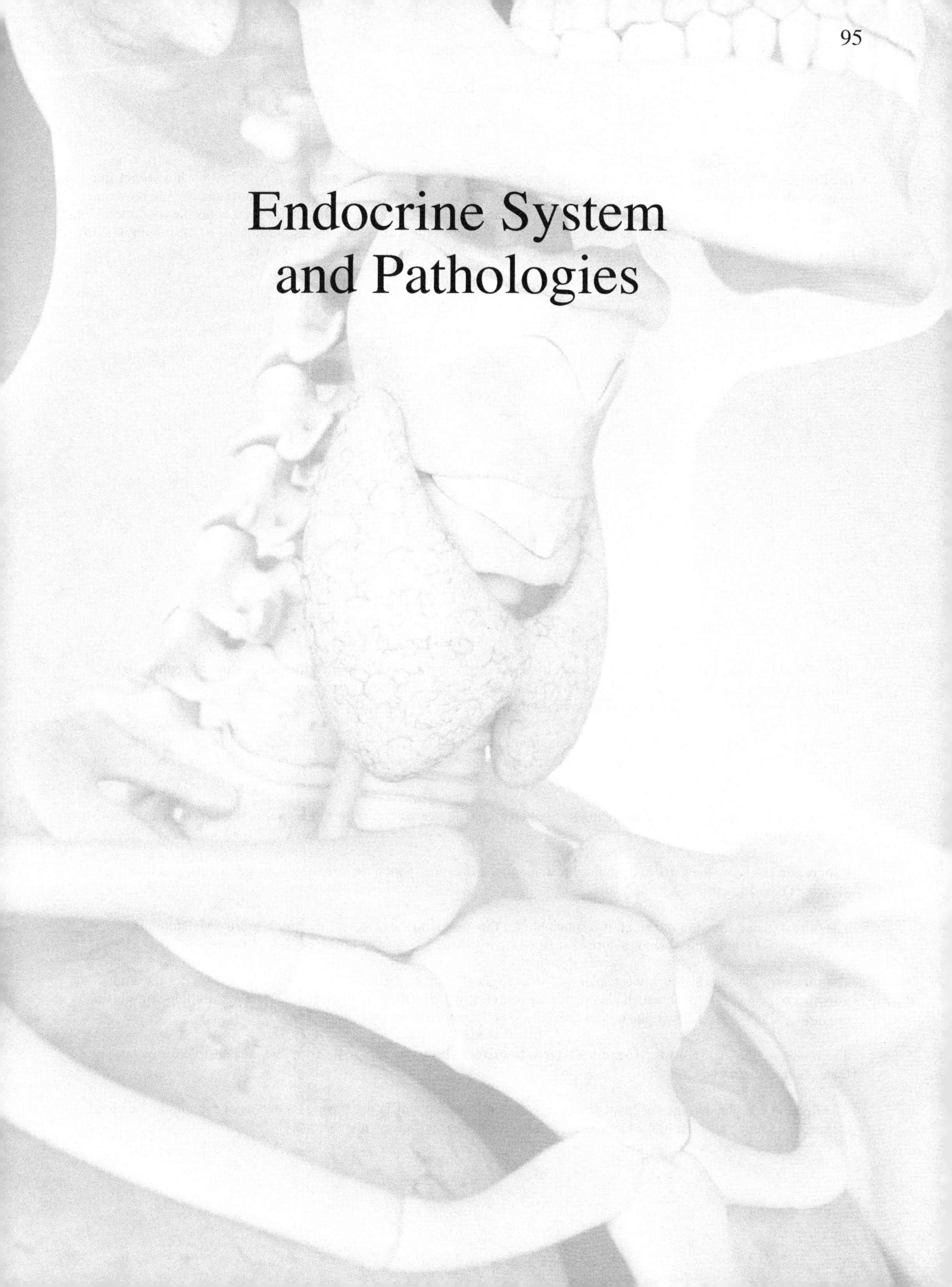

# Endocrine System

The Endocrine System is responsible for coordinating specific activities of cells and tissues by releasing **hormones** into the body. Endocrine glands differ from exocrine glands in two specific ways: endocrine glands create and secrete hormones, while exocrine glands create and secrete things like sweat, saliva, and oil. Endocrine glands secrete hormones directly into the **blood stream**, while exocrine glands secrete their substances onto a **surface**(such as the surface of the mouth or skin). Endocrine glands have many different functions that help regulate body function and homeostasis.

Endocrine gland

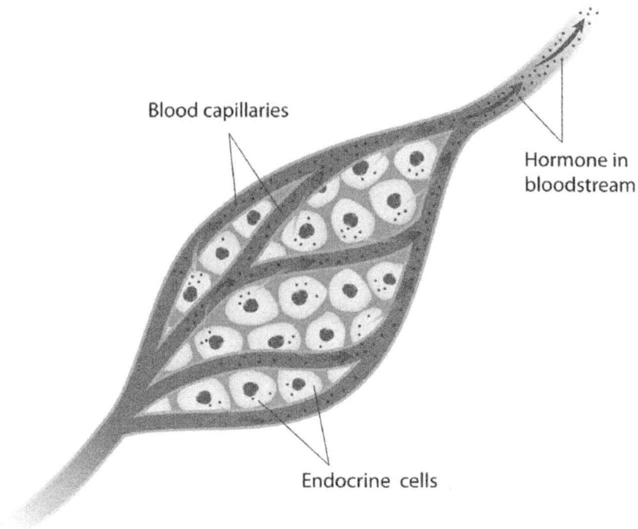


### Glands

The **adrenal** glands, located atop the kidneys(*ad-: towards; renal: kidney*), secrete **epinephrine** and **norepinephrine**. These hormones help to elevate blood pressure, heart rate, and blood sugar. They are considered stress hormones, and are secreted when the body is under stress, or in the sympathetic nervous response.

The **hypothalamus** produces **dopamine**, an important hormone that increases blood pressure and heart rate. It is considered the reward center hormone. If you win at a game or contest, your hypothalamus may release dopamine, which gives a sensation of excitement.

The **ovaries** are the female gonads, creating **estrogen** and **progesterone**, two hormones important to female development and bone growth.

**Pancreatic Islets** are the parts of the pancreas that create **glucagon**, which increases blood sugar levels, and **insulin**, which decreases blood sugar levels.

The **pineal** gland, found in the brain, is responsible for the production and secretion of **melatonin**. Melatonin is responsible for regulating a person's normal wake/sleep cycle, also known as the **circadian rhythm**.

The **pituitary** gland, which many consider the "master gland", secretes **growth hormone**, which regulates the amount of growth a person may experience. It also secretes **prolactin**, which stimulates milk production, and **follicle-stimulating hormone**, which influences production of female egg cells and male sperm cells.

The **testes** are the male gonads. The testes secrete **testosterone**, the primary male hormone, responsible for increasing bone and muscle mass.

The **thyroid** is a gland in the neck that produces **calcitonin**, which aids in decreasing the levels of calcium in the blood stream. Too much calcium in the blood may weaken the bones and cause kidney stones.

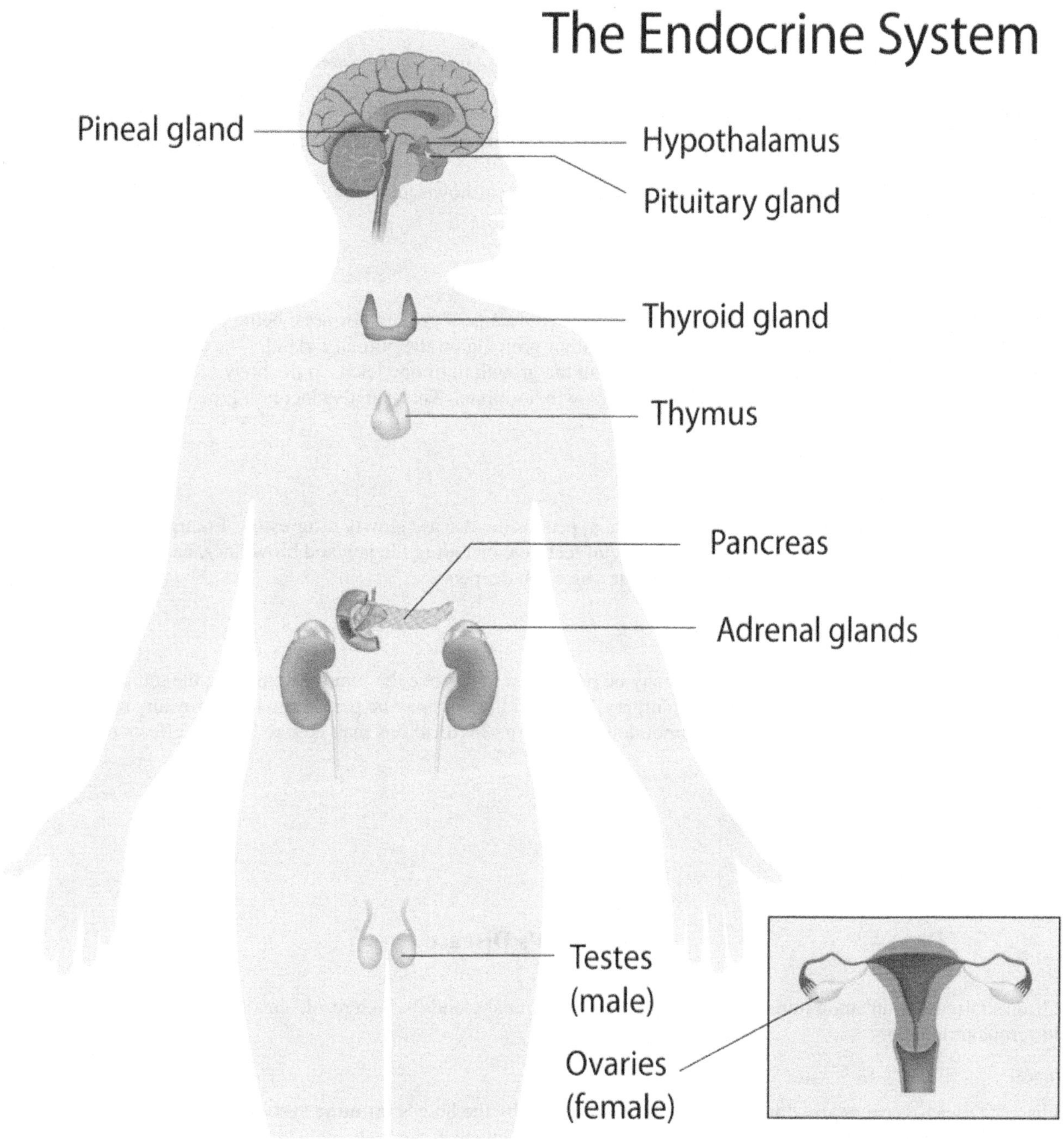
The Endocrine System
Pineal gland
Hypothalamus
Pituitary gland
Thyroid gland
Thymus
Pancreas
Adrenal glands
Testes
(male)
Ovaries
(female)

# Endocrine System Pathologies

## Acromegaly

*(acro-: extremity; -megaly: irregular enlargement)*

Acromegaly is **abnormal growth** during **adulthood**, resulting from the release of excessive amounts of growth hormone by the pituitary gland. This can cause bones to keep growing, increasing a person's size and changing their appearance.

Acromegaly can result in numerous severe health issues, such as cardiovascular issues, hypertension, sleep apnea, and arthritis.

***Causes***

As previously discussed, acromegaly is caused by increased amounts of growth hormone being produced by the pituitary gland. The most common reason for this to occur is a tumor growing on the pituitary gland. The tumor produces growth hormone and secretes it into the blood stream, increasing the growth hormone levels in the body. Rarely, a tumor elsewhere in the body, such as the adrenal glands, may produce growth hormone. This can also increase growth hormone levels in the body.

***Symptoms***

Symptoms of acromegaly generally take some time to appear as the disease slowly progresses. Enlarged hands and feet are an extremely common symptom. Enlargement of facial features, including the jaw and brow lines, can typically be seen in advanced stages. Skin can become thickened and the voice can deepen.

***Treatments***

If acromegaly is the result of a tumor, surgery may be performed to remove the tumor. Removing the tumor should stabilize the growth hormone levels in the body. After surgery, radiation therapy may be performed to destroy any remaining tumor cells in the body. This can help ensure the tumor does not return. Medications may help reduce the effects of growth hormone in the body.

***Contraindications***

Massage is indicated for acromegaly.

## Addison's Disease

Addison's Disease is an autoimmune disorder affecting the adrenal glands, which results in a lack of cortisol and/or aldosterone production.

***Causes***

Addison's Disease is caused by **damage** to the **adrenal cortex** by the body's **immune system**. Damage to these glands results in an inability to produce cortisol, which regulates stress levels in the body by helping control blood sugar, blood pressure, and metabolism, and aldosterone, which aids in reabsorption of water and sodium back into the blood stream.

***Symptoms***

Addison's Disease may result in fatigue, weight loss, low blood pressure, hair loss, hyperpigmentation of the skin, and nausea. It may become life-threatening if not treated.

Acute adrenal failure, also known as Addisonian Crisis, may result in severe vomiting and diarrhea, dehydration, low blood pressure, and pain in the low back, abdomen, and/or legs.

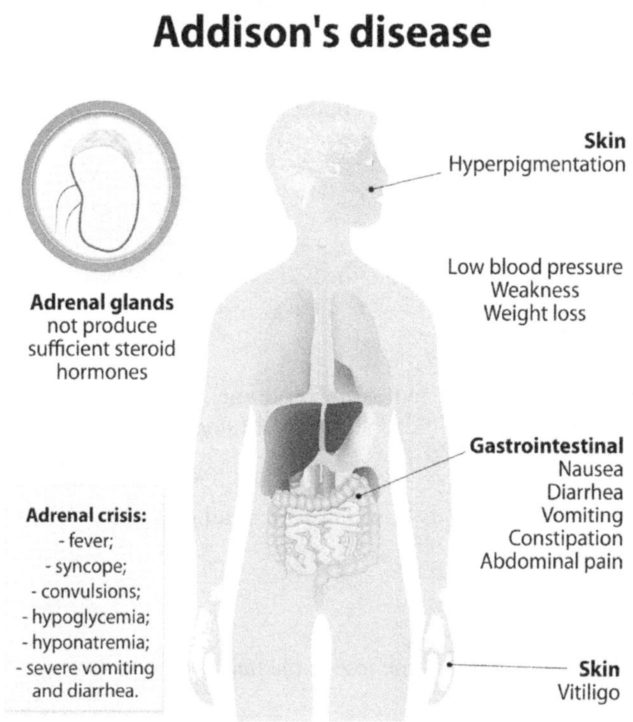


*Treatments*

Treatment primarily consists of hormone replacements, which may be taken orally or injected.

*Contraindications*

Massage is indicated for a client with Addison's Disease. However, the type and length of massage varies depending on how a client is feeling and their stamina. Clients with low stamina should receive shorter, lighter massages, while clients with increased stamina may receive longer and stimulating massages.

## Cushing's Disease

Cushing's Disease is a disease of the **pituitary** gland, which results in **hyper-production** of **adrenocorticotropic hormone(ACTH)**.

*Causes*

Cushing's Disease is the result of hyperplasia(excessive growth) of the pituitary gland, or development of a tumor. This causes too much ACTH to be released in the body, which stimulates hyper-production of **cortisol**.

*Symptoms*

Cushing's Disease may result in weight gain around the face and torso, weakening of bone, thinning of skin, fatigue, and acne, amongst other complications.

*Treatments*

Treatments for Cushing's Disease include surgery to remove a tumor, and hormone therapy to reduce the amount of cortisol being produced.

*Contraindications*

Massage is indicated for Cushing's Disease, but precautions may be taken in clients with weakened bones. Lighter massage is recommended for these clients to prevent damaging bone.

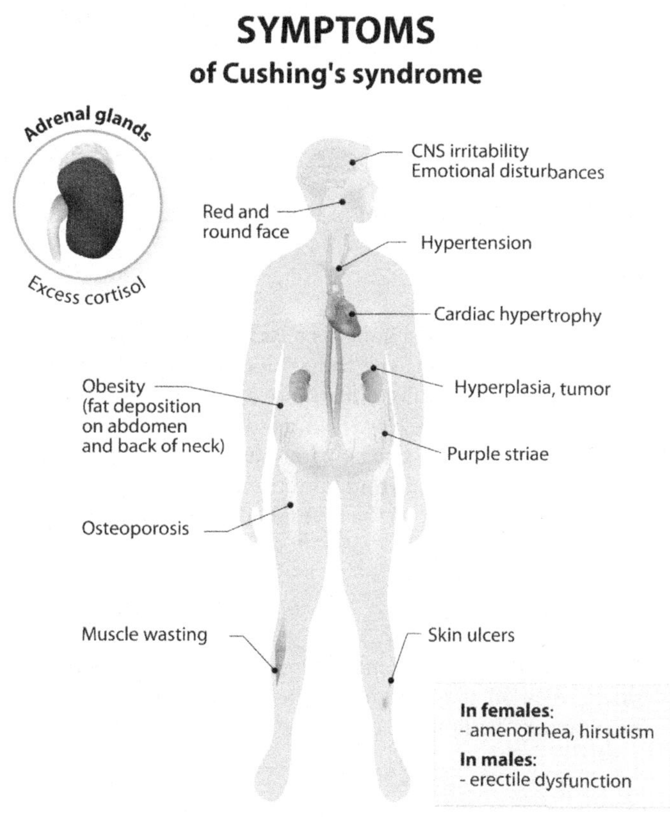

## Diabetes Mellitus

*(diabetes: to pass through; mellitus: sweet)*

Diabetes Mellitus is a condition of the endocrine system that affects **insulin** function in the body.

There are three types of diabetes: Diabetes Type I, Diabetes Type II, and Gestational Diabetes.

***Causes***

Diabetes Type I is often known as **juvenile diabetes**, as it begins in childhood. In Type I, the body's immune system attacks the pancreas, the organ that produces insulin. This results in the body not producing enough insulin, which the body needs in order to convert glucose to energy.

Diabetes Type II, the most common form of diabetes, is caused by the body having an **insulin resistance**. The insulin in the body is unable to break down glucose, which causes high levels of sugar in the blood stream. Obesity is a common cause of Diabetes Type II.

Gestational Diabetes is only present during **pregnancy**. Gestational Diabetes affects less than 10% of all pregnant women, and typically resolves after pregnancy ends.

***Symptoms***

Symptoms of diabetes include frequent urination, fatigue, weight loss, pain and/or numbness in the hands or feet, extreme thirst, and extreme hunger.

***Treatments***

Treatment for Diabetes Type I is primarily insulin injections. Treatment for Diabetes Type II includes medications, but exercise and dietary changes are most common. Treatment for Gestational Diabetes includes exercise, regulating weight gain during pregnancy, and possibly insulin medication depending on the severity.

***Contraindications***

Massage is indicated for a client with diabetes. If neuropathy is present, lighter massage in the affected area should be performed. If ulcers are present in areas afflicted with neuropathy, ulcers should be treated as local contraindications. If a client injects insulin, the injection site should also be avoided.

## Goiter

*(Latin "guttur": throat)*

A goiter is an **enlargement** of the **thyroid** gland, located at the base of the neck.

***Causes***

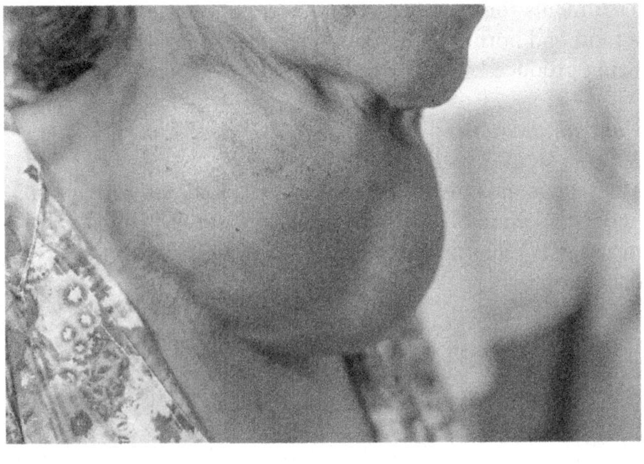

The primary cause of a goiter is a **lack of iodine** in the diet. If a person does not consume enough iodine, the body is unable to produce sufficient thyroid hormones. Other conditions, such as Graves' Disease or Hashimoto's Disease, can affect the levels of thyroid hormone being produced. Too much thyroid hormone or too little thyroid hormone being produced can have negative effects on the thyroid and could produce a goiter.

***Symptoms***

Goiters produce a bulge in the throat, which may place pressure on other structures such as the esophagus or trachea, making it difficult to eat or breathe.

***Treatments***

Treatment of a goiter typically depends on the cause. If it is caused by low levels of thyroid hormones, thyroid hormone replacement medications may be prescribed. If the thyroid is producing too much thyroid hormone, medications may be prescribed to stabilize the levels of thyroid hormone in the body. Surgery to remove the thyroid may be an option if the goiter causes any difficulty in breathing or swallowing, or causes discomfort.

Increasing iodine consumption may be all it takes to reduce the goiter. Iodized salt may be added to the diet, along with other foods high in iodine such as seafood.

***Contraindications***

A goiter is considered a local contraindication.

## Graves' Disease

Graves' Disease is an autoimmune disorder, in which the body's **immune system attacks** the **thyroid** gland, causing an increase in thyroid hormone production(**hyperthyroidism**).

***Causes***

The exact cause of Graves' Disease is unknown.

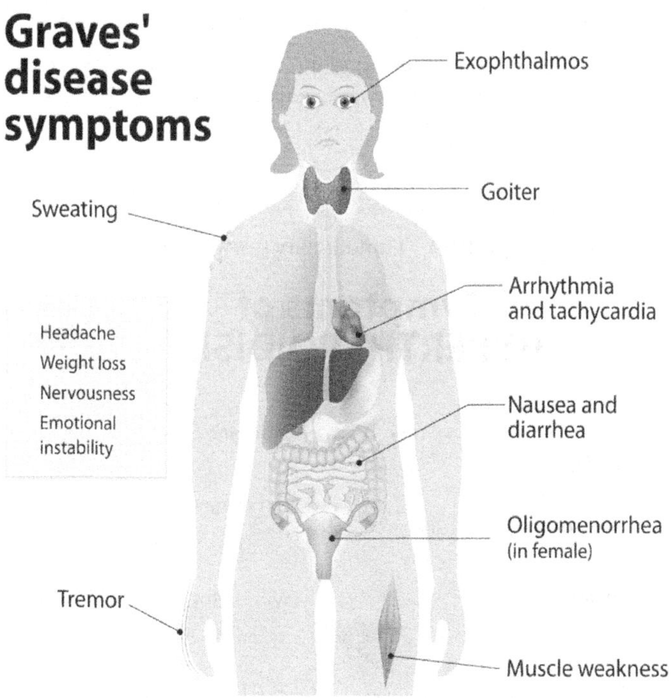


***Symptoms***

Graves' Disease can affect numerous parts of the body, resulting in sensitivity to heat, weight loss, the development of a goiter(enlargement of the thyroid), bulging of the eyes, and irregular heart rhythm. Women are more likely to develop Graves' Disease, as well as people under the age of 40.

***Treatments***

Treatment for Graves' Disease include medications such as beta blockers and anti-thyroid medications. If medication isn't helpful, surgical removal of the thyroid may be an option.

***Contraindications***

Graves' Disease is generally considered not contraindicated. However, a client with Graves' Disease may be sensitive to heat, so anything that uses heat in the massage treatment should be avoided. A goiter may also be present, which would be considered a local contraindication.

## Hyperparathyroidism

*(hyper-: excessive; parathyroid-: parathyroid; -ism: condition)*

Hyperparathyroidism is the result of **excessive production** of **parathyroid hormone**. This is usually the result of one of the body's four parathyroid glands becoming overactive.

***Causes***

Primary hyperparathyroidism is the result of a parathyroid gland enlarging. Causes for enlargement of a parathyroid gland vary, but is commonly caused by a tumor growing on the gland. This causes high levels of calcium to build in the blood, a condition known as hypercalcemia. Secondary hyperparathyroidism, much like other conditions, is the result of another disease of some sort decreasing the levels of calcium. This can cause the body to produce more parathyroid hormone.

***Symptoms***

Symptoms of hyperparathyroidism are often mild, but depending on the amount of damage caused to other structures or tissues, symptoms may be more severe. These symptoms may include the development of kidney stones, osteoporosis, body pain(specifically bones), increased urination, and pain in the abdomen.

***Treatments***

Treatment for hyperparathyroidism often depends on the cause and severity of the condition. If symptoms are mild, no treatment may be needed, but the condition should be closely monitored to determine if it is worsening. If hyperparathyroidism is the result of some sort of growth on a parathyroid gland, surgery to remove the gland may be performed. Medications to regulate calcium levels in the blood may be prescribed.

***Contraindications***

Generally, hyperparathyroidism is not contraindicated. However, if a client presents with associated symptoms such as osteoporosis, a lighter massage may be recommended.

## Hyperthyroidism

*(hyper-: excessive; thyroid: thyroid gland; -ism: condition)*

Hyperthyroidism is an **increase** in production of **thyroxine**, a hormone secreted by the thyroid gland. Thyroxine is primarily responsible for stimulating tissues to **consume oxygen.** Excessive amounts of thyroxine can significantly increase the body's metabolism, which can have numerous effects.

***Causes***

Hyperthyroidism is often caused by other conditions such as Graves' Disease(page 101). Tumors may grow in or on the thyroid, which can increase production of thyroxine.

***Symptoms***

Symptoms of hyperthyroidism are vast, and may be confused with other medical conditions. The main symptom of hyperthyroidism is sudden, rapid weight loss due to an increased metabolism. This may even cause an increase in appetite, despite the lost weight. Arrhythmia, specifically tachycardia, may also result. Heat sensitivity and sweating are other symptoms to be aware of.

***Treatments***

Treatments are often the same as those seen with Graves' Disease, including a prescription of oral radioactive iodine. Other medications may help lower the amount of hormones being produced by the thyroid. If a person has tachycardia as a result of hyperthyroidism, beta blockers may also be prescribed. In cases where these treatments aren't helpful, surgical removal of the thyroid may be performed.

***Contraindications***

Generally, hyperthyroidism is not contraindicated. However, conditions such as arrhythmia that can be caused by hyperthyroidism may be contraindicated if uncontrolled.

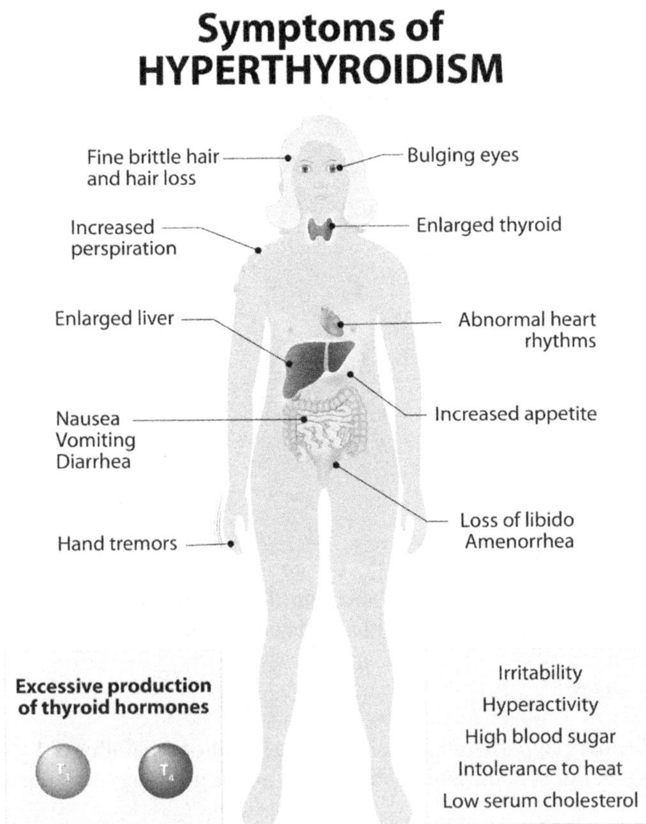

## Hypoparathyroidism

*(hypo-: below; parathyroid-: parathyroid; -ism: condition)*

Hypoparathyroidism is the result of the parathyroid glands secreting **low levels** of **parathyroid hormone**. This can lead to low levels of **calcium** and increased levels of **phosphorus** in the blood.

### *Causes*

Common causes of hypoparathyroidism include hereditary parathyroidism, in which the parathyroid glands don't work properly or a person is simply born without them, cancer or radiation treatment, which can damage the parathyroids, or most likely, damage to or removal of the parathyroids due to a surgical procedure.

### *Symptoms*

Symptoms of hypoparathyroidism may include fatigue, muscle spasms and cramping, and a tingling or burning sensation in the lips, fingers, and toes due to low levels of calcium.

### *Treatments*

Because hypoparathyroidism can lead to low levels of calcium in the blood, calcium supplementation is the main treatment given. Changing the diet may also help regulate the levels of calcium and phosphorus in the blood.

### *Contraindications*

Hypoparathyroidism is generally not contraindicated, however precautions should be taken in areas such as the fingers and toes which may experience tingling or burning sensations.

## Hypopituitarism

*(hypo-: below; pituitar-: pituitary gland; -ism: condition)*

Hypopituitarism is the result of the **pituitary** gland failing to produce enough of the hormones it regularly secretes. These hormones play an extremely important role in growth, and if they aren't being produced, a person may not grow normally.

### *Causes*

The primary cause of hypopituitarism is a **tumor** growth on the pituitary gland. Tumors may put pressure on the gland, restricting the secretion and production of hormones such as growth hormone and follicle-stimulating hormone. Other causes, although less common, may be stroke, an injury to the head, and meningitis.

### *Symptoms*

Symptoms of hypopituitarism vary based on the severity of the condition. These symptoms may include weight loss, low sex drive, anemia, cold sensitivity, an inability to produce breast milk, and a lack of body hair in males.

### *Treatments*

If hypopituitarism is the result of a tumor, surgery may be performed to remove the tumor. This could lead to the return of adequate hormone production. Hormone replacement drugs may be prescribed, including testosterone, estrogen, and growth hormone. These drugs give the body the amount of hormones it would normally get if the pituitary were functioning properly, but they do not cure the disease.

### *Contraindications*

Hypopituitarism is generally not contraindicated.

## Hypothyroidism

*(hypo-: below; thyroid-: thyroid; -ism: condition)*

Hypothyroidism is a most commonly an **autoimmune** disorder affecting the **thyroid** gland, resulting in a lack of **thyroid hormone** being produced.

***Causes***

When the body's immune system attacks the thyroid, it destroys healthy thyroid cells. When too many of these cells have been destroyed, the thyroid may not produce sufficient amounts of thyroid hormone. Hypothyroidism may also be the result of a previously inflamed thyroid, which can also damage thyroid cells.

***Symptoms***

Lack of thyroid hormone may result in weight gain, fatigue, hair loss, sensitivity to cold, and pain throughout the body.

***Treatments***

Synthetic thyroid hormones may be prescribed to increase thyroid hormone levels in the body.

***Contraindications***

Hypothyroidism is generally not contraindicated. A client with hypothyroidism may exhibit sensitivity to cold, so an extra blanket or increasing room temperature may be welcomed.

# Endocrine Pathologies

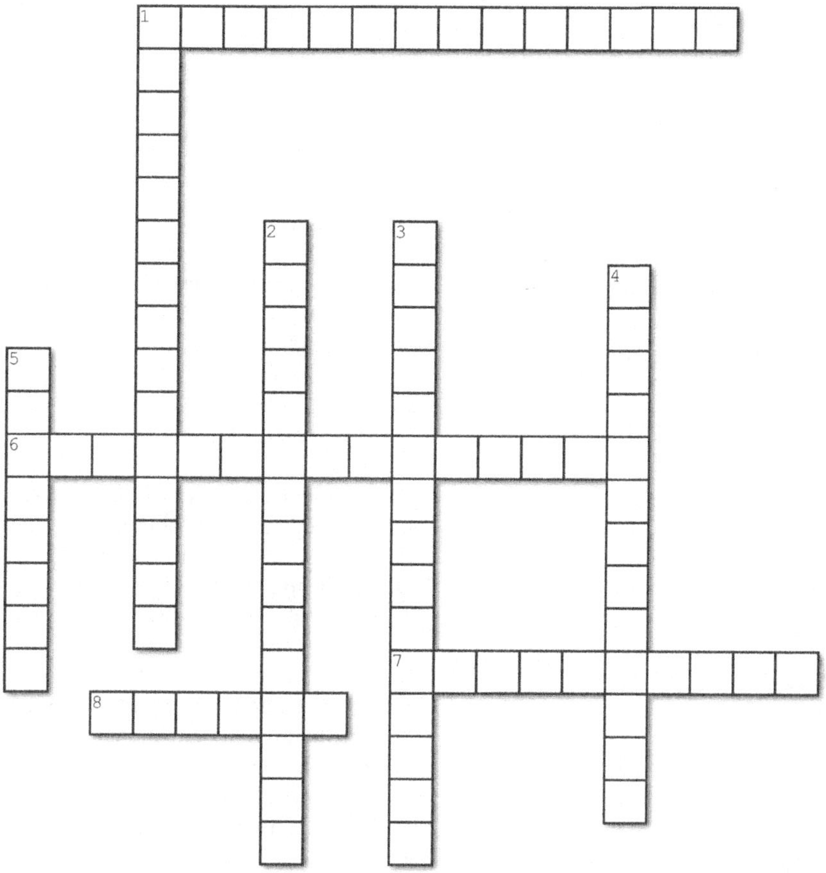

**Across**

**1.** Lack of thyroid hormone being produced

**6.** Damage to the adrenal cortex, causing a lack of cortisol production

**7.** Abnormal growth during adulthood caused by excessive growth hormone being produced

**8.** Enlargement of the thyroid, commonly caused by a lack of iodine in the diet

**Down**

**1.** Excessive production of thyroxine

**2.** Hyperplasia of the pituitary gland, causing excessive production of ACTH

**3.** Lack of adequate growth hormone being produced, commonly caused by a tumor on the pituitary gland

**4.** Autoimmune disorder affecting the thyroid, causing hyperthyroidism

**5.** Difficulty in the ability to break down sugar in the blood

Answer Key on Page 286

# Endocrine Quiz

1. Primary function of a gland
A. Secretion
B. Protection
C. Absorption
D. Contraction

2. Growth hormone, prolactin, and follicle-stimulating hormone are all produced by the
A. Thalamus
B. Pituitary
C. Testes
D. Thyroid

3. The adrenal glands are located atop which organs
A. Large intestine
B. Small intestine
C. Kidneys
D. Ureters

4. The pineal gland is located
A. In the neck
B. In the chest
C. In the abdomen
D. In the skull

5. Hormone responsible for increasing heart rate and moving blood from digestive organs into the muscles
A. Aldosterone
B. Oxytocin
C. Growth hormone
D. Norepinephrine

6. An enlargement of the thyroid results in
A. Goiter
B. Hypothyroidism
C. Lupus
D. Acromegaly

7. Overproduction of growth hormone can result in
A. Lupus
B. Myasthenia Gravis
C. Fibromyalgia
D. Acromegaly

8. Calcitonin is responsible for
A. Converting calcium into carbohydrates in the liver
B. Increasing calcium synthesis in the stomach
C. Converting calcium into insulin in the pancreas
D. Reducing calcium levels in the blood

9. The ovaries produce
A. Luteinizing hormone
B. Testosterone
C. Progesterone
D. Melatonin

10. Damage to the adrenal cortex, causing insufficient cortisol production
A. Addison's Disease
B. Graves' Disease
C. Cushing's Disease
D. Hyperparathyroidism

11. Low levels of calcium and increased levels of phosphorus in the blood can be attributed to
A. Hypoparathyroidism
B. Hyperpituitarism
C. Addison's Disease
D. Graves' Disease

12. Autoimmune disorder in which the immune system attacks the thyroid, causing an increase in thyroid production
A. Addison's Disease
B. Cushing's Disease
C. Graves' Disease
D. Diabetes Mellitus

13. Form of diabetes in which the immune system attacks the pancreas, limiting the production of insulin
A. Diabetes Type I
B. Gestational Diabetes
C. Pancreatic Diabetes
D. Diabetes Type II

14. A goiter is most commonly caused by a lack of
A. Insulin
B. Glucose
C. Iodine
D. Potassium

15. The most common form of diabetes, in which the pancreas produces insulin, but the insulin is unable to properly break down glucose in the blood
A. Diabetes Type II
B. Diabetes Type I
C. Pancreatic Diabetes
D. Gestational Diabetes

Answer Key on Page 289

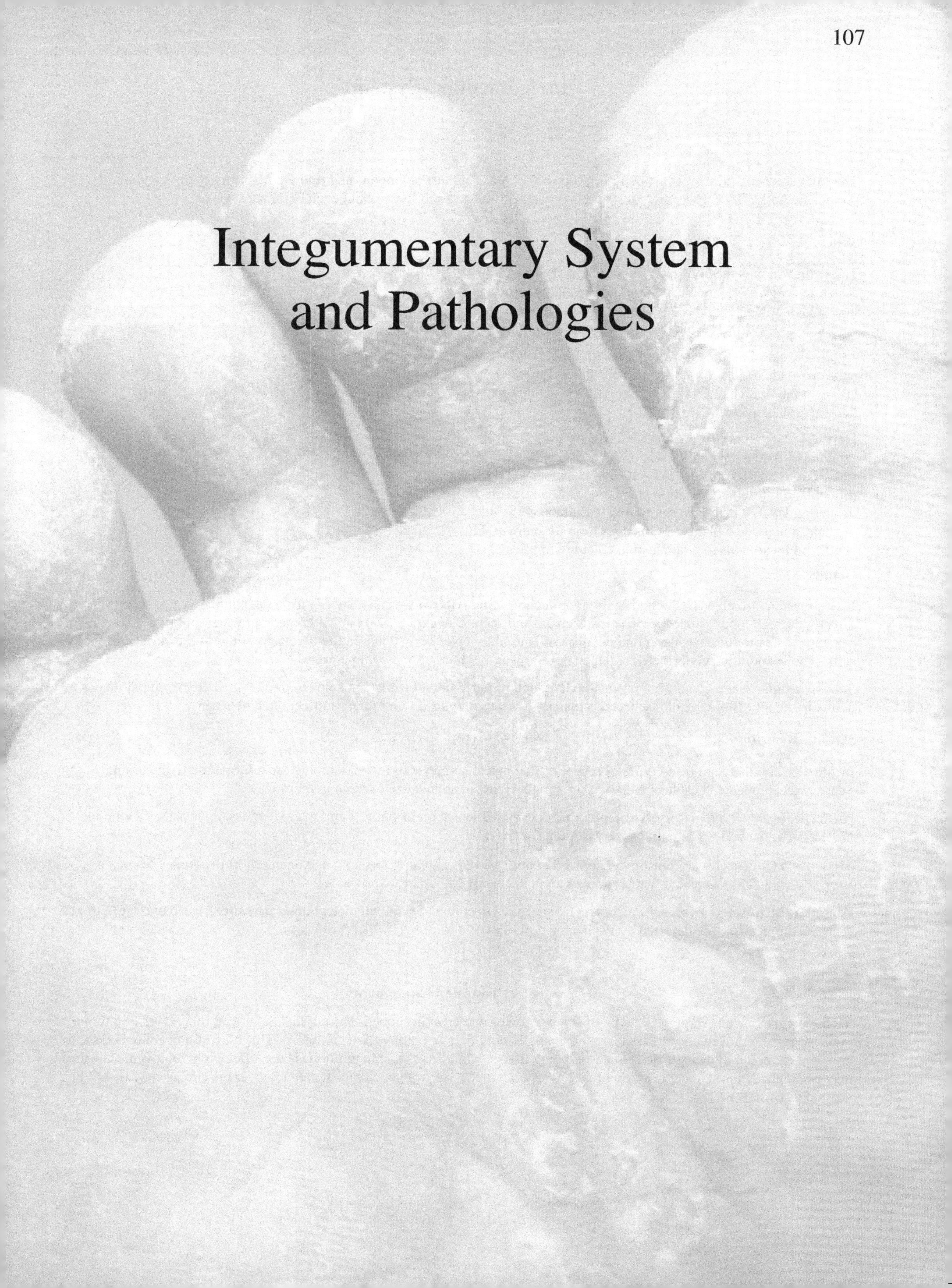

# Integumentary System and Pathologies

# Integumentary System

The Integumentary System is the body's first line of defense against pathogens and trauma. Its primary function is to protect the body. It also secretes substances, may absorb certain substances, and even eliminates waste.

### Skin

The **skin**, which is the body's largest organ, is the main structure of the Integumentary System. The skin **protects** the body by creating a thick barrier that prevents pathogens from entering, and helps to cushion the body from blunt trauma.

Aiding the skin in protection are the **nails**. Finger and toe nails are made of **keratin**, the same cells that create thick layers in the skin called calluses. The nails prevent damage to the distal phalanges.

**Hair** also aids in protection, but in a different way. Hair is used to regulate temperature. When body temperature drops, smooth muscle that attaches to each hair, known as **arrector pili**, contract, forcing the hair to stand up. This creates an insulating layer, which is meant to trap warmth underneath the hair, much like a blanket. This does little for humans, but is utilized by animals to retain heat in cold environments.

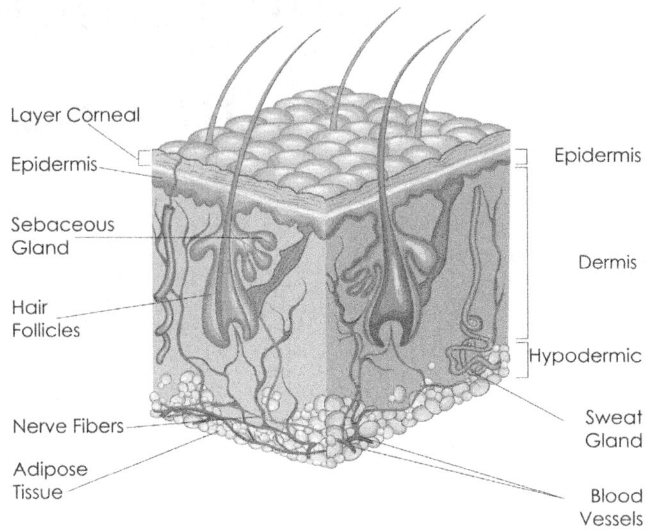


### Glands

Inside the skin are glands, which also aid in protection. **Sudoriferous** glands emerge from deep in the skin to the surface directly through tubes. Sudoriferous glands create and secrete **sweat**. Sweat is mostly made of water, but may also contain salt and waste products such as ammonia. Sweat is used to lower body temperature by evaporating off the surface of the skin. The evaporation cools the skin, which helps lower the internal body temperature.

**Sebaceous** glands are glands that connect to hair, and produce **oil(sebum)**. Oil helps to protect the body from pathogens and debris in the air. Blockage of a sebaceous gland, however, may lead to a bacterial infection, and acne.

### Sensory Receptors

Inside the skin, there are many types of receptors that detect certain sensations, relaying the information to the brain. Sensory receptors aren't exclusive to the skin, but there are an abundance of them in the skin.

**Nociceptors** are a type of sensory receptor that detects the sensation of **pain**. Pain, while unpleasant, is actually vital in protection of the body. The term "*noci-*" is Latin for "*hurt*".

**Meissner's Corpuscles** are sensory receptors that are very superficial in the skin, and detect **light pressure**. Massage strokes such as effleurage and feather strokes are detected by Meissner's Corpuscles.

**Pacinian Corpuscles** are sensory receptors that are very deep in the skin, and detect **deep pressure**. Deep massage strokes, such as compression, are detected by Pacinian Corpuscles.

## Medical Tests and Equipment

**Mohs Surgery**: Mohs surgery is a type of surgery performed on skin cancer. During this treatment, thin layers of a tumor in the skin are removed one at a time, until eventually nothing but healthy tissue remains. This type of procedure is done to reduce the amount of damage done to surrounding tissues while ensuring the tumor has been effectively removed. The area may be stitched closed, receive a skin graft, have skin pulled over from an adjacent area to cover the site, or may be left to heal on its own.

**Skin Graft**: A skin graft is transplanting skin from one location on the body to another where skin has been lost, commonly from burns or injuries. A thin layer of epidermis is removed using a shaver(similar to a potato peeler), then placed on the area where skin is needed. The area is covered in bandages to allow healing. Over time, the skin adheres to the injured area and becomes new skin for the area.

# Integumentary System Pathologies

## Acne

Acne is an infection of the skin, resulting from numerous factors. Acne may result in whiteheads, blackheads, or even cysts if left untreated.

***Causes***

Acne is caused by an increased production of sebum on the skin, which results in blocked pores. These blocked pores may become **infected**, which may develop into pustules. There are several contributing factors that lead to the development of acne, including **testosterone** production, stress, hormonal imbalances, and poor personal hygiene.

***Symptoms***

Acne may result in the development of whiteheads, blackheads, pimples, or even cystic lesions beneath the skin. These are often painful to the touch and may present with infection and inflammation.

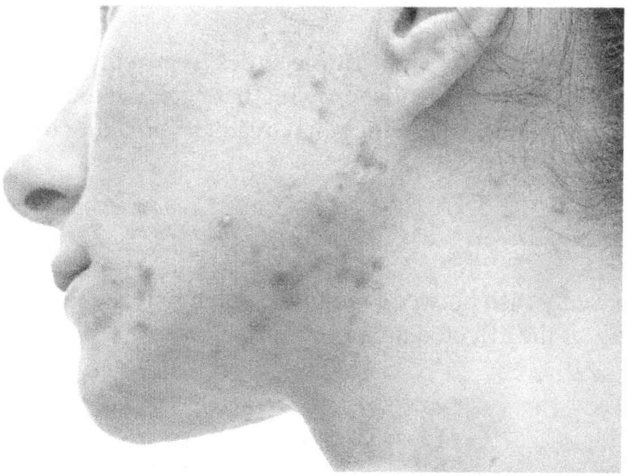

***Treatments***

Treatment includes over-the-counter skin care products for mild acne, or in the case of severe acne, medications such as birth control pills to regulate hormone levels in women, and antibiotics to eliminate bacterial growth. Other treatments include light therapy and chemical peels.

***Contraindications***

Whiteheads are considered local contraindications. Any part of the body experiencing inflammation from acne should also be considered a local contraindication.

## Albinism

*(albin-: white; -ism: condition)*

Albinism is a **genetic disorder**, causing little to **no melanin** to be produced. This results in the skin, hair, and eyes to appear extremely light. Albinism can affect people of all races.

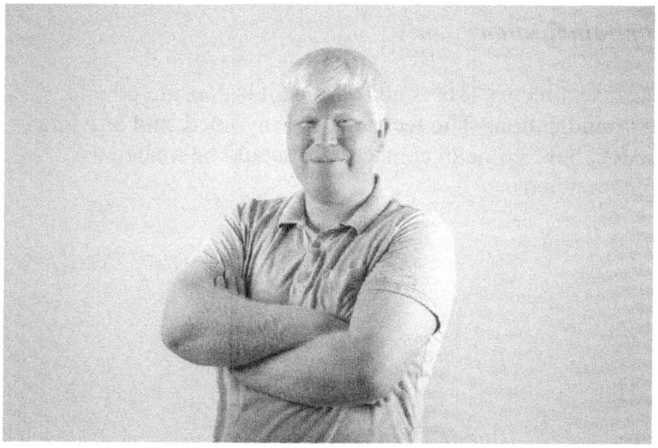

***Causes***

Albinism is a genetic disorder, and is the result of a person's genes being mutated in such a way that severely lessens or prevents the production of melanin all together.

***Symptoms***

People with albinism often appear to have white or pinkish skin, extremely light hair, and very light blue eyes. Changes in the appearance of any of these can occur. Albinism may lead to vision problems due to a lack of pigment in the iris of the eye, which usually helps to block light from entering into the eye.

***Treatments***

Treatment is limited due to the condition being genetic. Management of the condition, including the use of prescription lenses, may be advised. A person with albinism may need to be cautious of sunlight, as it may be easier for their skin to become damaged from the sun.

***Contraindications***

Albinism is not a contraindication for massage.

## Athlete's Foot

*(tinea: fungus; pedis: foot)*

Athlete's Foot(also known as Tinea Pedis) is a **fungal** infection of the **foot.** Despite the name, anyone may develop athlete's foot, not just athletes. Athlete's foot, like other fungal infections such as ringworm and jock itch, is highly contagious.

***Causes***

Athlete's foot is caused by exposure to fungus on the foot. When a person wears tight-fitting shoes, it provides an environment for the fungus to thrive: a warm, humid, dark space. The fungus spreads, growing between the toes, then expanding across the foot. The infection causes the skin to become dry and scaly, which may result in breaking of the skin and bacterial infection.

***Symptoms***

Symptoms of athlete's foot are typically the development of a red, scaly rash between the toes, which may spread proximally. Blisters and ulcers may be present in the area. Itching of the affected area is common.

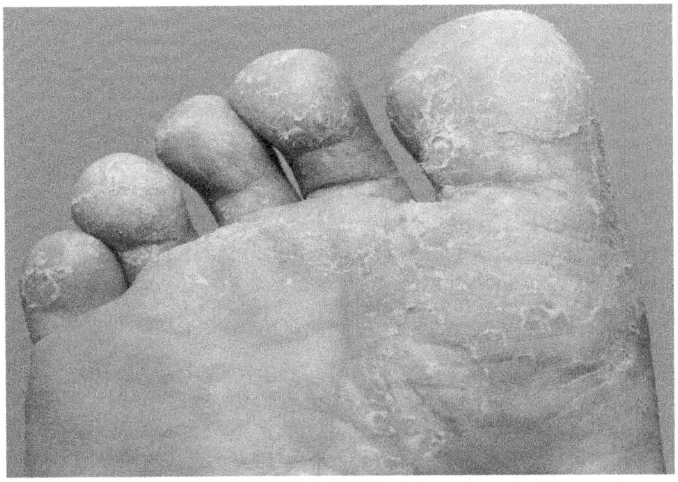

***Treatments***

Treatment of athlete's foot primarily consists of over-the-counter medications, in addition to self-care, such as ensuring the foot and footwear are dry as much as possible, wearing shower shoes in public bathing areas, etc.

***Contraindications***

Because athlete's foot is contagious, it is considered a local contraindication. The feet should be avoided, and any linens the feet have come in contact with should be treated as contaminated.

## Boil

A boil is a **bacterial** infection of a **hair follicle**, also known as a **furuncle**. A group of these infections together in one localized area is known as a carbuncle.

***Causes***

A boil typically results from small cuts in the skin(caused by things like shaving), allowing staphylococci bacteria to enter the body and reproduce. Boils can be red, inflamed, and painful to the touch. The lump initially produced by the infection begins to soften over a few days, and becomes much more painful. Pus develops on the affected area.

***Symptoms***

A boil may result in pain around the boil, the development of a fever, and swelling of lymph nodes. More boils may develop around the site of the original boil.

***Treatments***

Boils are treated by lancing(draining) the area with application of antibacterial soap and water, or in more severe cases, prescription of antibiotics to combat the bacterial infection.

***Contraindications***

A boil is considered a local contraindication for massage.

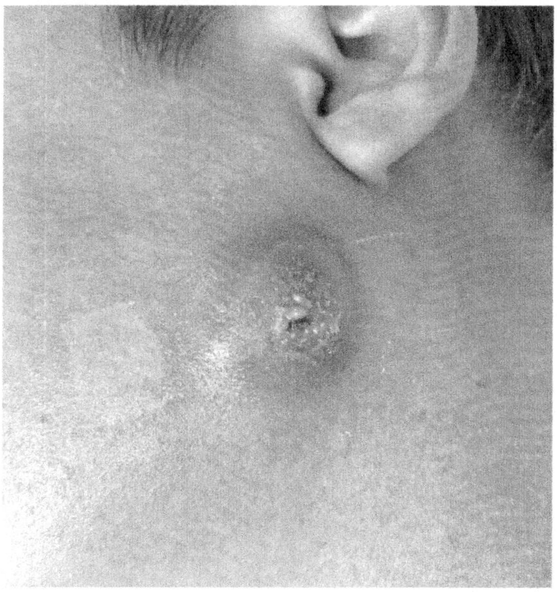

## Burns

Burns are a skin condition in which the skin is **damaged** due to exposure to **heat, chemicals,** or other means. This may result in inflammation, blister formation, or necrosis, depending on the severity of the burn.

Burns of the skin can be categorized as first, second, third, or fourth degree, with first being the least severe.

A first degree burn only affects the epidermis. It may lead to pain and inflammation of the skin, but nothing more. A common first degree burn is a sun burn. The pain and inflammation subsides in a day or two, and the skin returns to normal.

A second degree burn is more severe. In a second degree burn, the burn moves through the epidermis and into the dermis.

Because the burn goes deeper into the skin, it causes more damage, which can be seen by blistering. Blisters form to help repair the damage done by the burn. Second degree burns may result in scarring if they are too severe.

Third degree burns move even deeper into the skin, reaching the subcutaneous layer of the skin. Third degree burns often cause severe tissue damage and necrosis. Skin grafts may be needed to help repair an area damaged by a third degree burn.

While first, second, and third degree burns are most common, a fourth degree burn moves completely through all layers of the skin, and goes deeper into tissues beneath the skin, such as tendons, ligaments, muscles, and bones.

***Causes***

As stated, burns may be caused by many different factors, including heat(thermal burns), chemicals, electricity, radiation(such as sunburns), friction(rug burns), and even extreme cold temperatures.

***Symptoms***

Burn symptoms vary based on severity. First degree burns often present with inflammation and pain. Second degree burns present with pain, blistering, and discoloration of the skin as the body repairs the damaged tissue. Third degree burns may present with blackened, charred tissue, with the skin having a waxy appearance. Because tissue is destroyed in third and fourth degree burns, loss of sensation may occur resulting from nerves being destroyed.

***Treatments***

Treatment for burns often depends on the severity of the burn. Application of aloe vera may help reduce the pain in first degree burns. Second degree burns may require bandages with topical antibiotic cream to prevent infection. Third degree burns, again, may require surgery and skin grafts to repair the affected areas.

***Contraindications***

Burns are considered local contraindications for massage. Avoid any area experiencing inflammation, blistering, or has suffered necrosis.

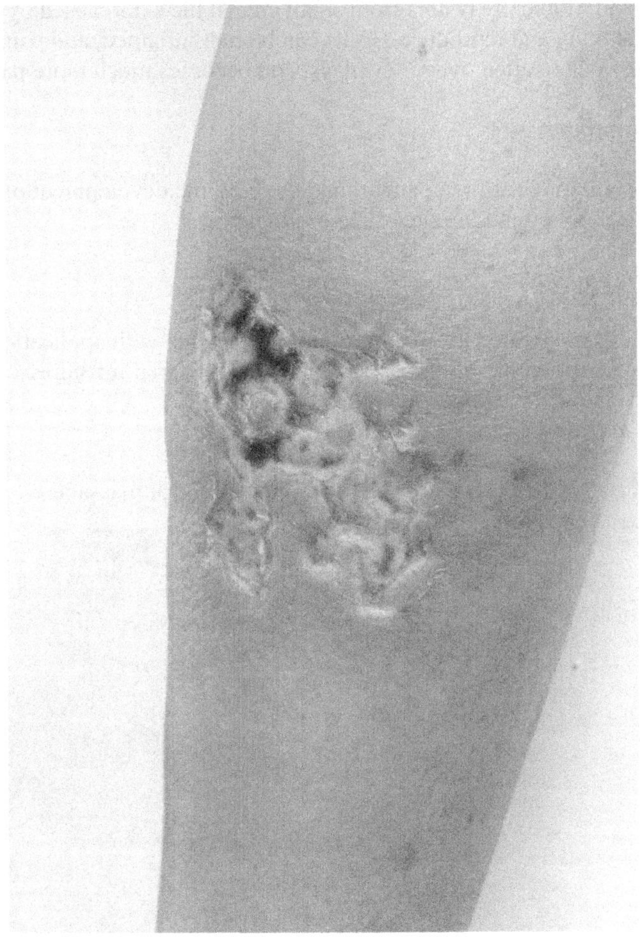

Third degree burn resulting from scalding

## Cellulitis

*(cell: cell; -itis: inflammation)*

Cellulitis is a **bacterial infection** of the skin, causing symptoms such as inflammation of the infected area, fever, pain, and blisters.

***Causes***

Cellulitis is caused by **staphylococci** bacterium entering the body through exposure to **wounds**, most commonly on the legs. The infection typically stays localized, but continues to spread to surrounding tissues as the bacteria grows. The infection can present with well-defined borders of infection. If the infection enters the blood stream, it may result in septicemia, a potentially life-threatening condition.

Spider or insect bites may also introduce the bacterium into the body. Any insect bite should be cleaned thoroughly to prevent infection.

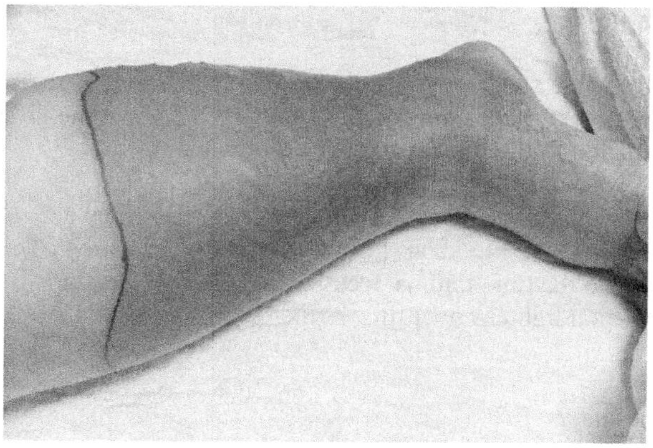

Defined borders commonly seen with cellulitis

***Symptoms***

Cellulitis may present with many symptoms, including a red area of skin that spreads and increases in size over time, swelling, pain, fever, and blisters on the infected area.

***Treatments***

Treatment for cellulitis includes antibiotic medication, taken orally. Cellulitis is not typically contagious.

***Contraindications***

Cellulitis is considered a local contraindication. Any open wounds should be avoided.

## Chickenpox

Chickenpox is a **viral infection**, resulting in **itchy rashes** with **small blisters**. Chickenpox is highly contagious, with symptoms usually appearing around two to three weeks after exposure to the virus.

***Causes***

A person contracts chickenpox by direct exposure to the virus. Coming into contact with a chickenpox rash may transmit the virus, as can breathing in air that has been exposed to the virus, primarily through an infected person sneezing or coughing. Those most at risk of contracting the virus are children, especially those who have not been vaccinated.

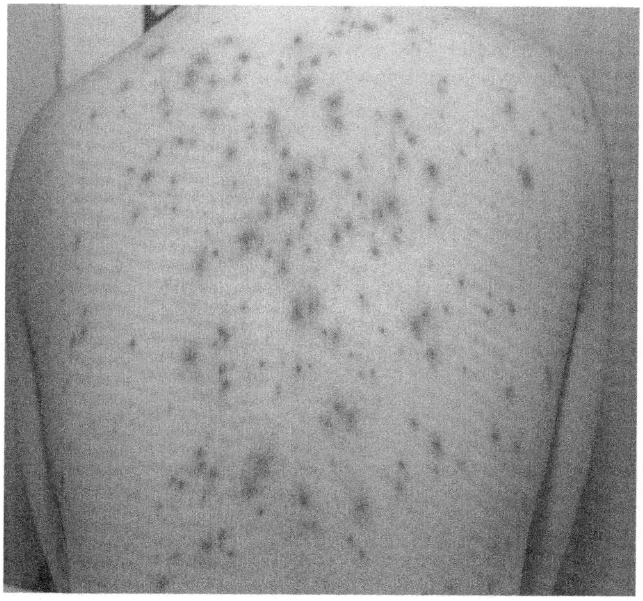

***Symptoms***

Raised red bumps in the skin are a main symptom of chickenpox. These can evolve into blisters, which eventually pop, allowing the fluid inside to leak out. The blisters then crust over, allowing the blister to heal. Other symptoms include fever and general malaise.

***Treatments***

As chickenpox is caused by a virus, there are no medications that can fight off the infection. Rest, increased fluid intake, and allowing the infection to run its course are the best ways to treat the symptoms of chickenpox.

***Contraindications***

Because chickenpox is highly contagious, it is considered an absolute contraindication to massage.

## Contusion

A contusion, also known as a **bruise**, is **damage** to **blood vessels** in the skin, resulting in **localized bleeding**. The bleeding usually stops quickly due to thrombocytes clotting the blood, but blood remains in a localized area until it can be slowly removed by the body over time.

***Causes***

Contusions are caused by trauma to an area damaging and breaking open capillaries in the skin. The trauma is usually caused by a direct blow to the skin.

*Symptoms*

In the acute stage, pain may be present in the area, as there is trauma. Inflammation may occur as a result of tissue damage. After the contusion has stopped bleeding, the inflammation usually subsides. There may be a dull ache in the contusion as the tissue is being repaired internally.

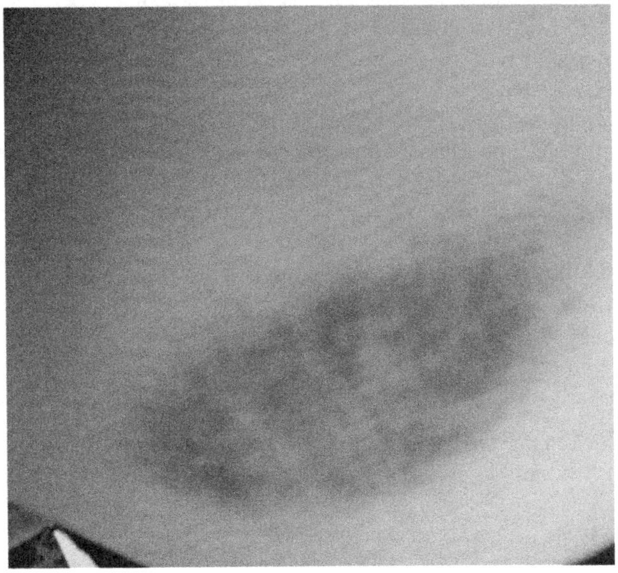

Contusions leave discoloration in the skin until they are healed and the blood has been removed from the area. The closer to the time trauma occurs, the darker the bruise is. The contusion lightens over time as the blood is removed from the area.

*Treatments*

PRICE is the best method of treating a bruise: protect the area from further damage, rest the area, ice the area to reduce pain and inflammation, compress the area to further decrease inflammation, and elevate the area to promote effective blood flow and limit inflammation. Over-the-counter pain medication may be used if the area is painful.

*Contraindications*

A contusion is considered a local contraindication to massage, due to the potential presence of blood clots in the contusion.

## Corn

A corn is a **built-up** area of **keratin** on the feet, usually **between the toes,** caused by **excessive friction** on the area. A corn is a type of callus. These may be asymptomatic, but some people may experience pain or discomfort with a corn.

*Causes*

The primary cause of the development of a corn is wearing shoes that don't fit properly. Tight-fitting shoes in particular may squeeze toes together, increasing friction between the toes. This can cause a corn to develop.

*Symptoms*

A corn feels thick, and may be painful. The corn is often raised off the skin, and may appear dry or waxy.

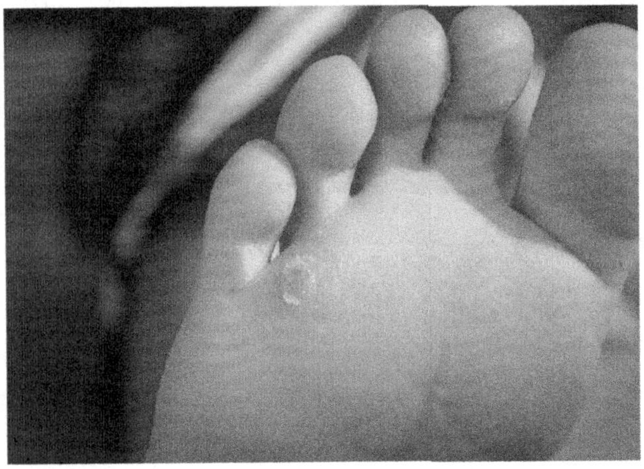

*Treatments*

Most commonly, correcting the cause of the corn results in the corn going away on its own. Sometimes, however, this may not completely get rid of the corn. Trimming the excess skin is helpful if there is far too much skin, and it still causes pain or discomfort. Other methods, such as the use of insoles may help relieve corns.

*Contraindications*

A corn is generally not considered a contraindication to massage. If the corn causes pain, however, it may be treated as a local contraindication, depending on the client's pain tolerance.

## Decubitus Ulcer

*(decubitus: the act of lying down; ulcer: open sore)*

A decubitus ulcer is a condition affecting the skin, resulting in the development of open sores.

***Causes***

Decubitus ulcers are also known as **bed sores** or **pressure ulcers**. When the body is in a static position for an extended period of time, such as when lying down, the parts of the body coming in contact with the bed, floor, or chair experience **ischemia**, a reduction of blood flow to the tissues due to pressure. When ischemia is present for too long, the tissue experiences **necrosis** due to a lack of oxygen. The dead tissue becomes ulcerated, and bacterial infection may occur.

People who are prone to decubitus ulcers are the elderly, disabled people, and people confined to a bed or wheelchair.

***Symptoms***

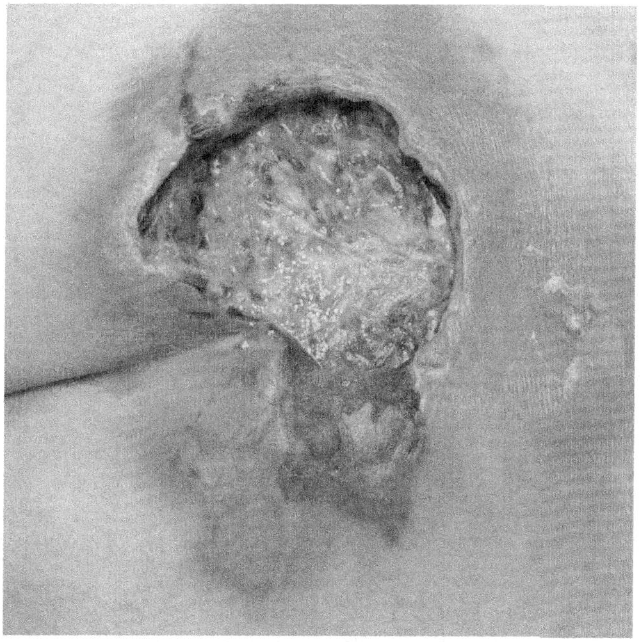

Symptoms of decubitus ulcers include discoloration of the skin, tenderness in the affected area, temperature variation in the affected area, and swelling. In severe cases, infection may result after ulceration has occurred.

***Treatments***

Treatments for decubitus ulcers vary, depending on the severity of the ulceration. If an infection is present, antibiotics may be prescribed. If there is an abundance of necrotic tissue, cleaning of the area(debridement) may be performed. If there is ischemia, but no ulcer, massage and application of heat may help bring blood back into the area.

***Contraindications***

A decubitus ulcer is considered a local contraindication if the skin has developed into an ulcer. If the skin has not opened, massage in the area is indicated to increase blood flow into the affected tissue. If the sore is present, massage up to two inches around the area is indicated to increase circulation and prevent further necrosis.

## Dermatitis

*(dermat/o: skin; -itis: inflammation)*

Dermatitis is **inflammation** of the **skin**. There are several types of dermatitis, including **contact** dermatitis, **atopic** dermatitis, and **seborrheic** dermatitis. Each has different causes, but each presents with some sort of inflammation of the skin.

***Causes***

Contact dermatitis results when the skin comes into contact with some sort of irritant or allergen, causing the skin to become inflamed. Atopic dermatitis, also known as **eczema**, can be caused by numerous factors, including an improperly functioning immune system, bacteria, dry skin, and the environment. Eczema usually begins in infancy. Seborrheic dermatitis is typically the result of a fungus growing on the skin, usually in regions that are more oily than others such as the scalp.

***Symptoms***

Contact dermatitis presents with inflammation and possible blistering where the skin has come into contact with an irritant. This is usually an acute condition, and will improve after the irritant has been cleaned or removed from the body. Atopic dermatitis presents with red, itchy patches on the body, usually near joints that flex and extend. This can be a chronic condition, and the patches may go away and come back later depending on factors such as the weather. Seborrheic dermatitis can cause itchy patches around the face, cheeks, nose, back, and chest.

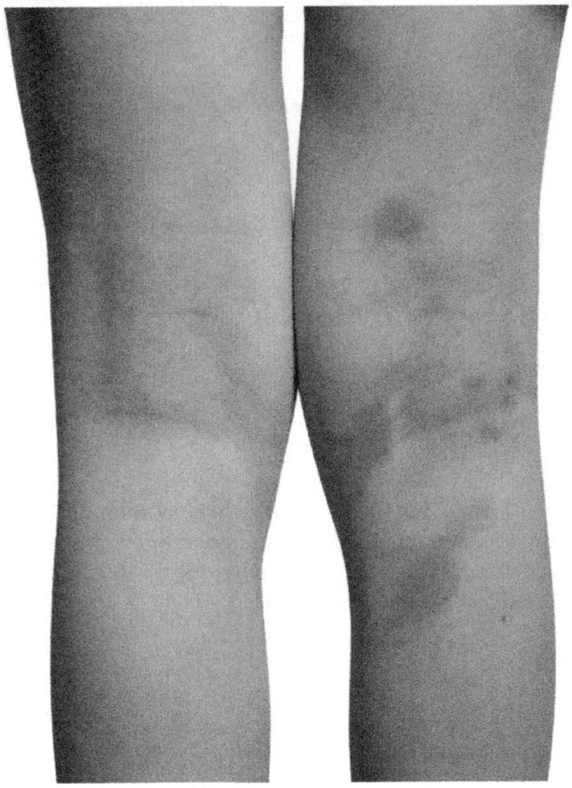

***Treatments***

Often times, application of an over-the-counter corticosteroid cream is all that's needed to alleviate dermatitis symptoms. If over-the-counter creams are ineffective, prescription strength corticosteroid creams may be administered, which usually take care of the dermatitis. Other treatments can even include exposure to sunlight.

***Contraindications***

Dermatitis is considered a local contraindication, as massage to the affected area will increase inflammation.

## Eczema

See: Dermatitis, Atopic.

## Folliculitis

*(follicul/o: follicle; -itis: inflammation)*

Folliculitis is **inflammation** of a **hair follicle**, usually the result of a **bacterial** or **fungal** infection. The infection may look like red bumps or acne. There are two types of folliculitis: superficial folliculitis and deep folliculitis. Superficial folliculitis affects only a small portion of the hair follicle, while deep folliculitis affects the entire hair follicle.

***Causes***

Superficial folliculitis is usually the result of small cuts on the skin, which allow staphylococci bacteria to enter the body. Ingrown hairs may also cause superficial folliculitis. Deep folliculitis, the more serious type of folliculitis, may be caused by certain types of medications being taken over prolonged periods, such as antibiotics, or infections not being properly treated and worsening. This can result in a boil(page 111).

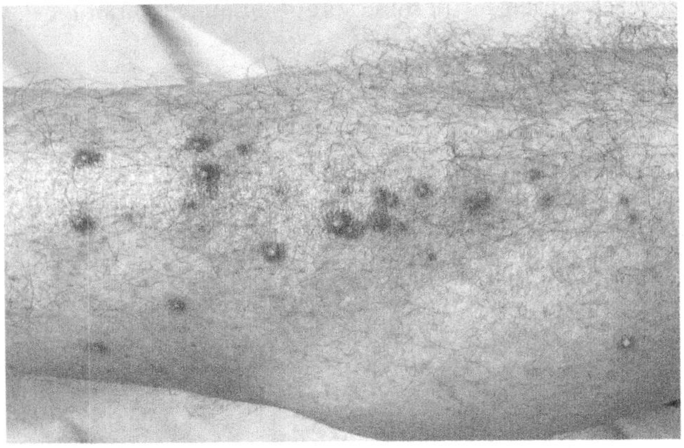

***Symptoms***

Symptoms of folliculitis include red bumps, pimples, blisters, painful skin, and itchy skin. The skin may feel swollen in addition.

***Treatments***

Treatment depends on the severity of folliculitis. If folliculitis is minor, antibiotics, antifungals, and/or steroid creams may be prescribed. If the infection is severe, surgery to drain the infection may be performed. Hair removal treatment may be an option if the condition does not improve with other treatments.

***Contraindications***

Folliculitis is considered a local contraindication to massage.

## Herpes Simplex

*(herpein: to creep; simplex: simple)*

Herpes Simplex is a **viral** infection of the skin. There are two types of herpes simplex: Herpes Simplex I, which causes sores around the mouth, and Herpes Simplex II, which causes sores around the genitals.

***Causes***

Herpes simplex is highly contagious, passing between people via direct contact. During an acute outbreak, a sore may appear on the skin, most commonly the mouth, face, or genitals. This sore disappears after a short time. Despite not having any sores present, a person may still be able to transmit the virus to another asymptomatically.

***Symptoms***

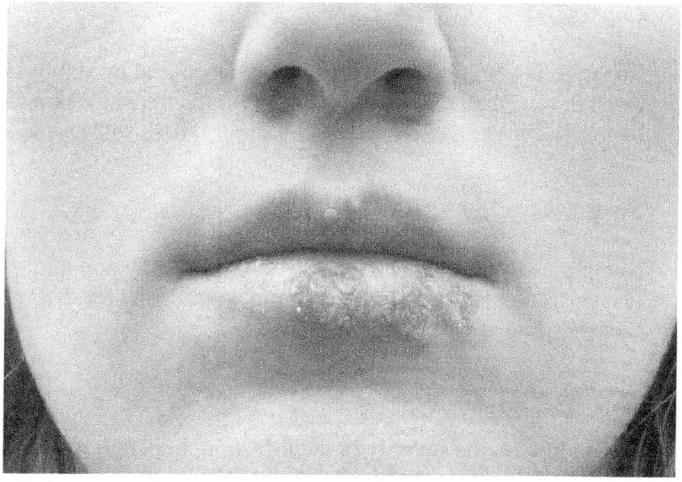

Symptoms vary depending on the type of herpes simplex a person has. Herpes Simplex I primarily presents with sores around the mouth, while Herpes Simplex II may cause painful urination. Both forms, however, may result in fever, headache, and swollen lymph nodes.

***Treatments***

While there is no cure for herpes simplex, medications may be prescribed to reduce the chance of spreading the infection to others.

***Contraindications***

In the acute stage, any sore caused by the herpes simplex virus is considered a local contraindication. In the post-acute stage, massage is indicated.

## Ichthyosis

*(ichthy-: dry, scaly; -osis: condition)*

Ichthyosis vulgaris is a skin condition causing the skin to develop **dry, thick scales**. Ichthyosis is a **genetic** disorder, usually appearing in early adolescence.

***Causes***

Ichthyosis is caused by inheriting a mutated gene from either one or both parents. If the gene is mutated in only one parent, the condition is typically more mild. If the gene is mutated in both parents, it can be more severe.

***Symptoms***

Ichthyosis is also known as fish scale disease, because it makes the skin resemble a fish's scales when dried. The skin becomes dry and scaly due to an excessive buildup of keratin in the skin. Fissures in the skin may also result, which can be painful.

***Treatments***

There is no cure for ichthyosis, and thus, managing symptoms is the primary goal of treatment. Creams that help exfoliate the skin may be useful. Medication may be prescribed that reduces the production of skin cells, which can help lessen the scaling seen on the skin.

***Contraindications***

Ichthyosis is generally not considered a contraindication. If fissures are painful, the massage may be altered depending on the client's pain tolerance. Body scrubs and application of lotion may help soften the built-up keratin in the skin.

## Impetigo

*(impetere: to attack)*

Impetigo is a **bacterial** infection of the skin, most commonly seen in **children**. Impetigo is often confused with Hand, Foot, and Mouth Disease, which is a viral infection.

***Causes***

Impetigo is a highly contagious infection, caused by staphylococci or streptococci, which most commonly enter the body through already damaged skin, but may affect healthy skin as well. When the bacteria enters the skin, it produces sores that blister and leak a yellow, crust-like fluid. These sores typically develop around the mouth, nose, and ears.

***Symptoms***

Symptoms of impetigo include red sores that may pop and leave a yellowish crust, swollen lymph nodes, and fluid-filled blisters. The affected areas may also itch.

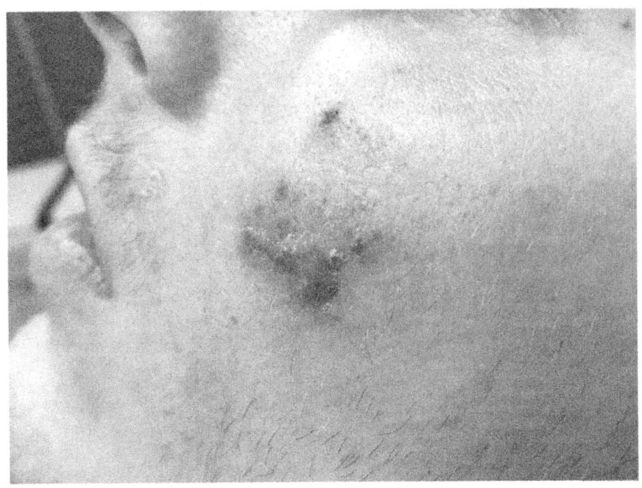

***Treatments***

Depending on the severity of the infection, impetigo may be treated with topical antibiotic cream for less severe cases, or with oral antibiotics for more severe cases. Recovery time is typically around one week with the use of medication.

***Contraindications***

Impetigo is a highly contagious bacterial infection, and therefore, is an absolute contraindication.

## Lice

Lice, plural for a head louse, are small **parasites** that live on the **head and scalp** that feed on **human blood**. Children are most likely to contract a lice infestation, also known as pediculosis capitis.

***Causes***

Lice are spread via direct contact. Lice do not jump or fly, and therefore must physically come into contact with a person to transfer to them. After lice have attached to a new host, they lay eggs on hair shafts. Once the eggs hatch, more lice are present.

***Symptoms***

The main symptom of lice is itching, caused by an allergy to the saliva of the lice.

*Treatments*

Over-the-counter or prescription medications may be prescribed to help kill the lice. Shampoos specifically designed to eliminate lice are often used.

*Contraindications*

Lice is a highly contagious parasitic infection, and is therefore an absolute contraindication.

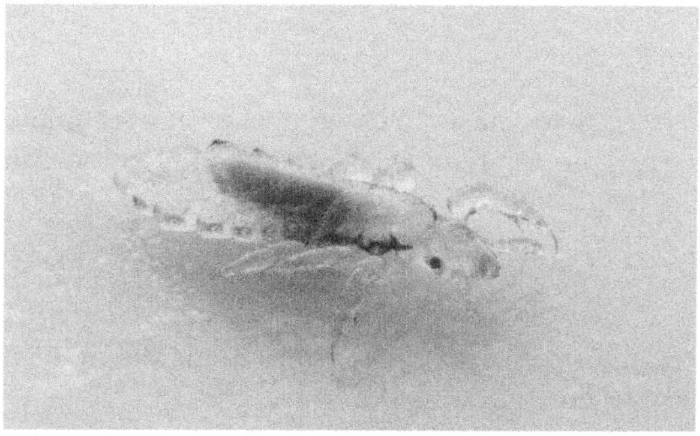

## Measles

Measles, also known as **rubeola**, is a highly contagious **viral infection**. Measles is most common in children, but is considered rare due to the development of a vaccine.

*Causes*

Measles is contracted by exposure to the virus in air droplets from a cough or sneeze. Once these droplets are inhaled, the virus can replicate in the nasal passages and throat.

*Symptoms*

Symptoms of a measles infection include the development of a **large rash** on the skin, fever, runny nose, sore throat, and a dry cough. Measles may also result in the development of pneumonia in people with weak immune systems, bronchitis, and bacterial ear infections. These conditions usually resolve when the measles clears up.

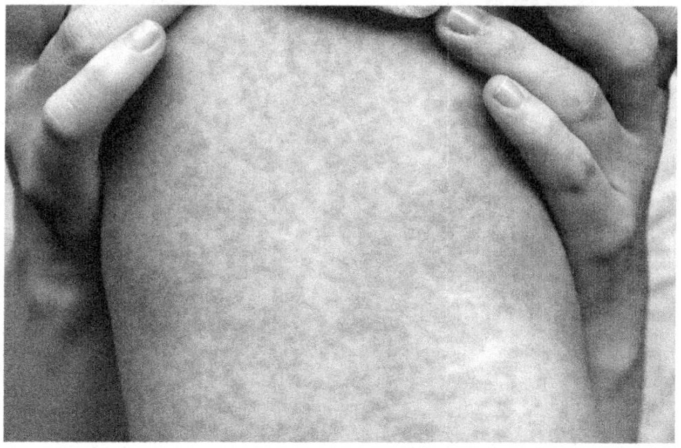

*Treatments*

Because measles is a viral infection, there is no cure, only ways to manage symptoms. Antipyretics may be used to reduce fever, and if there is some sort of bacterial infection such as ear infection or pneumonia, antibiotics may be prescribed. Increased rest and fluid intake is a key treatment with a measles infection.

*Contraindications*

Measles, despite its rarity, is caused by a contagious viral infection, and is considered an absolute contraindication.

## Mole

A mole, or nevus, is a **benign skin lesion**, often appearing as a small, brown spot. The color of the moles is caused by the amount of melanin in the lesion.

*Causes*

Moles are the result of melanocytes growing together in one localized area in the skin. Most people have several moles, which usually develop during childhood.

*Symptoms*

Moles typically all exhibit the same general symptoms, while there may be some variation: they are dark brownish in color, they usually have an oval shape, and they are usually less than ¼ of an inch in diameter. Of course, moles may be a different color or different shape or size.

***Treatments***

Treatment is not necessary for most moles. A doctor may recommend having a mole removed if they suspect it could be cancerous. In this case, surgical removal is performed. For more information on a mole that may be cancerous, see malignant melanoma(page 264).

***Contraindications***

A mole is not contraindicated for massage. Precautions should be taken with moles that rise up off the skin, which can be painful if pulled or pinched.

## Onychomycosis

*(onycho-: nails; myc-: fungus; -osis: condition)*

Onychomycosis is a **fungal infection** of the **nails**, most commonly the result of an infection by the dermatophyte fungi.

***Causes***

Onychomycosis is caused by fungi entering a nail, typically more common in older people due to the natural drying and cracking of nails that happens with age. The fungus enters into these cracks and begins growing, infecting the nail. Athlete's foot may also spread into the area and infect the nail.

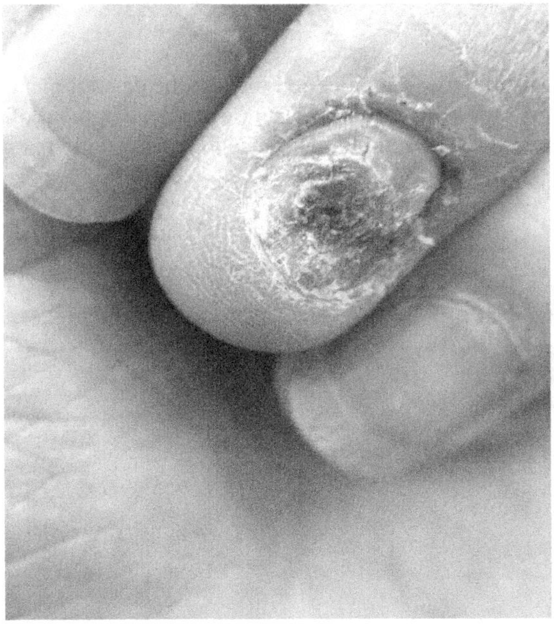

***Symptoms***

Symptoms of onychomycosis include thickening of the infected nail, change in the nail shape, discoloration of the nail turning it yellow or brown, and the nail becoming brittle.

***Treatments***

If symptoms are mild, treatment may not be necessary. When treatment is required, however, antifungal medications are the main form of treatment. Oral antifungals are used more often than topical creams, as they can work quicker. If the infection is severe, the nail may need to be surgically removed to allow antifungal cream to be applied directly to the nail bed.

***Contraindications***

Onychomycosis is a contagious fungal infection, and is considered a local contraindication.

## Psoriasis

*(psora-: to itch; -iasis: condition)*

Psoriasis is an **autoimmune** disorder of the skin, resulting in the production of **thick**, **dry**, **scaly patches**. Psoriasis has periods of exacerbation and remission, where the patches appear and then resolve themselves.

***Causes***

The exact cause of psoriasis is unknown. Certain triggers, such as stress, may cause the body's immune system to attack the skin. Normally, skin cells have a life span of 3-4 weeks, and ultimately flake off the body. When the immune system attacks the skin, the body responds by increasing production of epithelial cells at an extremely rapid pace, which is much faster than the cells are being destroyed. This rapid pace of cell production is what produces the patches on the skin.

***Symptoms***

Symptoms of psoriasis differ based on each person, but may include red, patchy skin covered in thick, silvery scales, dry skin that may crack and bleed, thickened finger and toe nails, and itchy skin.

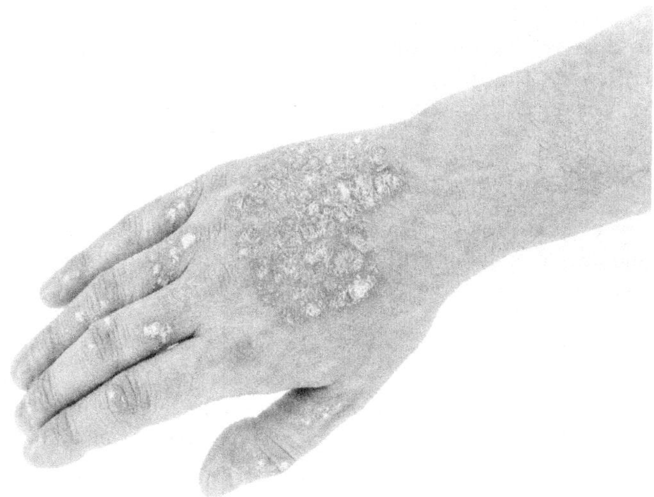

***Treatments***

There is no cure for psoriasis, but treatments are available to help manage the condition. Treatments include topical creams(which may contain steroids), exposure to sunlight, and application of aloe vera.

***Contraindications***

Psoriasis is not contraindicated for massage. Massage may be altered if the patches are painful or are scabbing, but otherwise, the patches may be massaged.

## Ringworm

*(dermato-: skin; phyt-: plant; -osis: condition)*

Ringworm(also known as dermatophytosis) is a **fungal infection** of the skin, similar to athlete's foot. Despite the name, it is not a parasitic infection. It results in a **ring-like** area of infection.

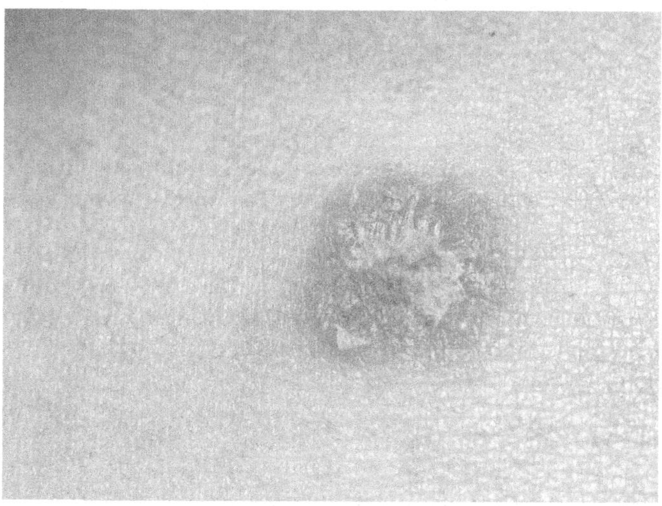

***Causes***

Fungus, like the kind found in ringworm, live on the dead cells of the body, such as the epidermis. When ringworm is contracted, it forms red blisters and a ring of infection begins to show, which then spreads as the infection grows through the skin.

Ringworm is contagious, and may be spread from person to person. It is especially common in athletes, whose bodies come in close contact with one another, such as wrestlers.

***Symptoms***

Ringworm typically presents with well-defined circular patches of infection on the skin, usually more red on the outer edges than inside. These patches can be itchy and develop blisters.

***Treatments***

Treatment includes good personal hygiene, and most commonly application of antifungal ointment to the affected area. More severe cases may require oral antifungal medication.

***Contraindications***

Ringworm is a highly contagious fungal infection, and is considered a local contraindication. Linens should be treated as contaminated.

## Rosacea

Rosacea is a condition in which the **skin in the face**, specifically around the nose and cheeks, can become **red** and **irritated**. The affected areas can present with visible blood vessels and small bumps filled with pus, similar to acne. Rosacea may be confused with other conditions that cause a rash on the face, such as lupus(page 134).

***Causes***

The exact cause of rosacea is unknown. People who are more likely to develop rosacea include women over 30 years of age and people with fair skin. Increasing blood flow to the skin may cause the rash to appear, so activities such as exercise or spending time in the heat could play a role.

***Symptoms***

Symptoms of rosacea include redness on the face, bumps that may contain pus similar to acne, and possibly enlargement of the nose. Occasionally, a person with rosacea may also develop eye irritation and dryness.

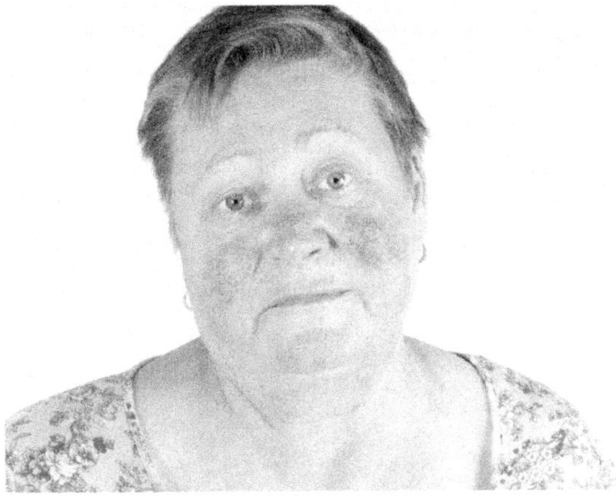

***Treatments***

While there is no cure for rosacea, there are ways to treat the symptoms. Medications such as brimonidine, which dilate blood vessels, are useful for reducing the redness of the face. To combat infections that may be seen with rosacea, antibiotics are used.

***Contraindications***

Rosacea may be considered a local contraindication if pain or pus-filled bumps are present in the area. Otherwise, it is not contraindicated.

## Scabies

Scabies is a **parasitic** infection caused by a **mite**, known as Sacroptes scabiei. This mite **burrows under the skin** and **lays eggs**, causing intense itching. The tunnels the mite creates are visible in the skin. Scratching due to a scabies infection may lead to an infection, and is not recommended.

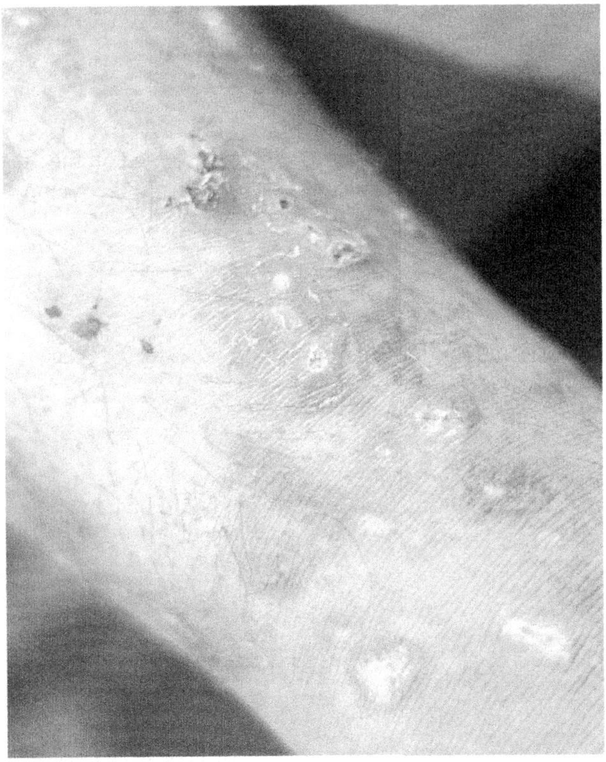

***Causes***

Scabies are extremely contagious, transmitting easily from one person to the next via physical contact, or sharing clothing or other linens.

***Symptoms***

The main symptoms of a scabies infection are severe itching and visible burrows in the skin where the mite has worked its way into the body.

***Treatments***

Topical creams that are specifically designed to kill mites are prescribed to treat scabies. They kill the mites quickly, but itching may persist for some time after treatment begins.

***Contraindications***

Scabies is a contagious parasitic infection, and is considered an absolute contraindication.

## Scar

A scar is a mark in the skin where the **skin** has **repaired itself** after trauma. Scars are formed by **collagen**, connecting the two sides of the damaged tissue together. This area forms a scab, and if the trauma was not mild, a scar may form when the scab falls off.

### *Causes*

Scars are caused by trauma to the skin. The body creates collagen to hold the damaged skin closed. If the skin has sustained too much damage, a scar may form from the collagen, permanently closing the wound.

### *Symptoms*

If excessive scar tissue forms, it can protrude off the skin, in what is known as a keloid.

### *Treatments*

Keloid scars may be surgically removed if the person desires. Topical creams may be used to lighten any scar, such as gotu kola cream.

### *Contraindications*

A scar is not a contraindication, and random collagen formation may be reduced as a result of massage.

## Scleroderma

*(sclero-: hard; -derma: skin)*

Scleroderma is a **hardening** of the **skin**. Scleroderma doesn't always only affect the skin, however. It can lead to damage of the heart, lungs, and kidneys.

### *Causes*

Scleroderma is the result of the body producing too much collagen, the same fibrous material that creates scars. The exact cause of this overproduction of collagen is unknown.

### *Symptoms*

In a person with scleroderma, the skin hardens and range-of-motion may be restricted, especially if it occurs around a joint. The fingers and toes may experience lack of blood flow due to damaged blood vessels. See Raynaud's Syndrome(page 65).

### *Treatments*

Medications are used to treat symptoms, but there is no known treatment for the exact cause of scleroderma. Medications that dilate blood vessels, such as statins, may be useful in returning blood flow to the fingers and toes. Immunosuppressants may help combat symptoms associated with scleroderma. The symptoms of scleroderma may disappear entirely after a few years.

### *Contraindications*

Generally, scleroderma is not considered contraindicated. Massage may help loosen collagen in the skin and increase blood flow into areas that may be affected.

## Sebaceous Cyst

A sebaceous cyst is a condition affecting the skin, but may affect other tissues as well. These are typically the result of a blockage in a sebaceous gland that causes a backup of sebum, which is then surrounded by a membrane to keep it or an infection from harming the rest of the body.

### *Causes*

A **sebaceous** gland produces oil, and secretes oil onto the surface of the skin. If a blockage of a sebaceous gland occurs, oil cannot escape the gland, and bacteria may infect the area. If too much bacteria is present, the body may develop connective tissue that surrounds the infected sebaceous gland, trapping it inside. This is a sebaceous cyst.

Sebaceous cysts may be large or small. They may be painful to the touch, or may lead to localized infections known as abscesses. Cysts may need to be removed surgically. If the entire cyst membrane is not removed, there may be a chance of the cyst returning in the future.

### *Symptoms*

Some cysts show no symptoms, but symptoms are more likely to appear the larger the cyst is. Small cysts usually do not cause pain, but large cysts may cause pain and discomfort in the surrounding area.

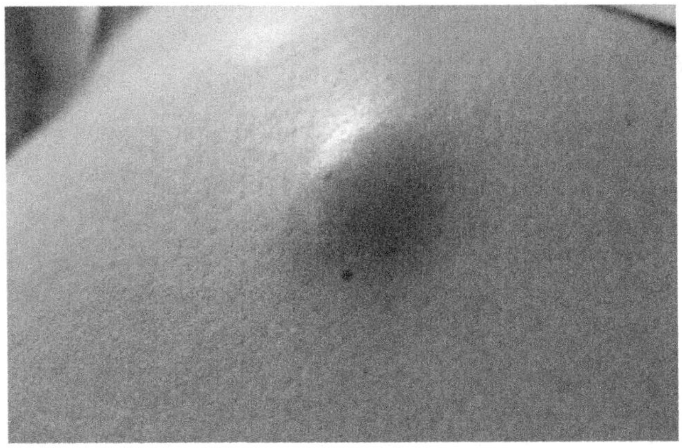

### *Treatments*

Treatment, if necessary, includes moist compresses on the area to help drain the cyst, or possible surgery if there is a risk of infection. Surgical removal may be required if the cyst is large, causes pain, or may be cancerous.

### *Contraindications*

Sebaceous cysts are considered local contraindications, and should be avoided to prevent damaging the cyst and allowing the fluid inside to affect the body. The area may also be painful.

## Shingles

Shingles, also known as **herpes zoster**, is a **viral** infection that results in a painful **skin rash**. The rash most commonly occurs on one side of the torso, although it can appear anywhere. The strain of herpes is not the same strain that causes cold sores or genital herpes(herpes simplex, page 117), but the same strain that causes chickenpox(page 113).

### *Causes*

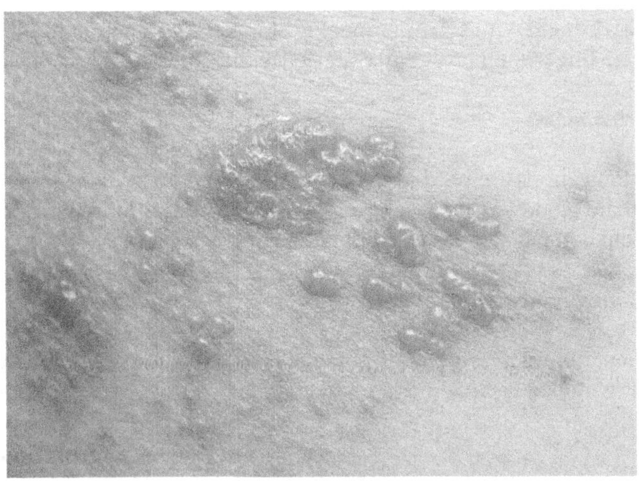

Shingles is the result of an infection of the varicella-zoster virus, the virus that causes chickenpox. Shingles occurs when the virus lies dormant in the nervous system after a chickenpox infection. The virus reactivates, but instead of causing chickenpox again, it causes a rash to appear in the skin. Not every person infected with chickenpox will have the virus reactivate and get shingles. Older adults and people with immune systems that may be weakened tend to develop shingles more commonly than others.

### *Symptoms*

Painful, burning rashes appear on the skin, usually on one side of the body. These rashes may contain blisters that can break open.

### *Treatments*

Although there is no cure for shingles, treatments are available to help with symptoms. These treatments include antiviral medications to prevent the virus from reproducing, and medications that relieve pain that may be associated with the infection. The condition should resolve after no longer than six weeks.

***Contraindications***

Much like chickenpox, shingles should be treated as an absolute contraindication until the condition resolves.

## Urticaria

Urticaria, also known as hives, is a condition that results in welts, known as **wheals**, appearing on the skin. Wheals are raised areas that typically itch. Wheals can appear anywhere on the body.

***Causes***

Urticaria is caused by the release of **histamines** into the blood. The body may release histamines in response to the body coming into contact with a substance it is allergic to, in response to insect or bug bites/stings, scratches, and even certain infections. Histamines dilate blood vessels, which bring leukocytes into the area to help destroy any substance that may be causing the reaction.

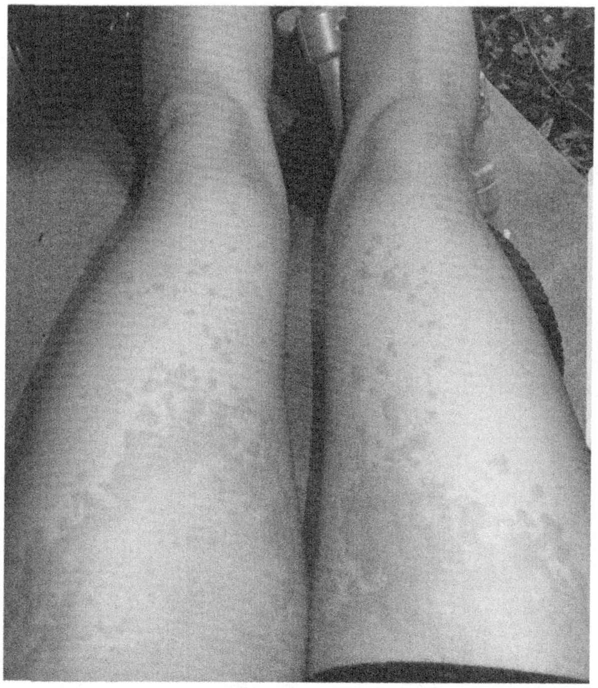

***Symptoms***

Typically seen in the skin, wheals form that are usually itchy. These can be raised off the skin, discolored, and possibly painful.

***Treatments***

Over-the-counter antihistamines are likely the first treatment recommended. If the condition does not resolve, prescription antihistamines may be given. Immunosuppressants, anti- inflammatory medication, and even oral corticosteroids such as prednisone may also be given to help with the reaction.

***Contraindications***

In the acute stage, the cause of the hives should be determined before massage can be performed. Once the cause is determined, massage on the area should be avoided, or if it's a more serious reason for hives, massage should be avoided completely.

## Vitiligo

Vitiligo is a condition resulting in the **skin losing melanin**, usually in **spots** or **blotches**. Vitiligo can occur in any person of any race, but is more noticeable in people with darker skin.

***Causes***

In vitiligo, the body stops producing melanin in certain areas. Reasons for this vary, from damage to melanocytes from things like a sunburn, to autoimmune disorders, where the body's immune system may attack the melanin.

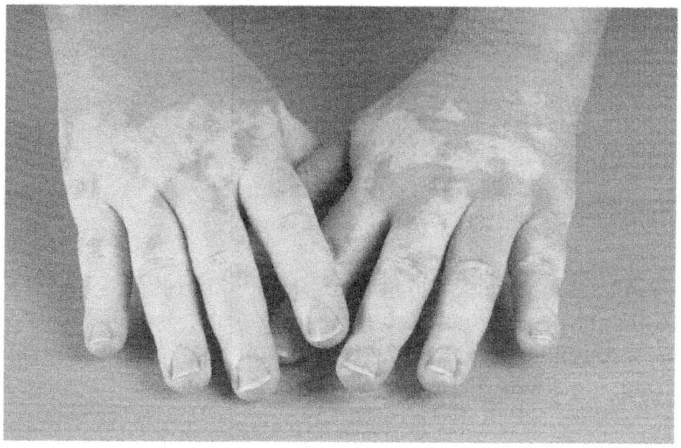

***Symptoms***

Loss of pigment is the main symptom of vitiligo. Pigment is mostly lost in the skin, but can also be lost inside the mouth. Hair may turn grey earlier than normal.

***Treatments***

While treatment is not necessary, it may be desired if the person affected is self conscious about the appearance of their skin. Self-tanning lotion may be used to cover spots. Certain medications may be prescribed to try to slow the progression of discoloration, including immunosuppressants and anti-inflammatory drugs. Light therapy may be used to increase melanin production. If a person wishes, they can have the remaining pigment in their skin removed by using depigmenting substances.

***Contraindications***

Vitiligo is not contraindicated for massage.

## Wart

Warts(also known as verrucae), are small benign growths on the skin, caused by the **human papilloma virus(HPV)**.

***Causes***

Warts are contagious, and may be spread by direct skin contact. The human papilloma virus stimulates the skin to produce more **keratin**, which causes a hard, thick overgrowth on a small localized area. This is a wart.

Warts may be located in numerous locations on the body, including the hands, feet(plantar warts), and genitals(genital warts).

***Symptoms***

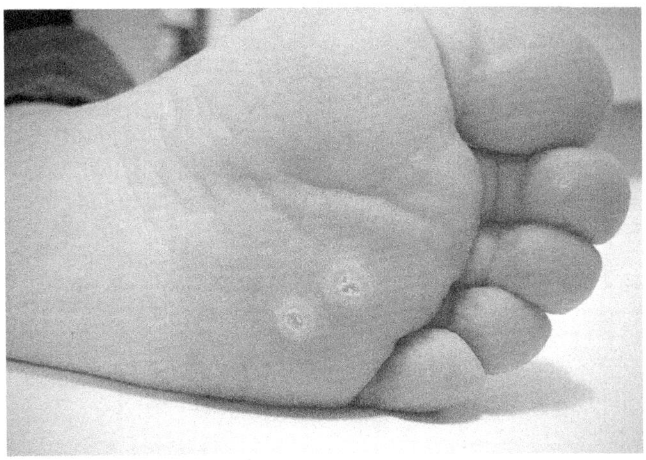

Warts are typically rough, grainy bumps, which may be a range of colors, from the color of the person's skin to white, tan, or even pink. Often, warts may have black spots in them, which is nothing more than blood clots.

Depending on the location of the wart, such as plantar warts, the wart may be painful due to calluses forming over them, pushing them deeper into the skin.

***Treatments***

Warts often go into remission on their own, and treatment is not necessary. Treatment options include cryotherapy to freeze the wart, excising(cutting out) the wart, or electrosurgery to burn the wart.

***Contraindications***

Warts are contagious, and should be treated as a local contraindication.

## Wounds

Wounds are the result of a **breakage** in the skin, which exposes underlying tissues. There are several different types of open wounds.

An **abrasion** is a scraping off of layers of the skin, such as a skinned knee from falling. An **avulsion** is when the skin or another structure, such as a finger or toe nail, is pulled and ripped. An **incision**, such as produced during surgery, is a **clean cut** through tissue. A **laceration** is a cut that produces **jagged edges**. A **puncture** is caused by an object **piercing** the skin, producing a **hole**.

***Causes***

Wounds can be caused by many different factors. Ischemia may cause wounds in cases such as decubitus ulcers(page 115). Infections may cause wounds to appear in the skin as well. Damage to blood vessels, like those seen in diabetes mellitus(page 100) can result in wounds.

Trauma is usually the main cause of wounds, however. These include abrasions, lacerations, incisions, and punctures.

***Symptoms***

Wounds in the acute stage often present with bleeding, pain, and redness in the area. These symptoms usually resolve with the healing process. If a wound is not properly treated, infection may occur, along with fever if the infection becomes systemic. A wound that becomes infected and results in necrosis is known as gangrene, caused by a severe lack of blood flow in the area.

***Treatments***

Wounds should be cleansed with soap and water, and a sterile bandage should be applied to stop bleeding. If a wound is caused by a bite from an animal or insect, medical attention may(and probably should) be recommended.

***Contraindications***

Wounds should be treated as local contraindications until healed.

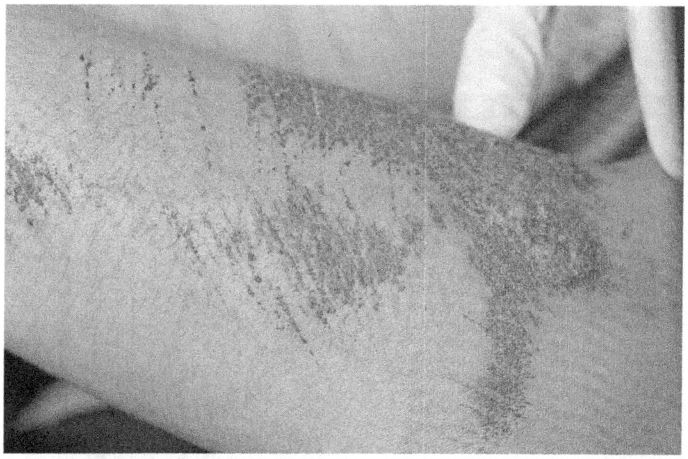

Abrasion

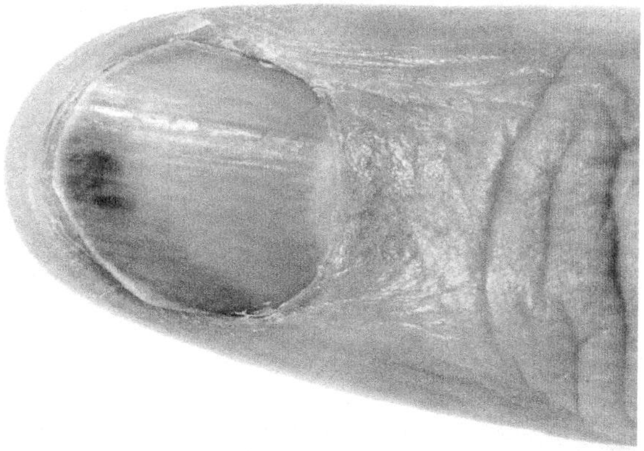

Avulsion

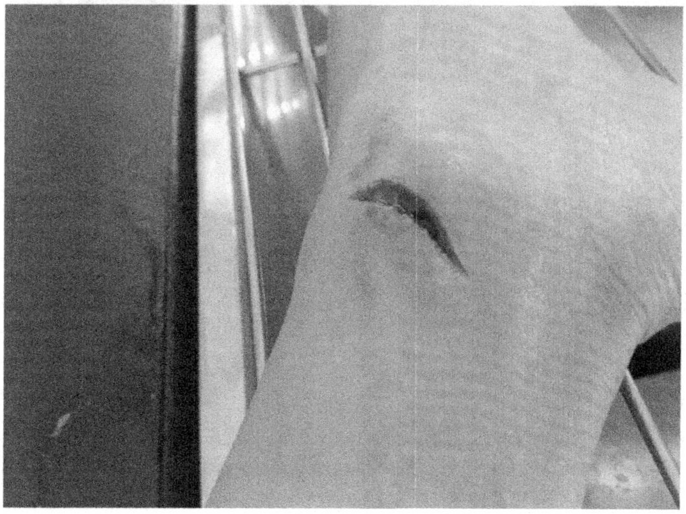

Laceration

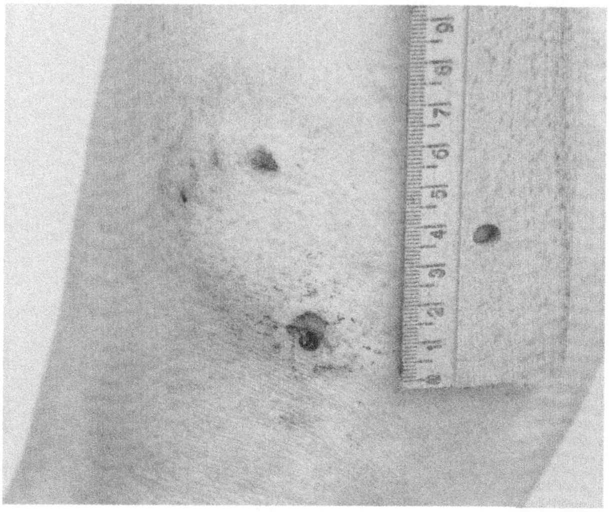

Puncture

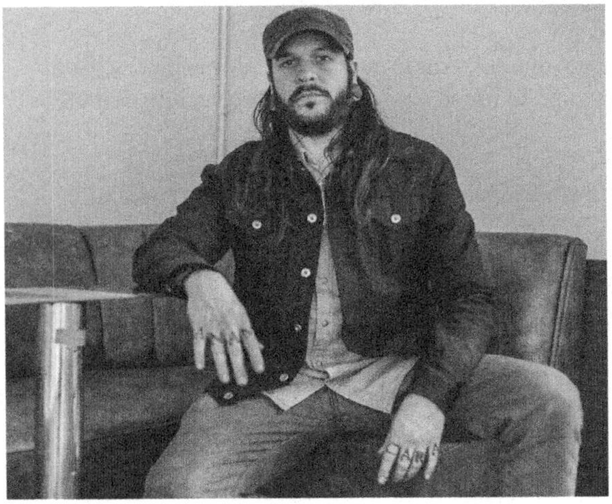

**Shawn James, Musician, Laceration**
ShawnJamesMusic.com
Facebook.com/ShawnJamesSoul
@ShawnJamesMusic

Tell me about the night the laceration happened.

*We were playing a festival in Germany, and it was one of the biggest crowds we had ever played. I turned to the boys before the set started and said something along the lines of, "Let's give them a show they won't forget."*

How did you get the laceration?

*There's a long intro for the first song, "Lost" from the album The Gospel According to Shawn James and the Shapeshifters. After the intro, everything hits at once. I jumped up before it hit and landed on my feet, while also bring the guitar down and my head down as well. I miscalculated the distance, which resulted in me hitting the edge of the guitar on my eyebrow.*

What was your initial reaction to it?

*I honestly didn't even notice it until the band noticed it.*

What was your band's reaction?

*They were shocked, and told me that my face was covered in blood. I still just kept going, paying no mind to it.*

Was it serious enough to require medical attention?

*I didn't think so, but everyone else made me go to the hospital. I got three stitches.*

How does the scar look? Awesome, right?

*Totally. Hahaha.*

How long did you have the stitches in?

*A couple weeks? I can't remember exactly.*

Did you receive any type of medication?

*A numbing shot right above my eyebrow.*

Did you play the entire set with blood pouring into your face, or did you stop and clean up at all?

*Yes, and no I didn't clean it up. When I roared and got louder, I could feel the blood spurting out from the pressure, haha.*

Would you do it all over again if you could?

*Absolutely!*

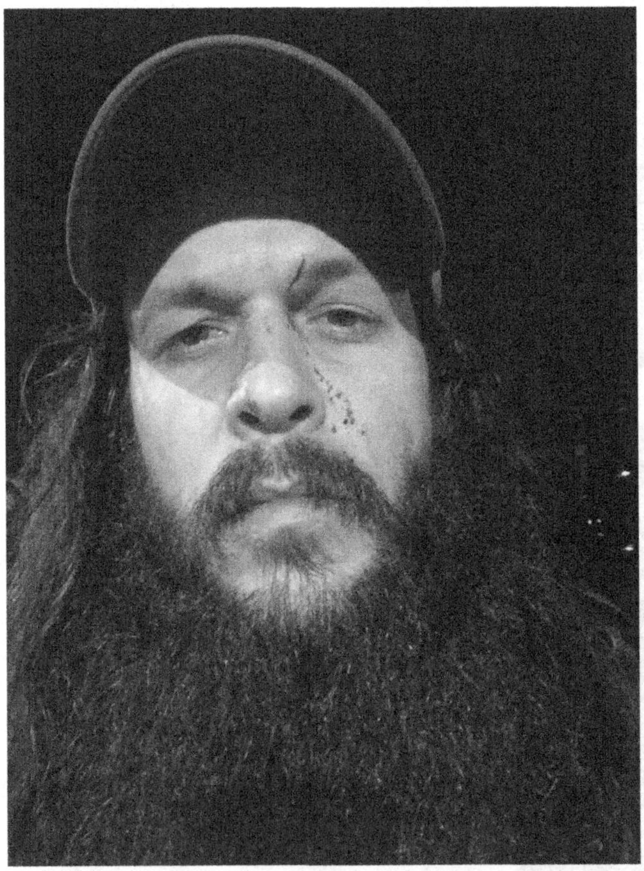

# Integumentary Pathologies

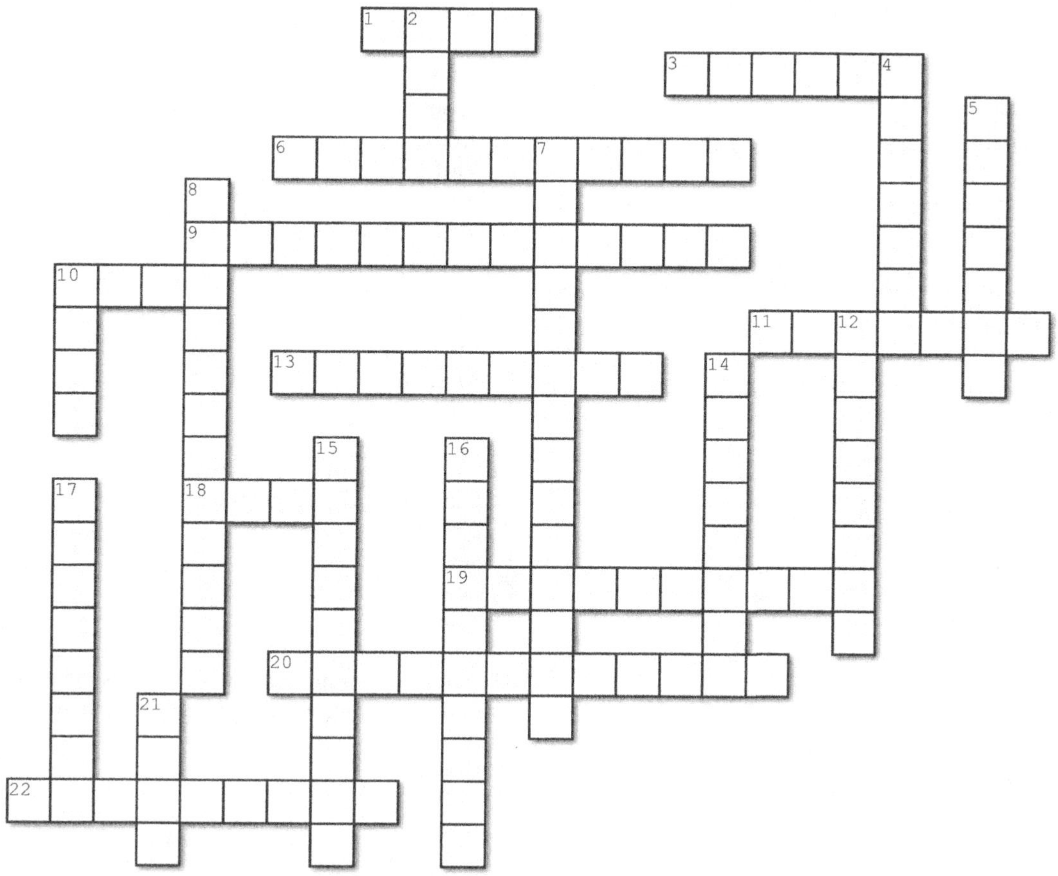

**Across**

1. Raised patch of keratin caused by the human papilloma virus
3. Viral infection of the skin that results in cold sores around the mouth
6. Excessive collagen formation in the skin, causing the skin to harden
9. Fungal infection of a nail
10. Bacterial infection of a hair follicle, also known as a furuncle
11. Rare viral infection, most commonly seen in children that can cause a rash on the body
13. Damage to blood vessels in the skin that result in bleeding inside the skin
18. Parasites that live on a person's head that feed on human blood
19. Bacterial infection of the skin that presents with well-defined borders of inflammation
20. Fungal infection affecting the foot
22. Autoimmune disorder causing an excessive build-up of epithelial cells

**Down**

2. Skin infection caused by excessive sebum production
4. Parasitic infection in which a mite burrows under the skin and lays eggs, which results in severe itching
5. Reddening and irritation of the skin on the nose and cheeks
7. An open sore caused by excessive pressure, resulting in ischemia and necrosis in the area
8. Inflammation of a hair follicle, commonly caused by an infection
10. Damage to the skin by exposure to things such as heat and chemicals
12. Genetic disorder causing the body to lack melanin
14. Highly contagious bacterial infection of the skin, most commonly seen in children
15. Inflammation of the skin
16. Viral infection causing itchy rashes and blisters all over the body
17. Herpes zoster infection, causing painful skin rash
21. A built-up area of keratin on the feet or between the toes, caused by friction

Answer Key on Page 287

# Integumentary Quiz

1. Psoriasis
A. Inflammation of skin resulting from skin coming into contact with an irritant
B. Autoimmune disorder resulting in thick, dry, silvery patches of skin
C. Blockage of sebaceous glands, resulting in pustules
D. Skin irritation caused by exposure to cold, affecting blood vessels and hair follicles

2. An injury that tears skin, producing jagged edges
A. Laceration
B. Incision
C. Puncture
D. Abrasion

3. Herpes simplex is a
A. Bacteria
B. Virus
C. Fungus
D. Parasite

4. Fungal infection affecting the epidermis, resulting in a circular rash
A. Cordyceps
B. Athlete's foot
C. Ringworm
D. Whitlow

5. A dermatologist is a doctor who specializes in the
A. Heart
B. Kidneys
C. Skin
D. Brain

6. In a client with herpes simplex, exposure to sunlight, stress, or hormonal changes may result in the development of
A. Impetigo
B. Decubitus ulcers
C. Cold sores
D. Acne

7. Which type of gland is found in the skin
A. Adrenal
B. Mammary
C. Pineal
D. Sebaceous

8. Nociceptors detect which sensation
A. Temperature
B. Pain
C. Light pressure
D. Deep pressure

9. A contusion is also known as
A. Bruise
B. Wart
C. Fracture
D. Hives

10. Tinea is a form of
A. Virus
B. Fungus
C. Bacteria
D. Parasite

11. Which type of gland plays an important role in maintaining body temperature
A. Pineal
B. Sebaceous
C. Sudoriferous
D. Adrenal

12. Streptococci infection which enters the body through wounds, resulting in infection of the skin and surrounding tissues
A. Cold sore
B. Boil
C. Rosacea
D. Cellulitis

13. During the course of a massage, the massage therapist notices a pre-existing contusion on the client's leg. The massage therapist should
A. Avoid the contusion, notify the client where the contusion is located, and document the contusion in SOAP notes
B. Work over the contusion to help break up potential blood clots that may have formed during the course of healing
C. Apply a cold compress to the affected contusion to reduce blood flow to the contusion
D. Reschedule the massage until the contusion has resolved

14. The most common form of papilloma
A. Wart
B. Acne
C. Psoriasis
D. Cyst

15. A furuncle is a
A. Bacterial infection of hair follicles
B. Bacterial infection of mucous membranes
C. Viral infection of mucous membranes
D. Bacterial infection of bone

Answer Key on Page 289

# Lymphatic System and Pathologies

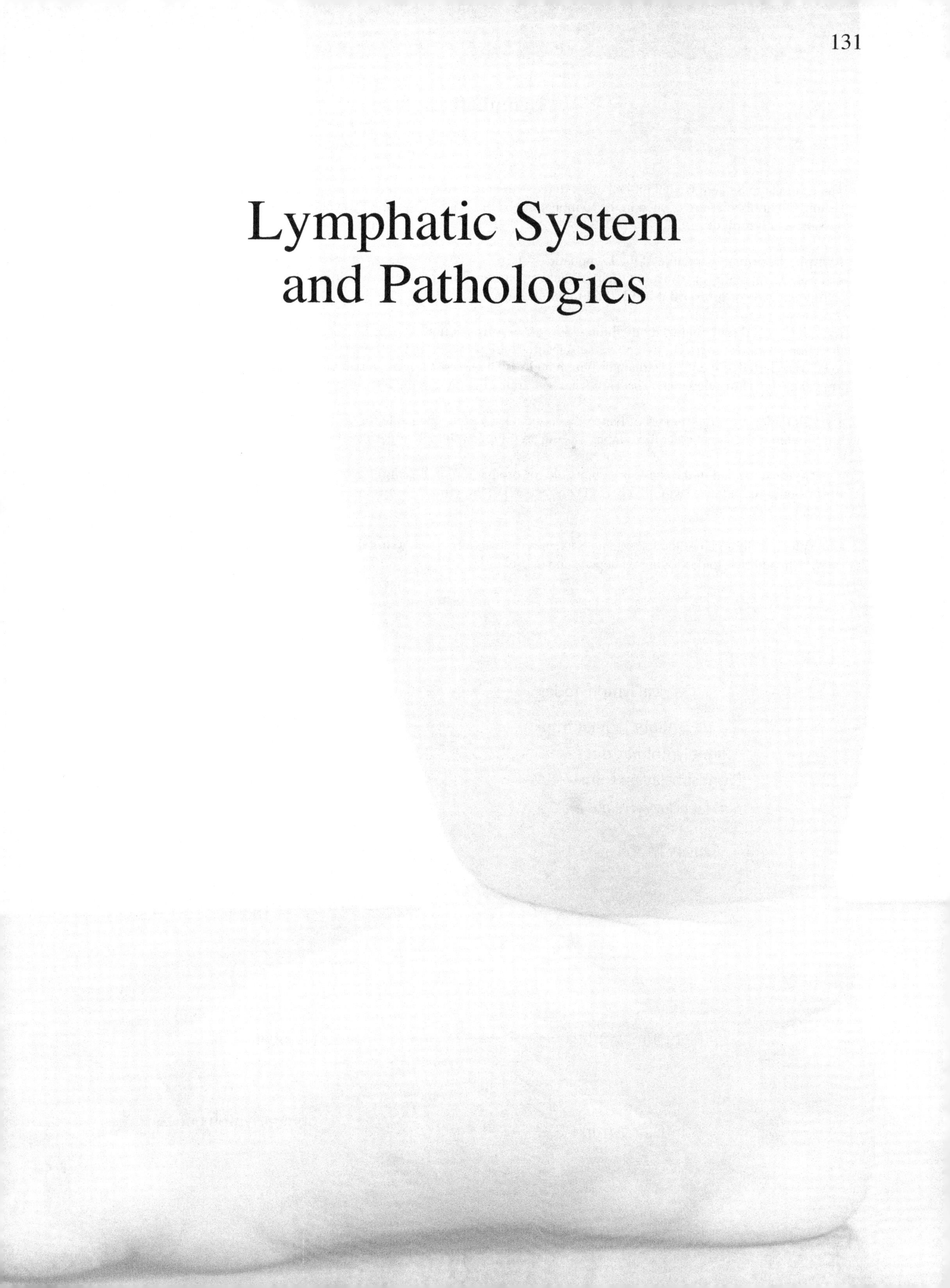

# Lymphatic System

The Lymphatic System is vital in the body's **defense** against pathogens and disease. Not only are leukocytes abundant in lymph, but antibodies are created in the Lymphatic System. The Lymphatic System contains **lymph**, **lymph nodes**, **lymph vessels**, and **lymph organs**.

**Lymph**, the primary structure of the Lymphatic System, is a fluid composed of **water**, protein, leukocytes, urea, salts, and glucose. Lymph allows **transport** of all of these substances through the body, ultimately dumping into the blood stream. Lymph is made of **interstitial fluid**, fluid found between cells.

Lymph travels throughout the body through **lymph vessels**. Lymph vessels are similar to blood vessels, but only flow in one direction, towards the heart. Lymph vessels absorb foreign bodies and nutrients from tissues, bringing them into the lymph to be transported to the blood stream or lymph nodes. The **largest lymph vessel** in the body is located in the trunk. It is known as the **Thoracic Duct**. The Thoracic Duct drains lymph into the **left subclavian vein**, where it joins with blood.

**Lymph nodes** are large **masses** of lymphatic tissue. They are responsible for production of **antibodies**, and help destroy any foreign objects that enter the lymph. During an infection, lymph nodes may become tender and swollen.

The **thymus**, located in the chest, is responsible for production of **T-lymphocytes**, or T-cells. T-cells are vital in regulation of the body's immune system. If a person contracts HIV, the virus destroys the T-cells, which essentially disables the immune system.

The **spleen** is an organ of the Lymphatic System responsible for **destroying** dead or dying **red blood cells** from the blood stream, in addition to destroying pathogens and debris.

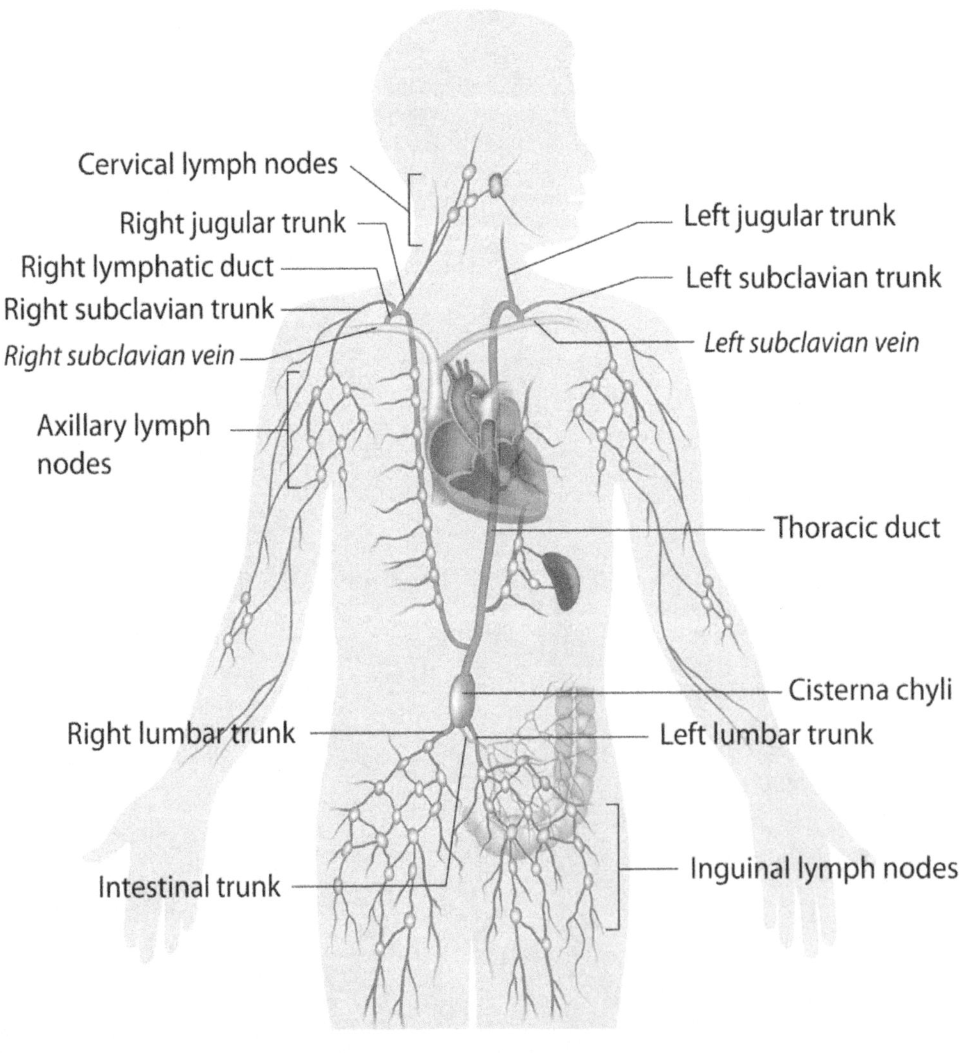

**Medical Tests and Equipment**

**Compression Devices:** Compression devices are used to mimic the Lymphatic System, and rhythmically compress the legs to increase the flow of lymph. This can decrease lymphedema. Typical compression devices may also include compression socks, and cuffs that wrap around the legs.

**Cryotherapy**: Cryotherapy is the use of cold or ice in a treatment. Cryotherapy can be used to reduce inflammation, increase circulation after a short period of application, destroy tissues such as warts, or even destroy nerves that may be causing pain. Cryotherapy can be applied many different ways, from the use of cold packs, to ice baths.

# Lymphatic System Pathologies

## Acquired Immunodeficiency Syndrome

Acquired Immunodeficiency Syndrome, also known as AIDS, is a chronic condition caused by infection by **HIV**, the human immunodeficiency virus. Once in the body, HIV **destroys** the body's **T-cells**, which function to regulate the response of the body's immune system to antigens. When HIV destroys too many of the body's T-cells, the immune system is considered compromised, and a person is then diagnosed with AIDS. While most people who are infected with HIV in the United States are properly treated and don't develop AIDS, a small portion of people do get AIDS after HIV infection, typically around ten years after initial infection.

***Causes***

HIV is spread though unprotected sex, through needles that have been shared by an infected person, as a result of a mother passing HIV on to their unborn child, or even through blood transfusions if the blood has not been properly screened beforehand. HIV cannot be spread through skin contact, water contact, through the bites of insects such as mosquitoes, or breathing in the air of an infected person.

***Symptoms***

Close after the initial infection has occurred, a person may experience fever, fatigue, body aches, headache, and swollen lymph nodes. As the infection spreads, symptoms emerge such as diarrhea and weight loss in conjunction with previously mentioned symptoms.

Complications caused by infection by HIV include being more prone to infection of other conditions such as pneumonia. A type of cancer known as Kaposi's Sarcoma(page 262) may develop. Severe wasting of the body may occur, in which a person loses at least ten percent of their total body weight.

HIV Entry to T Cell

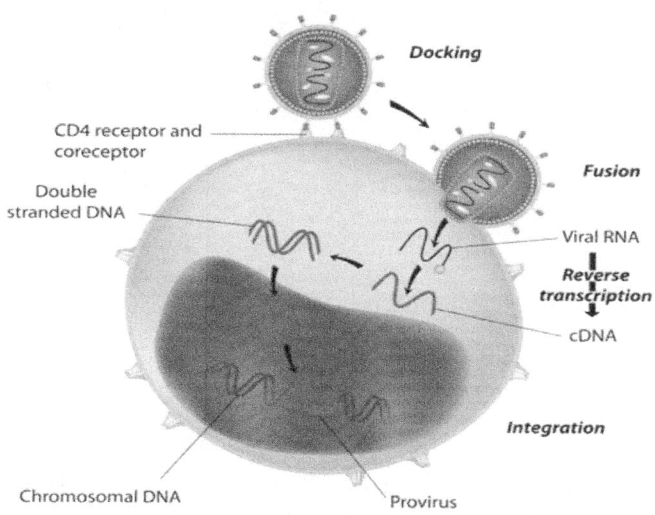


***Treatments***

A person infected with HIV should be prescribed antiretroviral therapy to help prevent the virus from further replicating.

***Contraindications***

AIDS is not a contraindication to massage. Any open sores should be treated as a local contraindication. If the client isn't feeling well, the massage should be rescheduled.

## Allergy

An allergy is a reaction of the body's immune system in response to substances that normally **do not affect people**. Common substances people may be allergic to include dust, pollen, mold, certain foods, pet dander, and medication.

***Causes***

Allergies occur when a substance enters the body that the body's immune system thinks is dangerous. The body produces **antibodies** for that specific substance. When the substance enters the body, the body releases the antibodies and other substances such as **histamines** to attack the substance. The release of histamines is what gives people allergy symptoms.

***Symptoms***

Allergies may be mild, or may be severe and result in serious conditions such as anaphylactic shock. Anaphylactic shock requires the use of an epinephrine shot to reverse the effects of the allergen. Less severe allergies may result in a runny nose, itchy eyes or skin, and hives.

***Treatments***

Typical treatments of allergens include the use of antihistamines, decongestants, and steroid nasal sprays. Avoiding the allergen is advised.

***Contraindications***

Allergies should be determined prior to massage to avoid using any allergens in massage lubricant. If a client develops any signs of contact with an allergen during the massage, massage should be stopped. If essential oils are the cause of the allergic reaction, effects can be managed with the application of vegetable oil.

## Lupus Erythematosus

*(lupus: wolf; erythemat-: red skin; -osus: pertaining to)*

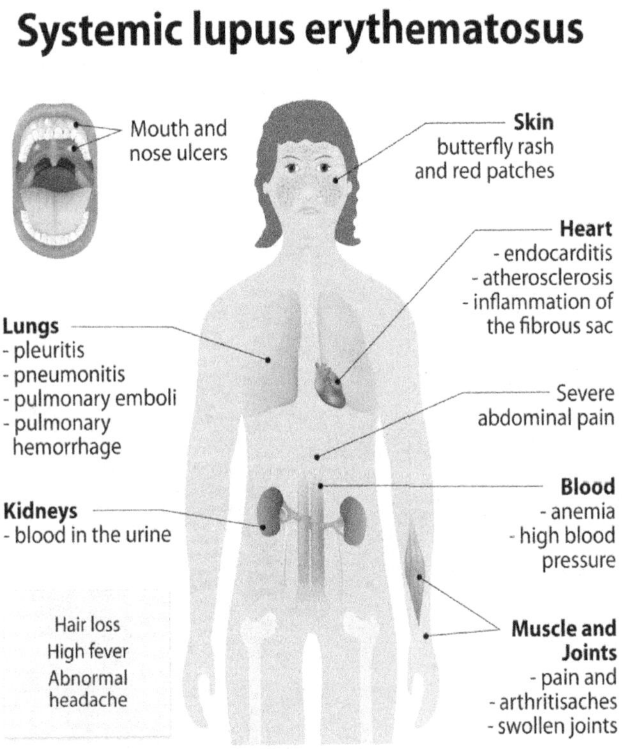


Lupus Erythematosus is an **autoimmune disorder** affecting the **connective tissues** of the entire body, but can be physically seen in the skin by the formation of a **butterfly rash** that appears on the face during flare-ups. This rash is similar in shape to the markings found on the face of a wolf, which is where lupus gets its name.

***Causes***

The exact cause of lupus is unknown. Some experts believe it is a genetic disorder that influences the immune system's function. Lupus may also be triggered by smoking, sunlight, infections, and medications.

***Symptoms***

Symptoms of lupus erythematosus include fever, the formation of a butterfly rash, joint pain, discomfort, fatigue, and sensitivity to sunlight. It may also contribute to the development of other medical conditions, such as Raynaud's Syndrome.

***Treatments***

There is no cure for lupus erythematosus, but treatment is available to help manage the condition. Non-steroidal anti-inflammatory drugs may help with systemic inflammation in non-severe cases. Topical corticosteroid creams may help alleviate rashes. Blood thinners may also be used in more severe cases.

***Contraindications***

During flare-ups, lupus may cause extensive pain over the body, and massage would likely be postponed until the condition has gone into remission. If there are no symptoms, lupus is not contraindicated.

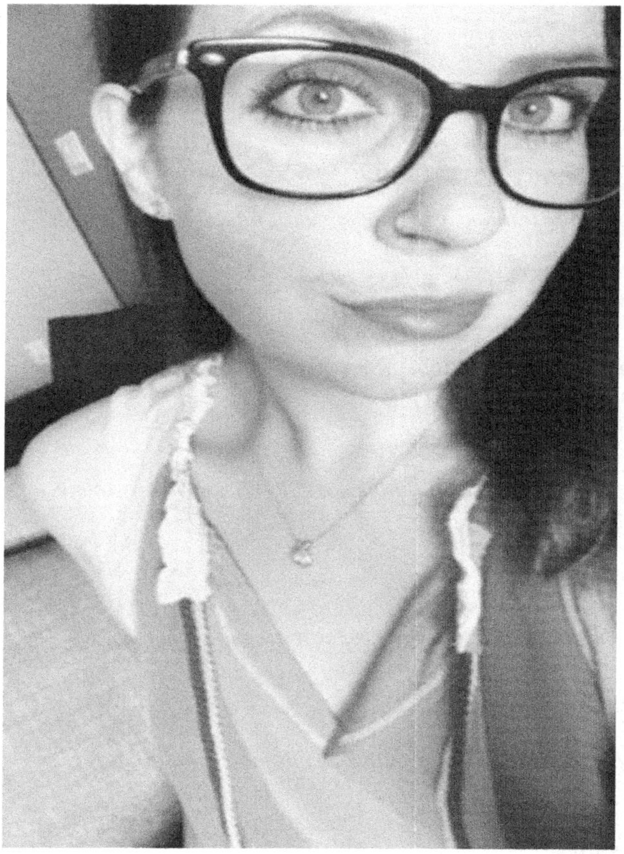

**Ashley, Lupus**

When were you diagnosed with lupus?

*2010.*

What kind of symptoms were you experiencing that led you to getting checked out?

*Joint pain, fatigue, and constant infections. If I got a cold, it turned to pneumonia or bronchitis, also pleurisy, and sores inside my mouth and nose.*

How long had you been experiencing these symptoms?

*About six years.*

What kind of tests, if any, were performed to help the diagnosis?

*Blood work, and x-rays of my hips and spine.*

What did the tests show?

*Elevated ESR(erythrocyte sedimentation rate), elevated CRP inflammatory and the x-rays showed joint damage on my spine and hips.*

What was the prognosis the doctor gave you?

*He didn't really. Just told me it was manageable with medication but sometimes complicated to find the right combination of meds.*

What kind of medications were you prescribed?

*Plaquenil, Mobic, Tramadol, and Flexeril.*

What are they for?

*Plaquenil is a anti-malaria drug that is supposed to help lupus symptoms, Mobic and Tramadol are bone and joint pain, and Flexeril is a muscle relaxer.*

Did you find any of them helped?

*Not so much. Probably just the Flexeril. It helped me sleep.*

Did you have any side effects with these medications?

*The pain medication bothered my stomach and made my reflux worse.*

Did you get any other medication prescribed as a result?

*Not from that doctor.*

What impact has lupus had on your everyday life?

*Trigger question! Hahah I just started crying.*

Sorry 'bout that one!

*It's ok! It's impacted my everyday life greatly. I always feel sick, I always hurt, it's just to what degree. I can't work full time, and I have to pick and choose when I can go out and have a personal life, because I only have so much energy on any given day.*

What hurts?

*My bones and my muscles. I also have cyclic migraines that my neurologist thinks is a side effect of lupus. Sometimes I'll have a migraine for 4-5 days.*

Have you been to other doctors for lupus?

*My next doctor after that one was in California and he thought I had ankylosing spondylitis.*

But you don't?

*I have the majority of the symptoms but the genetic factor was negative, so he doesn't think so. I do have arthritis in my spine.*

Is it assumed that it's caused by lupus?

*Yes, although this idiot I have now has no idea what I have, even though I have literally every single lupus factor.*

Has the lupus caused any other health problems you're aware of?

*Inappropriate sinus tachycardia, gastric motility issues, IBS, osteoarthritis, Raynaud's Disease, dysautonomia, Sjogren's Syndrome, pleurisy, and possibly another autoimmune disease.*

Does your lupus ever go into remission, where you don't feel like garbage?

*Never. It's been years since I woke up and haven't felt some kind of sick. Some days are better than others.*

Are there any medications you take that seem to help?

*Enbrel helps my joints a little bit, and Zofran helps with the constant nausea.*

Are there any medications you take that don't help, or make things worse?

*Naproxen helps, but really aggravates my stomach issues.*

Have you ever received massage since being diagnosed?

*No.*

Why not?

*I have pressure points on my lower back and near my shoulder blades that hurt when they're touched. I'd try it, though!*

## Lymphangitis

*(lymph-: lymph; ang-: vessel; -itis: inflammation)*

Lymphangitis is **inflammation** of the **walls** of the **lymphatic ducts**, most commonly the result of an **acute bacterial infection**.

***Causes***

Lymphangitis is most commonly the result of a **bacterial infection from the skin** entering into the lymphatic channels. The bacteria causes the lymph vessels to become inflamed, which can usually be seen in the skin, appearing as red streaks on the limbs moving proximally towards the trunk.

***Symptoms***

Symptoms depend on the severity of the infection. Fever and chills may present, and the lymph nodes may be enlarged. A person suffering from lymphangitis may experience general malaise or body aches. If the infection progresses, it can become a blood infection known as septicemia, which may be life threatening.

***Treatments***

Because lymphangitis is most commonly caused by bacterial infection, antibiotics are prescribed to destroy the bacteria. If pain is present, pain relievers may also be prescribed.

***Contraindications***

In the acute stage, lymphangitis is contraindicated for massage because massage increases the flow of lymph, and may push the infection further throughout the body.

## Lymphedema

*(lymph: lymph; -edema: swelling)*

Lymphedema is a condition of the Lymphatic System that results in increased **interstitial fluid** in a limb, which causes **swelling**.

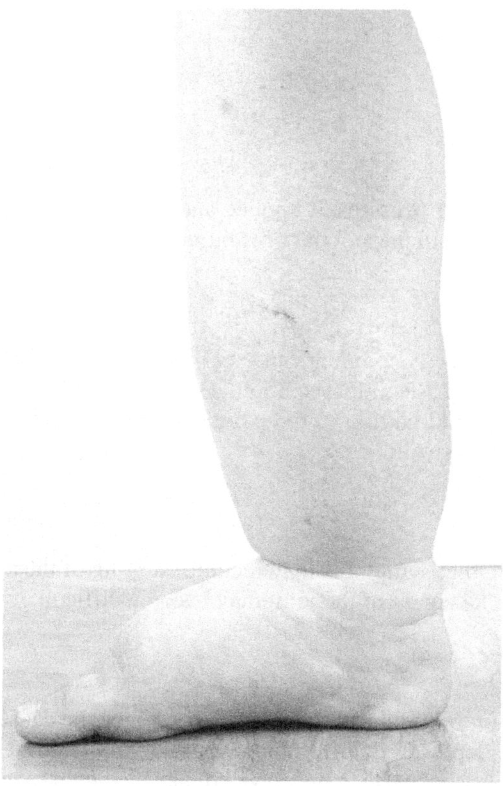

***Causes***

Causes of lymphedema vary. Most commonly, it results from damage to the lymph nodes and vessels during treatment for cancer(such as a mastectomy, where breast tissue and lymph channels may be completely removed). This results in lymph not draining properly. Other causes include obesity and advanced age.

***Symptoms***

Symptoms of lymphedema include swelling in the limbs, restricted range-of-motion, discomfort in the affected area, and thickening of the skin.

***Treatments***

While there is no cure for lymphedema, treatments may help reduce the amount of fluid in the area by stimulating lymph circulation. Massage therapy is highly effective at increasing lymph circulation. Compression clothing may help move lymph. Exercise is also extremely helpful in increasing lymph flow.

***Contraindications***

Lymphedema is not contraindicated for massage. Lymphatic drainage may help move lymph out of the area. When performing lymphatic draining, light strokes moving towards the trunk should be performed on the proximal end of the affected limb, then distal areas may be worked on, again with strokes moving towards the trunk.

## Mononucleosis

*(mono-: one; nucle/o: nucleus; -osis: condition)*

Mononucleosis is a systemic infection of the body, caused by exposure to the Epstein-Barr virus. Most people who contract mononucleosis develop antibodies for it, and symptoms do not appear again.

***Causes***

Mononucleosis is mainly spread through saliva, which is why it is often known as the "kissing disease". Coughing and sneezing, however, can also spread the virus. Sharing drinking glasses or utensils may also help spread the virus.

***Symptoms***

Mononucleosis may present with fever, fatigue, swollen lymph nodes, and sore throat. The disease typically lasts for six weeks at the most, with the most intense stages of infection occurring in the first two weeks.

***Treatments***

Because mononucleosis is caused by a virus, there are no medications that destroy the virus, and treatment consists of rest and staying hydrated.

***Contraindications***

In the acute stage, massage is an absolute contraindication. In the post-acute stage, massage may be performed.

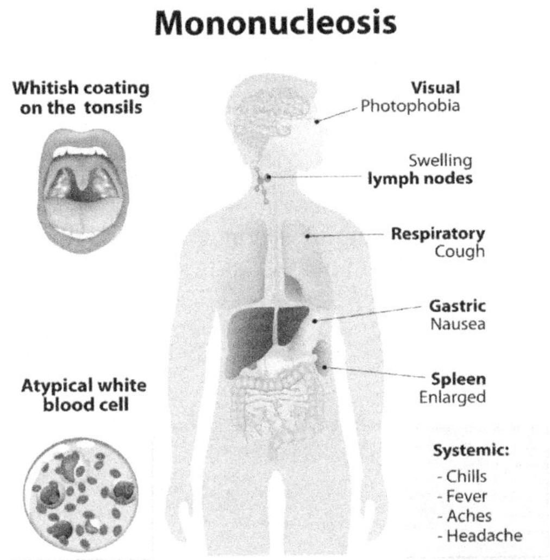


## Pitting Edema

*(edema: swelling)*

Pitting edema is a form of lymphedema that produces **pits** in the skin after **pressure** is applied and released. Lymphedema does not leave pits, and the skin rebounds immediately due to the amount of fluid in the area.

***Causes***

Pitting edema may be non-serious, or may have severe underlying causes. A common cause of pitting edema is pregnancy, due to the body creating much more fluid than it normally has. This increases fluid retention. Other more serious causes include heart failure, liver failure, or most commonly amongst these, **renal** failure. If these organs are not functioning properly, fluid is not effectively drained from the body, which increases swelling.

***Symptoms***

Pitting edema results in pits left in the skin after applying pressure. Other symptoms may include swelling of the area, pain, numbness, and cramping in the area. If the swelling is near a joint, movement of the joint may become difficult.

***Treatments***

For serious cases of pitting edema, it is recommended to visit a doctor to find the underlying cause. Once the cause is determined, a proper treatment plan may be developed. Typically, if a person is suffering from organ failure, diuretics may be prescribed to help drain excess fluid from the body. Keeping limbs such as the legs elevated may also help reduce swelling.

***Contraindications***

Massage on a client with pitting edema should not be performed until the cause of pitting edema is established. If the cause is something such as pregnancy and not organ failure, massage of the limb may be performed as it would be done with lymphedema.

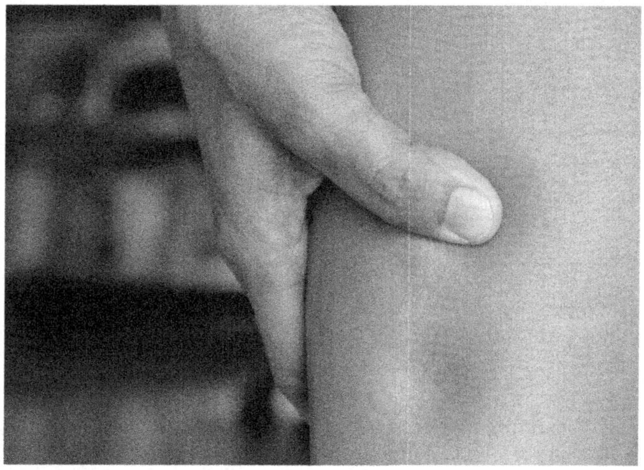

Palpation of swollen area

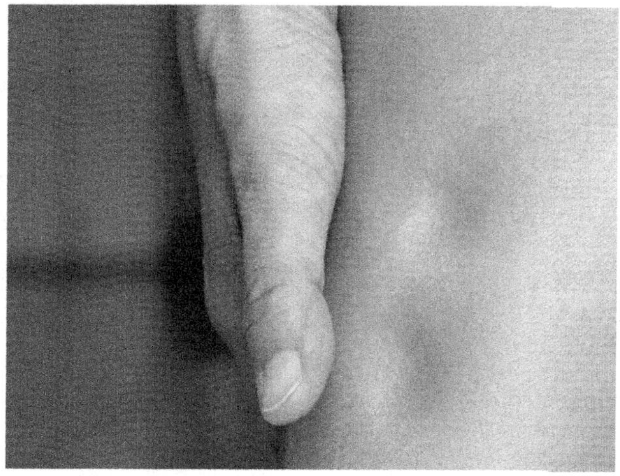

Release of pressure, pitting of edema occurs

## Tonsillitis

*(tonsill/o: tonsil; -itis: inflammation)*

Tonsillitis is **inflammation** of the **tonsils**, usually caused by some sort of **infection**. The tonsils are responsible for trapping things like bacteria. If the tonsils become too saturated by bacteria or viruses, they may become infected.

***Causes***

Streptococcus bacteria, discussed during strep throat, is a primary cause of tonsillitis. Tonsillitis may occur with strep throat. Viruses that may contribute to inflammation of the tonsils include influenza, herpes simplex, and adenoviruses.

***Symptoms***

Symptoms of tonsillitis include pain in the throat, painful difficult swallowing, fever, a coat on the tonsils that appears yellow or white, and swollen lymph nodes in the neck.

***Treatments***

Because tonsillitis is often a secondary illness caused by another condition, identifying the root cause is the start of treatment. If it is caused by a bacterial infection, antibiotics will be prescribed to destroy the bacteria. If it is caused by a virus, a person will have to manage symptoms until the body fights off the infection itself. Rest, lozenges, and gargling with salt water can all help reduce the effects of the infection.

***Contraindications***

Tonsillitis is commonly caused by an infection that is contagious, and is therefore an absolute contraindication until the condition has resolved.

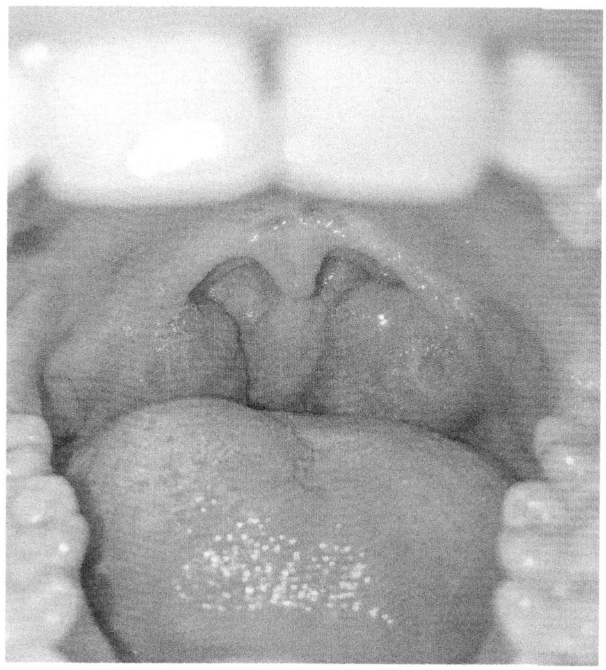

Inflamed tonsils at back of mouth

# Lymphatic Pathologies

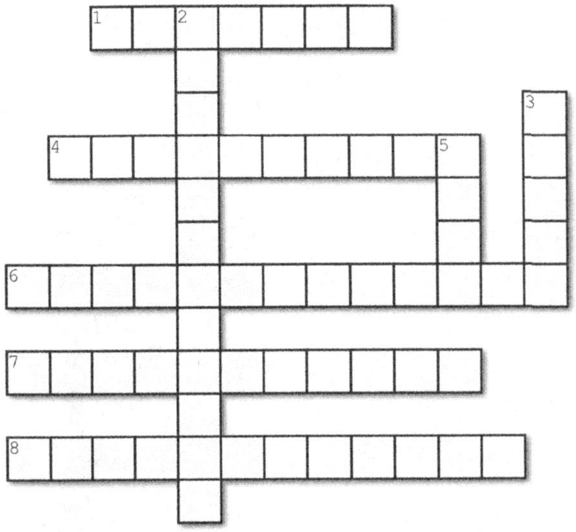


**Across**

1. Reaction of the body to substances that are usually harmless in most people
4. Swelling of a limb due to excessive accumulation of lymph
6. Systemic infection caused by the Epstein-Barr virus
7. Inflammation of the tonsils due to bacterial or viral infection
8. Swelling of an area that leaves pits upon pressure application

**Down**

2. Inflammation of the walls of the lymph ducts, commonly caused by bacterial infection
3. Autoimmune disorder affecting the body's connective tissues
5. Excessive destruction of T-cells, essentially disabling the body's immune system

Answer Key on Page 287

# Lymphatic Quiz

1. Type of cell broken down inside the spleen
A. Osteocyte
B. Leukocyte
C. Thrombocyte
D. Erythrocyte

2. T-lymphocytes are produced by which gland
A. Thymus
B. Thalamus
C. Pituitary
D. Pineal

3. Allergic reactions in the body may be controlled with use of
A. Vasodilators
B. Statins
C. Antihistamines
D. Beta-blockers

4. The largest lymph vessel in the body
A. Thoracic duct
B. Subclavian vein
C. Superior vena cava
D. Aorta

5. An increased amount of interstitial fluid in an area results in
A. Aneurysm
B. Inflammation
C. Edema
D. Thrombus

6. Lupus is an autoimmune disorder that attacks the following type of tissue
A. Nervous
B. Connective
C. Muscular
D. Epithelial

7. Infection caused by the Epstein-Barr virus that causes fever, fatigue, and swollen lymph nodes
A. Mononucleosis
B. Lupus
C. Herpes Simplex
D. Tonsillitis

8. Swelling that leaves indentations in the area after pressure is placed on the area
A. Lymphedema
B. Lupus
C. Pitting Edema
D. Mononucleosis

9. A butterfly rash, while not common, may appear on the face of a person with
A. Lymphangiitis
B. Pitting Edema
C. Mononucleosis
D. Lupus

10. Lymph vessels travel in which direction relating to the heart
A. Towards the heart
B. Laterally from the heart
C. Distally away from the heart
D. Medially towards the midline

11. Lymph contains all of the following except
A. Urea
B. Salts
C. Water
D. Erythrocytes

12. A lymph node is
A. A mass of lymph tissue
B. A collection of lymph
C. The site of lymph production
D. Where lymph drains into the blood

13. Lymph from the thoracic duct drains into which vein
A. Aortic
B. Left subclavian
C. External iliac
D. Right brachial

14. Devices used to mimic the lymphatic system by rhythmically squeezing the legs
A. Lymphatic devices
B. Tapotement devices
C. Compression devices
D. Dialysis devices

15. All of the following are part of the lymphatic system except
A. Thyroid
B. Spleen
C. Thoracic duct
D. Thymus

Answer Key on Page 289

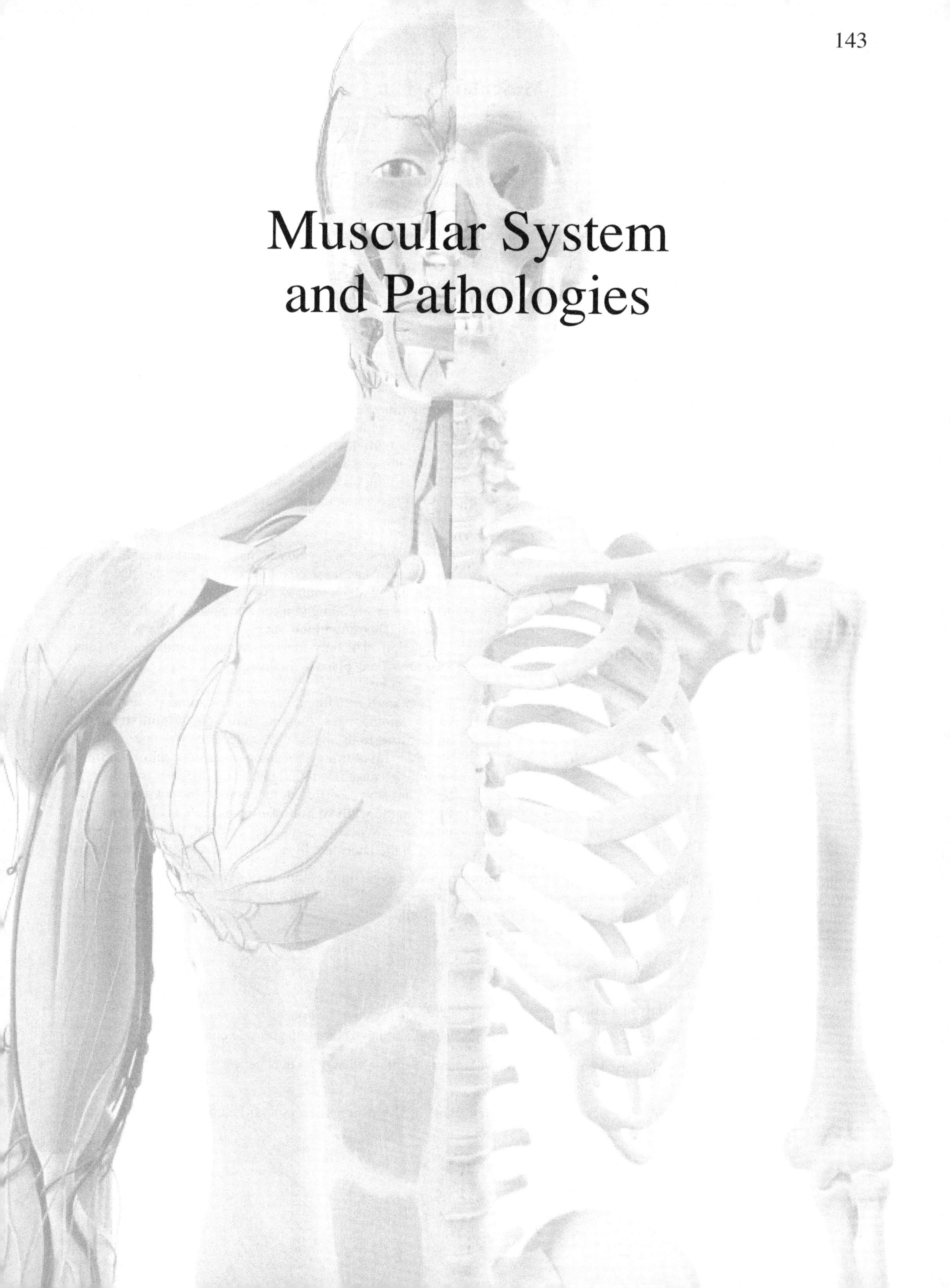

# Muscular System and Pathologies

# Muscular System

Muscles have numerous actions in the body, primarily **producing body heat**, contracting to allow **movements**, and constricting **organs** and **blood vessels**.

Muscles can all be categorized under three main types: **Skeletal**, **Cardiac**, and **Smooth**.

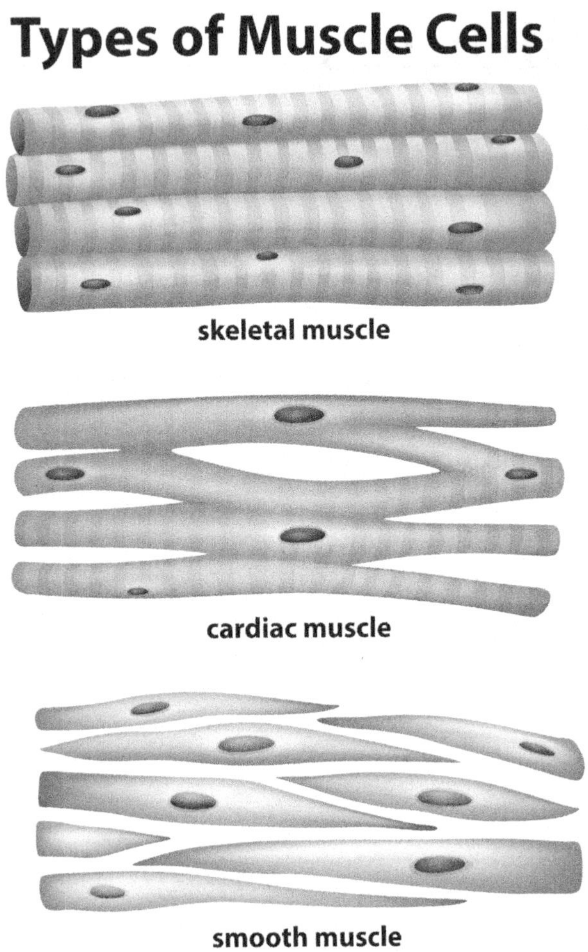


**Skeletal** muscles, as the name implies, attach to the **skeleton**. Another name for skeletal muscle is "**striated**" muscle, due to its appearance under a microscope. These muscles are **voluntary**, meaning you can control them. When these muscles contract, they pull on the bones they attach to, which allows **movement**.

Skeletal muscles are always in a state of **twitching**, even if you can't feel it. It's this twitching, very fine contractions, that produces **body heat**. When body temperature drops, the skeletal muscles increase the amount of contraction, which produces high body temperature, with the twitching of the muscles becoming more apparent. This is what happens when you shiver!

**Cardiac** muscle is the muscle that makes the **heart**. Another name for cardiac muscle is "**branching**" muscle, due to its appearance under a microscope. Cardiac muscle is **involuntary**, meaning you can't control it. Cardiac muscle is powerful, shooting **blood** out of the heart with each contraction. The only function of cardiac muscle is to send blood from one place to another.

**Smooth** muscle is found in several locations throughout the body. Another name for smooth muscle is "**non-striated**" muscle, due to its appearance under a microscope. Smooth muscle is **involuntary**, meaning you can't control it. Smooth muscle, because it is found in several different regions of the body, has several different functions. Smooth muscle can be found in the **walls** of **hollow organs** such as the stomach and intestines. When these muscles contract, they force food through the Digestive System, which is known as **peristalsis**.

Other locations smooth muscle can be found are in the **skin**, and in the **eyes**. In the skin, smooth muscle attaches to hair. When these muscles contract, they stand hair up, producing goosebumps. These muscles are known as the **arrector pili** muscles. In the eyes, smooth muscles help to **dilate** the **iris** and **pupil**.

## Muscle Structure

Skeletal muscles are broken down into the following components:

- **Sarcomeres** are the functional units of skeletal muscle. When they shorten, the muscle contracts.
- **Actin** is part of a sarcomere, known as the **thin** filament. Actin is what myosin attaches to during a muscle contraction.
- **Myosin** is part of a sarcomere, known as the **thick** filament. Myosin resembles a golf club head, and attaches to actin during a muscle contraction.

- **Tropomyosin** is a protein that **covers** the attachment sites myosin attaches to actin on during a contraction. **Calcium ions** are responsible for removing the tropomyosin from the actin, allowing the myosin to attach to the actin and initiate a contraction.

The working unit of muscles are known as sarcomeres. A sarcomere contains thick filaments, known as myosin, and thin filaments, known as actin. When a muscle isn't in a state of contraction, the myosin and actin do not interact due to the presence of tropomyosin preventing myosin from attaching to actin. When the body wants to allow the muscle to contract, calcium ions bind to tropomyosin, causing them to reveal the attachment sites on the actin for the myosin. Once the tropomyosin is removed, the myosin attaches to the actin, pulling the Z-lines closer together. This causes the sarcomere to shorten. The shortening of all the sarcomeres in a muscle fiber result in the entire muscle contracting.

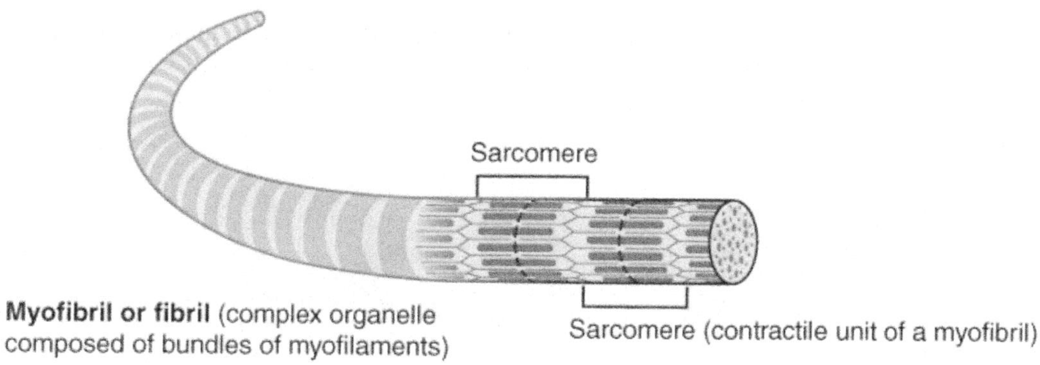


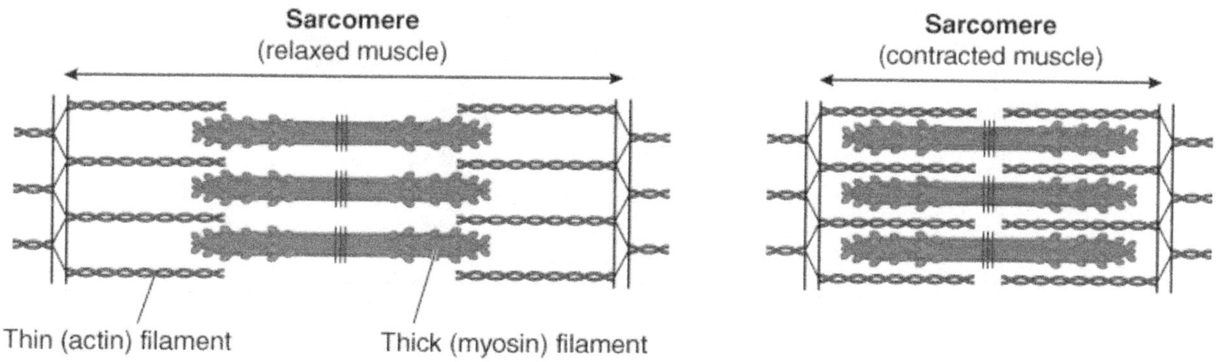


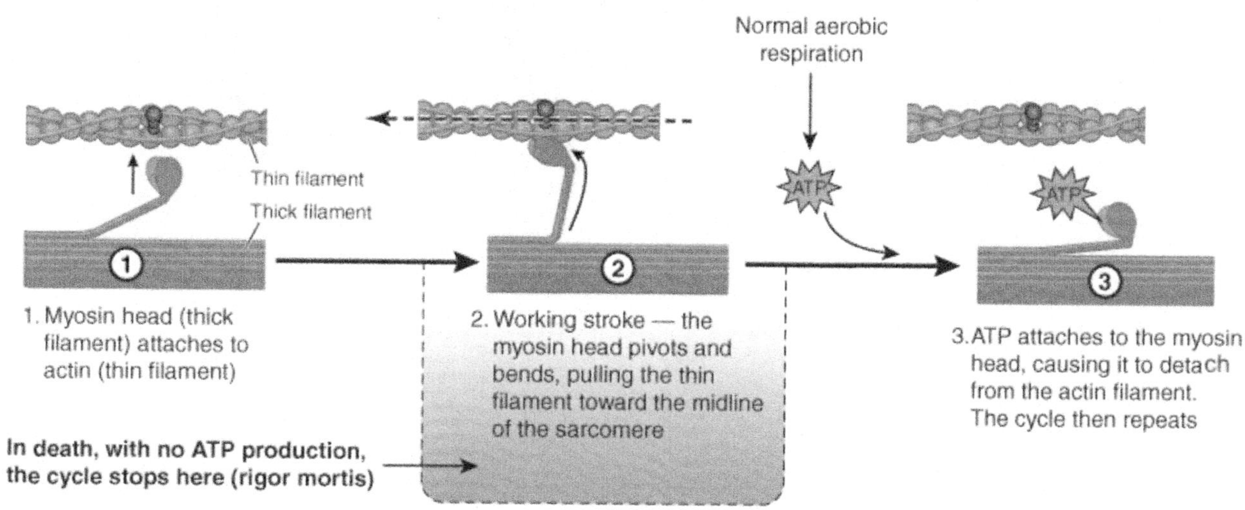

### Muscle Shapes

Muscles have numerous different shapes. These include:

**Circular**: Circular muscles are arranged in a **circular** manner. Examples include Orbicularis Oris and Orbicularis Oculi.

**Convergent**: Convergent muscles are **spread out** on one end and **merge** together at another end. An example is Pectoralis Major.

**Parallel**: Parallel muscles have muscle fibers that all run in the **same direction**. Examples include Sartorius and Coracobrachialis.

**Pennate**: Pennate muscles have an appearance resembling a **feather**. These muscles can be **unipennate**(one feather), **bipennate**(two feathers), or **multipennate**(multiple feathers). Examples include Flexor Pollicis Longus(unipennate), Rectus Femoris(bipennate), and Deltoid(multipennate).

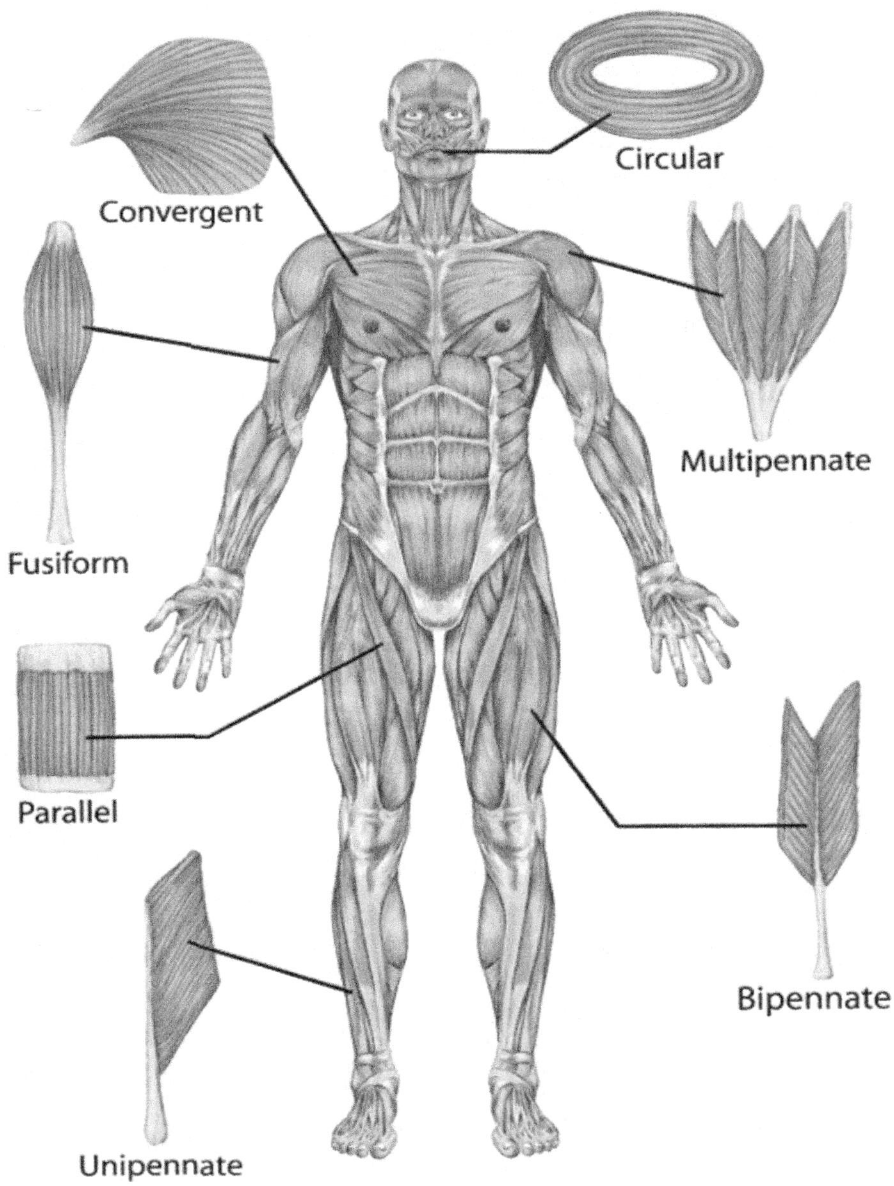

## Muscle Contractions

When there is **tension** in a muscle, it is **contracting**. A muscle can contract without moving, though. There are four types of muscle contractions.

**Isometric Contraction**: Iso means "**Same**" or "**Equal**". Metric means "**Length**". When an isometric contraction occurs, as the name implies, the length of the muscle **stays the same**, but tension in the muscle **changes**. An example: imagine trying to lift something that is too heavy for you to lift. The muscle required to lift the object increases in tension, but because the muscle isn't strong enough, the length of the muscle doesn't change.

**Isotonic Contraction**: Iso means "**Same**" or "**Equal**". Tonic means "**Tension**". When an isotonic contraction occurs, as the name implies, the tension in the muscle **stays the same**, but the muscle length **changes**. There are two separate types of isotonic contractions:

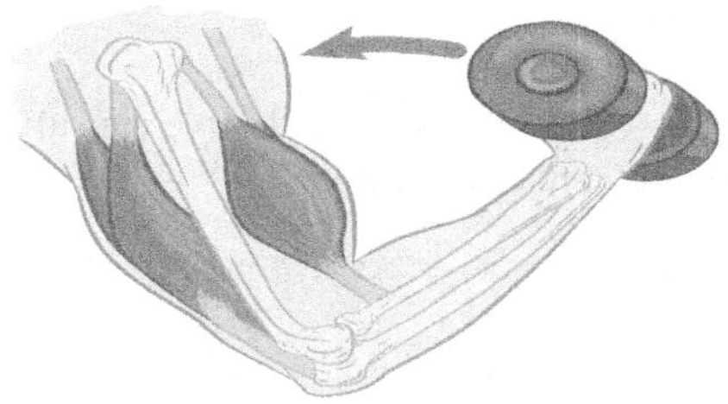

Concentric Contraction

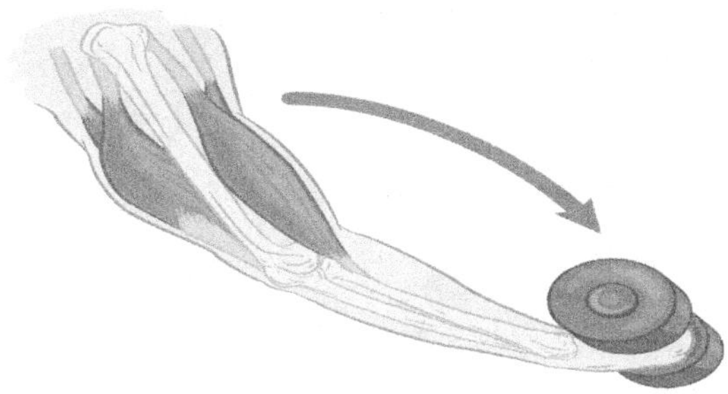

Eccentric Contraction

**Concentric Contraction**: When a concentric contraction occurs, several things take place. The tension in the muscle **initially increases** until the amount of tension required to perform the action is reached, then the tension **remains constant**. While the tension remains constant, the muscle **length decreases**. An example is performing a Biceps curl.

**Eccentric Contraction**: When an eccentric contraction occurs, several things take place. The tension in the muscle **initially decreases** until the amount of tension required to perform the action is reached, then the tension **remains constant**. While the tension remains constant, the muscle length **increases**. An example is extending the elbow and lowering the weight down after the Biceps curl in a concentric contraction.

## Medical Tests and Equipment

**Electromyography**: Electromyography(EMG) is a test used to detect the proper functioning of muscles and the nerves that innervate the muscles. This is done to assess any nerve or muscle damage that may be present, or if communication between the nerve and muscle has been impaired. Electromyography is performed by several different means. A needle may be placed directly into the muscle to read electrical activity. Adhesive pads may be placed on the skin above the muscle to detect nervous conduction as well.

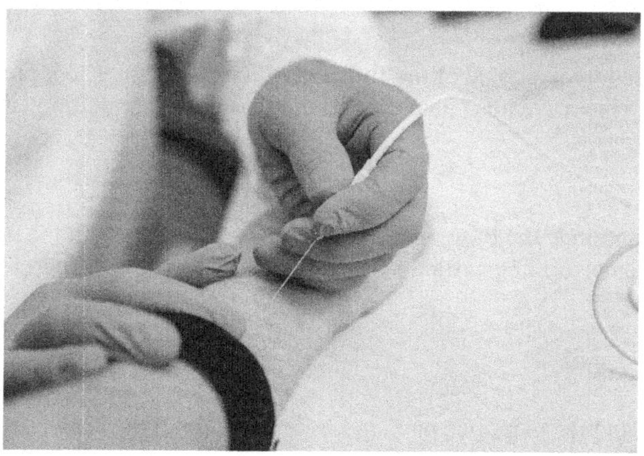

# Muscular System Pathologies

## Adhesive Capsulitis

*(capsul-: capsule; -itis: inflammation)*

Adhesive capsulitis is a condition of the Muscular System, which results in **restricted range-of-motion** at the **shoulder joint**. Another name for adhesive capsulitis is "**Frozen Shoulder**".

***Causes***

Surrounding the glenohumeral joint is connective tissue known as the joint capsule. This joint capsule holds everything in the joint in place, such as the bones themselves, synovial membrane, synovial fluid, etc. If there is irritation or over-use of the shoulder joint, **adhesions** may form between the joint capsule and the head of the humerus. These adhesions can decrease range-of-motion in the joint, and make movement in the joint uncomfortable.

The **subscapularis** muscle is often called the "Frozen Shoulder Muscle", due to its possible role in adhesive capsulitis. If the subscapularis is hypertonic, it may pull back on the humerus, which can restrict range-of-motion.

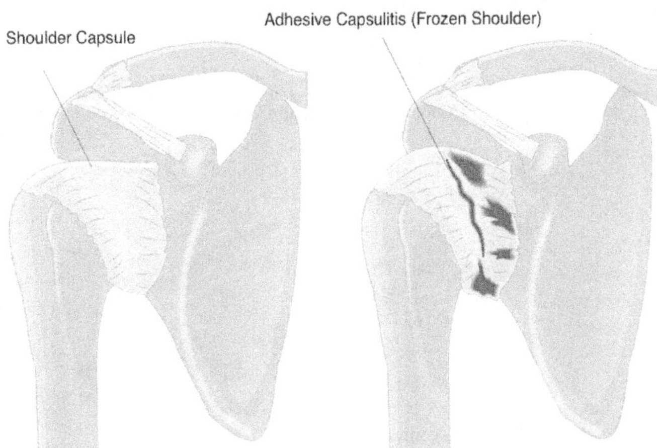


***Symptoms***

As adhesive capsulitis progresses, symptoms vary. In beginning stages, pain may be present, with a gradual decrease in the range-of-motion. As the condition advances, pain may subside, with a severely reduced range-of-motion.

***Treatments***

Treatments include stretching exercises and massage therapy to help break up the adhesions restricting range-of-motion, or to relax the subscapularis.

***Contraindications***

Adhesive capsulitis is not a contraindication. Massage may help loosen adhesions and increase range-of-motion. Stretching should be performed, as well as compression in the joint.

## De Quervain's Tenosynovitis

*(teno-: tendon; synov-: synovial; -itis: inflammation)*

De Quervain's Tenosynovitis is a form of tenosynovitis(page 154) that specifically affects the **thumb**.

***Causes***

De Quervain's Tenosynovitis is caused by **over-use** of the **thumb**, which contributes to straining of the tendons around the thumb and their protective sheaths. This may cause pain around the thumb, inflammation, and difficulty in moving the area.

***Symptoms***

Symptoms include pain and inflammation at the base of the thumb, loss of sensation in the posterior thumb, and difficulty moving the thumb and/or wrist while performing certain actions. Pain may gradually increase and radiate to other areas, such as the posterior forearm.

***Treatments***

Treatments primarily consist of rest and ice to reduce pain and inflammation in the area. Any repetitive actions that are causing the inflammation should be stopped to allow irritation to subside.

***Contraindications***

Massage is a local contraindication for De Quervain's Tenosynovitis, as it may increase inflammation and pain. Application of cold may be performed to decrease inflammation around the thumb.

## Dupuytren's Contracture

Dupuytren's Contracture is a condition that results in **deformation** of the **hand**, due to tissues under the skin **hardening**, **thickening**, and **shortening**. These tissues pull the fingers into flexion, and don't allow the fingers to completely straighten.

***Causes***

There are no known causes of Dupuytren's contracture. Men over the age of 50 are more likely to develop the condition, but exact reasons why are still not understood.

***Symptoms***

Deformity of the hand, specifically in the pinky finger, can occur. The skin on the palm of the hand can thicken, and the fascia under the skin thickens, pulling the pinky and ring finger towards the palm. This causes the affected fingers to lose the ability to fully extend, impairing function of the hand.

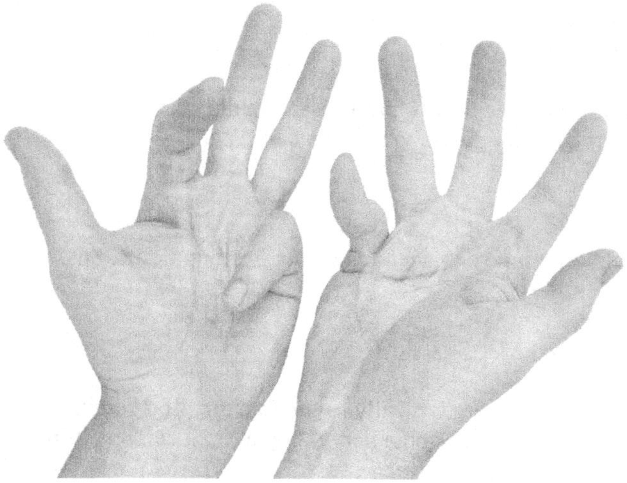

***Treatments***

Treatments include injecting enzymes into the cords to help soften them, a technique called needling in which needles are inserted into the cords that help to break them, or surgery to partially or completely remove the cords from the hand. Each treatment has varying degrees of success, and the contracture may return.

***Contraindications***

Dupuytren's contracture is indicated for massage, although massage is unlikely to help loosen the tendon and help the finger return to its normal position.

## Fibromyalgia

(*fibro-: fibrous; my-: muscle; -algia: pain*)

Fibromyalgia is a condition causing **pain** throughout the **body**, in conjunction with **fatigue**. Trouble with memory may also be present. Fibromyalgia may occur suddenly, or may worsen over time. Fibromyalgia typically affects women much more often than men. Diagnosis involves first ruling out other conditions that may be causing symptoms. If these other conditions are ruled out, then the duration of pain(over three months) and location of pain(using the Widespread Pain Index) are taken into account.

***Causes***

The exact cause of fibromyalgia is unknown. Many theories state the cause could range from hereditary to environmental factors, such as stress or trauma.

***Symptoms***

Symptoms of fibromyalgia primarily include widespread pain, usually a dull ache, in specific regions of the body for longer than three months, general fatigue, and issues with memory.

***Treatments***

Medications are important in the treatment of fibromyalgia. Pain relievers help to reduce the pain a person may be experiencing, while antidepressants can help treat depression that may result due to the fatigue a person can experience.

***Contraindications***

Fibromyalgia is indicated for massage, working within the client's pain tolerance.

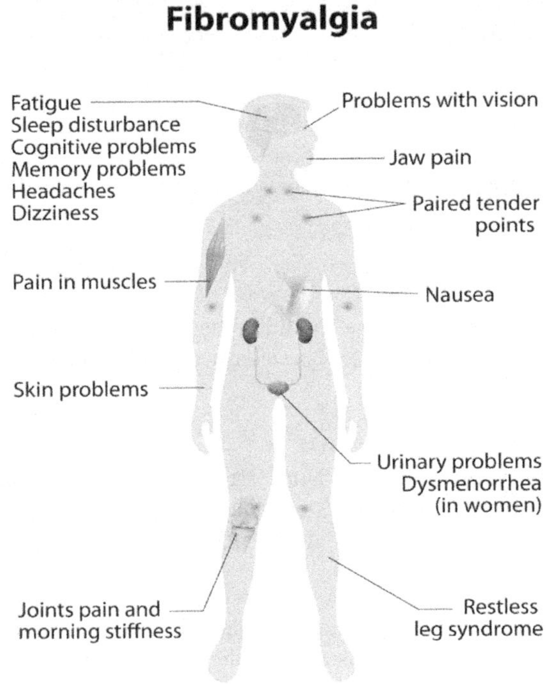


## Ganglion Cyst

*(ganglion: anything gathered into a ball)*

A ganglion cyst is a small, **fluid-filled sac** that forms along the **tendons** in the **hands** and **wrists**. While normally nothing to worry about, a ganglion cyst may place pressure on a nerve running by it, which can cause pain.

***Causes***

There is no known cause of ganglion cysts. They may be the result of an injury to a tendon or surrounding tissue, but commonly form for unknown reasons.

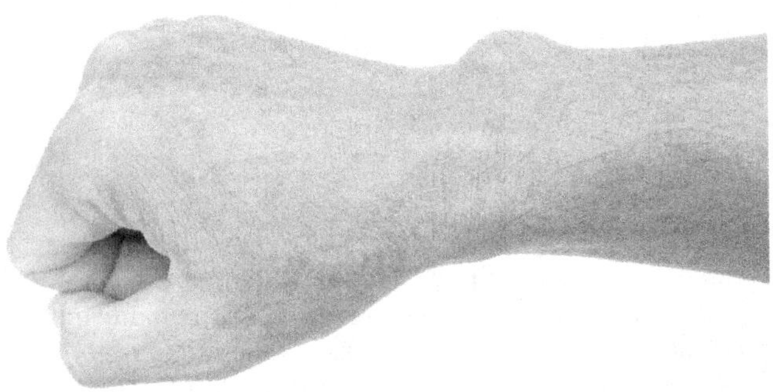

***Symptoms***

Ganglion cysts are typically asymptomatic. If a ganglion cyst places pressure on a nerve, however, it can result in pain.

***Treatments***

Most commonly, ganglion cysts do not require treatment, as they do not cause any side effects. If there is pain, or if a person is self-conscious about them, treatment may include immobilizing the area to reduce friction between the cyst and the tendon, or surgery to either drain the fluid from the cyst or to completely remove the cyst from the body.

***Contraindications***

Ganglion cysts should be treated as a local contraindication.

## Golfer's Elbow

Golfer's Elbow is a form of tendonitis that affects and weakens the **flexors** of the wrist. Golfer's Elbow is also known as Medial Epicondylitis, inflammation of the **medial epicondyle**.

### *Causes*

Golfer's Elbow is caused by repetitive motions such as elbow flexion, which put strain on the tendons connecting the flexors of the wrist to the humerus, at the medial epicondyle.

### *Symptoms*

Golfer's Elbow may present with pain and inflammation at the medial epicondyle of the humerus, weakness in the elbow joint, and numbness in digits four and five.

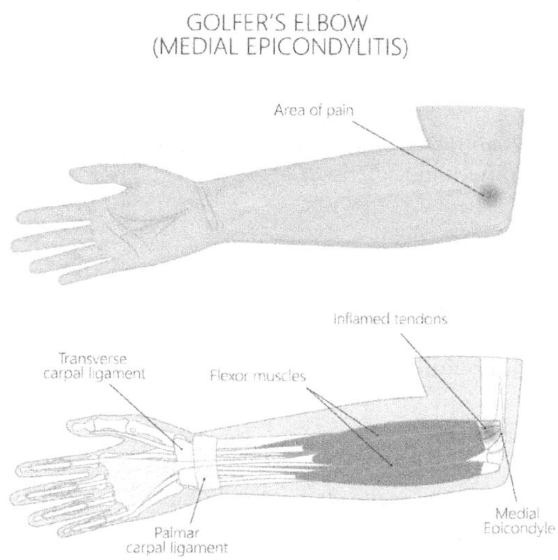


### *Treatments*

Treatment typically involves rest and ice on the medial epicondyle to reduce inflammation. Any repetitive actions that are causing the inflammation should be stopped to allow irritation to subside.

### *Contraindications*

Golfer's Elbow should be treated as a local contraindication. Application of cold may help reduce pain and inflammation at the medial epicondyle of the humerus.

## Headache

A headache is **pain** in the **head**. The pain felt can vary depending on the cause. The pain can be unilateral, bilateral, involve the entire head, or only affect a portion of the head. There are many different types of headaches, ranging from muscular tension headaches to migraines. Each type of headache may have its own cause.

### *Causes*

Causes vary extremely between different types of headaches. Muscular tension headaches, for example, may be caused by hypertonicity of a muscle placing too much pressure on a part of the head. Migraine headaches are caused by extracranial blood vessels dilating, which puts pressure on the meninges and reduces the flow of fluid in the skull. Diet may play a role in the development of headaches, such as blood sugar or a chemical dependence like caffeine.

Headaches may also be caused by other conditions. Examples include encephalitis(page 170), meningitis(page 171), dehydration, hypertension, etc. These are known as secondary headaches.

### *Symptoms*

Pain in the head is the main symptom of headaches, although symptoms may vary between differing types of headaches. Migraine headaches may also present with visual problems and sensitivity to sound or light.

### *Treatments*

Over-the-counter pain medications, such as aspirin or ibuprofen, are incredibly useful for treating acute headaches. To prevent headaches from occurring, a doctor may prescribe muscle relaxants or antidepressants.

*Contraindications*

Headaches are not contraindicated for massage. If muscular tension headache is suspected, massage should be performed on areas around the location of pain to try to ease tension and reduce pain. Application of heat or cold may be performed, depending on a client's specific needs.

## Muscle Cramp

Muscle cramps are **involuntary contractions** of the muscle, and are usually **painful**.

*Causes*

Dehydration and overusing a muscle are prime causes of muscle cramps. However, a cramp may develop due to other factors, including a low supply of blood which reduces oxygen intake in the muscle, or compression of nerves. Loss of electrolytes, such as sodium or potassium, may also lead to muscle cramping.

*Symptoms*

Pain in the location of the cramp is the prime symptom of muscle cramps. A person may also be able to visibly see the muscle cramping under the skin.

*Treatments*

Cramps are typically not serious, and only require minimal treatment to fix. Stretching and utilizing reciprocal inhibition(contracting the opposing muscle of the muscle cramping) can help calm the cramping in the acute stage. Keeping hydrated and providing the body with nutrients such as potassium may help prevent muscle cramping.

*Contraindications*

Muscle cramps in the acute stage should be considered a local contraindication. Reciprocal inhibition should be performed to stop the cramp. After a cramp has subsided, massage may be performed on the area, bringing fresh blood and nutrients into the area. The client should increase water intake after the massage as a preventative measure.

## Muscular Dystrophy

*(dys-: difficult; -trophy: nourishment)*

Muscular dystrophy is a **genetic disorder** resulting in **weakness** and **wasting** of **muscle tissue**. The disease typically appears in childhood, affecting males more commonly than females. The disease progresses slowly, usually affecting muscles of the lower limbs, making walking difficult. As the disease progresses, a person may lose the ability to walk, have issues breathing, develop spinal conditions such as scoliosis, and formation of contractures.

*Causes*

Muscular dystrophy is caused by a genetic defect, causing a weakness in muscle fibers that eventually causes the fibers to break down. The most common cause is a lack of the gene that produces dystrophin, a protein in muscle fibers that provide strength and structure to the fiber.

*Symptoms*

Symptoms usually seen in a person with muscular dystrophy include problems walking, breathing, staying up-right, and possible heart complications. Most symptoms appear in childhood.

*Treatments*

Although there is no cure for muscular dystrophy in any of its forms, treatments may help manage the symptoms, including corticosteroids and physical therapy. Exercise is recommended to maintain muscle mass.

### *Contraindications*

Muscular dystrophy is indicated for massage. Precautions should be taken regarding pressure used. The therapist should expect to help a client with muscular dystrophy onto and off of the table. Massage can help bring nutrients into tissue and eliminate waste, which may not be sufficiently achieved if the muscles aren't being used.

## Strain

A strain is an injury to a **tendon** or **muscle**, usually caused by over-exertion or over-use.

### *Causes*

Activities such as exercise are a common cause of strains. Much like burns, there are three grades of strains: grade 1, grade 2, and grade 3. The less severe the strain, the lower the grade.

A grade 1 strain results in slight tearing of a tendon or muscle. An example could be a person's muscles being sore after exercise. The muscles have experienced slight tears during exercise, but will heal after a day or two.

A grade 2 strain results in more tearing of a muscle or tendon. Grade 2 strains may require surgery to repair, or may heal on their own with rest. There may be accompanying bruising and inflammation around the strain.

A grade 3 strain results in complete tearing of a muscle, or more commonly, a tendon. Surgery is required to repair a grade 3 strain. The quadriceps and biceps brachii are two muscles prone to grade 3 strains more than others. Grade 3 strains will inhibit movement involved with the muscle involved, due to its inability to pull on the bone.

### *Symptoms*

Strains may result in pain, inflammation, and an inability to move the injured muscle or tendon.

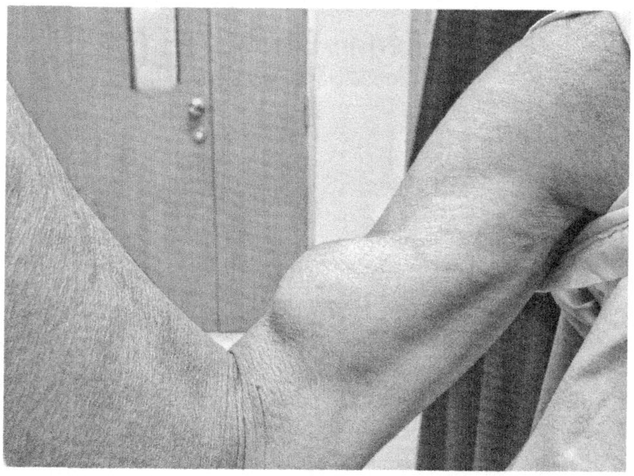

Grade 3 strain of the tendon of the long head of biceps brachii

### *Treatments*

Treatment varies depending on the severity of the strain. Grade 1 strains should be able to receive massage and heat therapy after 24-48 hours to increase circulation and promote healing. Grade 2 strains may need to rest longer before treatment. Grade 3 strains would require surgery to repair.

### *Contraindications*

Acute strains are considered a local contraindication, and should be avoided to prevent increasing pain and inflammation in the area. Contrast therapy, utilizing alternating cold and heat, ending with cold, may be performed to decrease inflammation and bring fresh blood to the area.

## Tendonitis

*(tendon-: tendon; -itis: inflammation)*

Tendonitis is an injury that results in **inflammation** of a **tendon**.

### *Causes*

Tendonitis is a mostly repetitive strain injury, caused by repeated use of one specific muscle, which can over-exert the tendon. When the tendon is over-exerted, it may tear slightly, which causes pain and inflammation.

There are several different types of tendonitis, including Golfer's Elbow(inflammation of the tendon at the medial epicondyle of the humerus), Tennis Elbow(inflammation of the tendon at the lateral epicondyle of the humerus), and Jumper's Knee(inflammation of the patellar tendon). All these conditions are caused by repetitive movements.

***Symptoms***

Symptoms may include pain upon moving a muscle connected to an affected tendon, and inflammation.

***Treatments***

Treatment for tendonitis is primarily rest and application of ice to reduce any inflammation. Repetitive actions causing the inflammation should be stopped until the irritation subsides.

***Contraindications***

Tendonitis should be treated as a local contraindication. Alternating application of cold and heat, ending with cold, can assist in decreasing inflammation and associated pain.

## Tennis Elbow

Tennis Elbow is a form of tendonitis that affects and weakens the **extensors** of the wrist. Tennis Elbow is also known as Lateral Epicondylitis, inflammation of the **lateral epicondyle**.

***Causes***

Tennis Elbow is caused by repetitive motions such as elbow extension, which put strain on the tendons connecting the extensors of the wrist to the humerus, at the lateral epicondyle.

***Symptoms***

Tennis Elbow commonly presents with pain that radiates distally to the posterior forearm. Weakness may result, especially when performing actions that require grasping.

***Treatments***

Treatment typically involves rest and ice on the lateral epicondyle to reduce inflammation. Any repetitive actions that are causing the inflammation should be stopped to allow irritation to subside.

***Contraindications***

Tennis Elbow should be treated as a local contraindication. Alternating application of cold and heat, ending with cold, can assist in decreasing inflammation and associated pain at the lateral epicondyle of the humerus.

Tennis Elbow
Right arm, lateral (outside) side

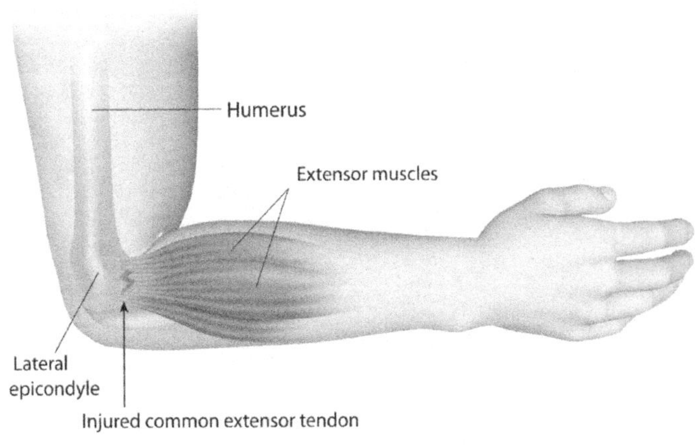


## Tenosynovitis

*(teno-: tendon; synov-: synovial; -itis: inflammation)*

Tenosynovitis is a repetitive strain injury that results in **inflammation** of a **tendon** and its **protective sheath**.

***Causes***

Tenosynovitis primarily affects the hands, wrists, and feet due to the length of the tendons in these areas. The longer the tendon is, the easier it becomes to strain. Because there may be inflammation, pain may be present, and it may be difficult to move the affected area.

A common type of tenosynovitis is known as De Quervain's Tenosynovitis, which causes inflammation around the thumb due to over-use.

***Symptoms***

Tenosynovitis may produce pain and inflammation in affected joints, making it painful to move these joints. The area of the inflamed tendon may also be red.

***Treatments***

Tenosynovitis is typically treated the same as any strain, with rest and ice to reduce pain. Less commonly, tenosynovitis may be the result of bacterial infection, which may produce a fever. If a fever is present, medications such as antibiotics and antipyretics may be prescribed to combat bacterial growth and fever.

***Contraindications***

Massage is a local contraindication for tenosynovitis, as it may increase inflammation and pain. Application of cold may be performed to decrease inflammation in the tendon and reduce pain.

## Torticollis

*(torti-: twisted; collis: neck)*

Torticollis, also known as **wry neck**, is a condition causing the neck to **twist to one side**, which tilts the head.

***Causes***

Trauma to the cervical region may cause torticollis. Often an injury to the sternocleidomastoid is the prime cause. Spasms of the sternocleidomastoid may cause a type of torticollis known as spasmodic torticollis, and is usually a chronic condition. An injury to the trochlear nerve may cause a separate type of torticollis known as trochlear torticollis, in which a person must adjust the position of their head to see properly due to the trochlear nerve, which provides stimulation to muscles controlling the eye, no longer functioning as effectively.

***Symptoms***

A person affected by torticollis will have their head tilted to one side. This can be uncomfortable or painful, especially when trying to move the neck or head back to a normal position. This can also lead to pain in the back and shoulders, and headaches.

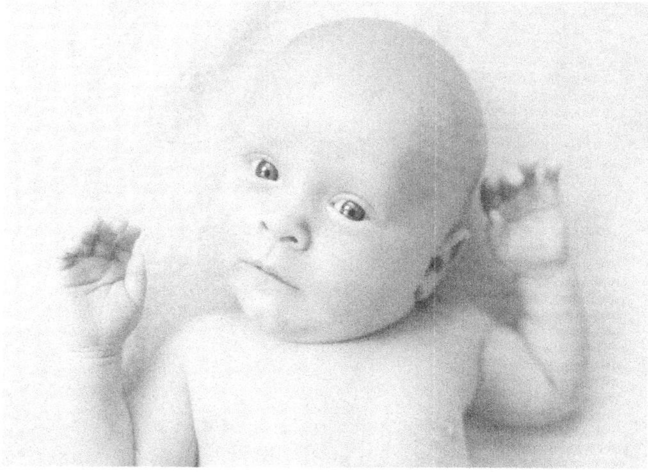

***Treatments***

Because torticollis is the result of a spasm or contraction of neck muscles, treatments aim to relax the affected muscles. These treatments may include physical therapy, prescribing muscle relaxants, or possible surgery to correct any structural issues that may arise. Torticollis usually resolves itself within a few days, unless there is a more severe cause.

***Contraindications***

Torticollis is generally not considered a contraindication, but precautions should be taken if damage to a muscle or nerve is the cause.

# Muscular Pathologies

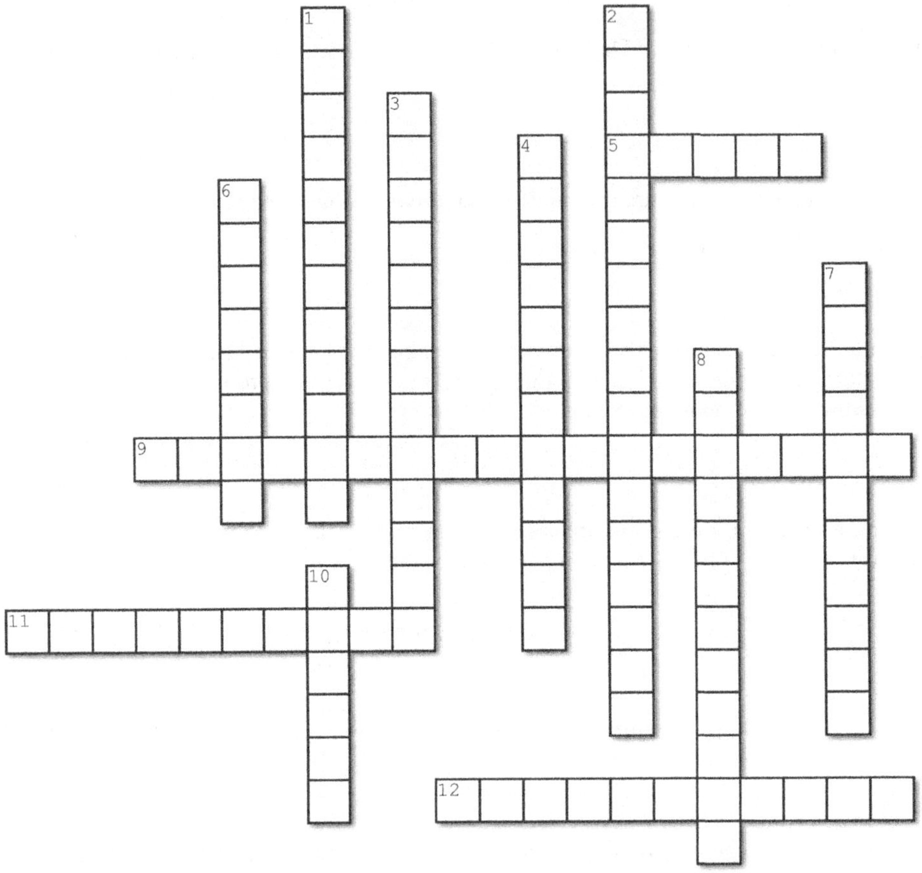

**Across**

**5.** Involuntary contraction of muscle, commonly caused by dehydration
**9.** Restricted range-of-motion at the shoulder joint, due to adhesions forming between the joint capsule and head of the humerus
**11.** Inflammation of a tendon
**12.** Twisting of the head and neck to one side

**Down**

**1.** Fluid-filled sac forming at a tendon in the hand or wrist
**2.** Genetic disorder causing weakness and wasting of muscle tissue
**3.** Repetitive strain injury that causes inflammation of a tendon and its protective sheath
**4.** Widespread pain throughout the body, typically at specific points
**6.** Pain in the head
**7.** Inflammation at the lateral epicondyle of the humerus
**8.** Inflammation located at the medial epicondyle of the humerus
**10.** An injury to a muscle or tendon

Answer Key on Page 287

# Muscular Quiz

1. Cryotherapy treatment used for an acute strain or sprain
A. PPALM
B. SOAP
C. PRICE
D. CAR

2. Adhesive capsulitis
A. Adhesions forming in the liver, causing decreased bile production and blood detoxification
B. Joint capsule surrounding the glenohumeral joint adhering to the head of the humerus, reducing movement
C. Tearing of fascia along the medial tibia, causing increased pain upon walking
D. Autoimmune disorder causing degeneration of myelin sheaths in the central nervous system, resulting in scarring of an axon

3. Movement of the limbs is controlled by which type of muscle tissue
A. Cardiac
B. Skeletal
C. Smooth
D. Hyaline

4. Involuntary painful contraction of a muscle caused by lack of oxygen or dehydration
A. Cramp
B. Spasm
C. Twitch
D. Strain

5. Inflammation of a tendon and its surrounding sheath is known as
A. Tendonitis
B. Carpal Tunnel Syndrome
C. Sprain
D. Tenosynovitis

6. Torticollis
A. Inflammation of a tendon and its sheath
B. Degeneration of muscle tissue
C. Spasm of muscles in the neck that causes the head to tilt to one side
D. Inflammation located at the lateral epicondyle of the humerus

7. An injury to a muscle or tendon
A. Sprain
B. Strain
C. Fracture
D. Break

8. Muscular Dystrophy
A. Genetic disorder causing degeneration of muscle tissue
B. Autoimmune disorder causing hyper-sensitivity in various spots of the body
C. Bacterial infection causing intense muscle cramping
D. Cyst formation on a tendon

9. Inflammation located at the medial epicondyle of the humerus is known as
A. Tennis Elbow
B. Bowler's Shoulder
C. Jumper's Knee
D. Golfer's Elbow

10. Lateral epicondylitis affects the following muscle group
A. Wrist extensors
B. Shoulder flexors
C. Hip adductors
D. Neck rotators

11. The functional unit of a muscle fiber
A. Z Line
B. Sarcomere
C. Epimysium
D. Myofibril

12. Chemical required to produce a muscle contraction
A. Dopamine
B. Potassium
C. Calcium
D. Phosphorus

13. Deformation of the hand, the result of tendons in the hand becoming extremely tight, which pulls in the fingers into permanent flexion
A. Ganglion Cyst
B. Tennis Elbow
C. Dupuytren's Contracture
D. Muscular Dystrophy

14. Lateral epicondylitis is also known as
A. Tennis Elbow
B. Golfer's Elbow
C. Bowler's Shoulder
D. Racquetball Wrist

15. Complete rupture of a tendon, which requires surgery to successfully repair
A. Grade I strain
B. Grade III strain
C. Grade IV strain
D. Grade II strain

Answer Key on Page 289

# Nervous System and Pathologies

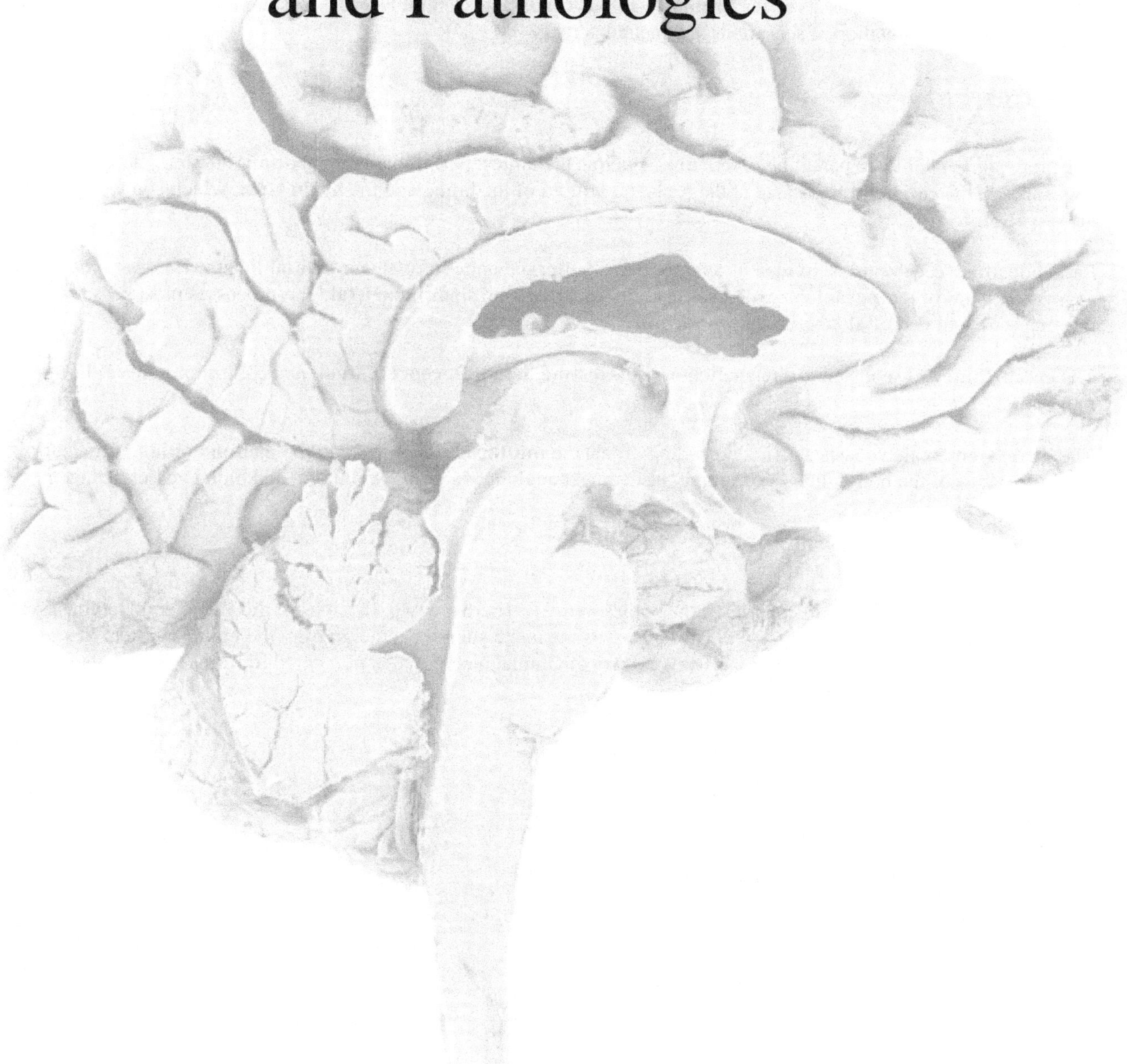

# Nervous System

Nerves are structures in the **Nervous System**, made of nervous tissue. Nerves have many functions, from regulating vital functions within the body, to controlling muscles.

There are two divisions of the Nervous System: the **Central Nervous System**, and the **Peripheral Nervous System**. The Central Nervous System consists of the **brain** and **spinal cord**. The Central Nervous System is under involuntary control, responsible for interpretation of sensations and mental activity.

## Central Nervous System

The brain consists of three parts: the **cerebrum**, which is the largest part of the brain and split into left and right hemispheres, the **cerebellum**, located at the back and bottom of the brain, and the **brain stem**, which connects the brain to the spinal cord.

Each side of the **cerebrum** is divided into **lobes**, named after the bones atop them: **frontal** lobe(processes motivation, aggression, mood), **temporal** lobe(processes memory, hearing, and smell), **parietal** lobe(processes most sensory information), and **occipital** lobe(processes vision).

The **cerebellum** is responsible for regulation of **muscle tone**, **balance**, **coordination**, and control of **general body movements**.

The **brain stem**, which consists of(in descending order) the **midbrain**, the **pons**, and the **medulla oblongata**, controls the **vital functions** of the body, such as breathing, heart rate, coughing, sneezing, vomiting, and blood vessel diameter.

## Peripheral Nervous System

The Peripheral Nervous System consists of the body's **nerves**. There are two divisions of the Peripheral Nervous System: **Cranial Nerves** and **Spinal Nerves**. Cranial Nerves, as the name suggests, emerge from the brain, and help to regulate the functions of the head and face. There are **twelve pairs** of Cranial Nerves, each numbered in Roman Numerals:

- Olfactory(I)
- Optic(II)
- Oculomotor(III)
- Trochlear(IV)
- Trigeminal(V)
- Abducens(VI)
- Facial(VII)
- Vestibulocochlear(VIII)
- Glossopharyngeal(IX)
- Vagus(X)
- Accessory(XI)
- Hypoglossal(XII)

Spinal Nerves are much more numerous than Cranial Nerves. There are **31 pairs** of Spinal Nerves. The Spinal Nerves, as the name suggests, emerge from the spinal cord, and are responsible for controlling skeletal muscle.

A bundle of Spinal Nerves that emerge from the spinal cord is known as a **Plexus**. There are three plexi in the body: **Cervical Plexus**, **Brachial Plexus**, **Lumbosacral Plexus**. The Cervical Plexus emerges from the spinal cord in the range of **C1-C4**. The primary nerve of the Cervical Plexus is known as the **Phrenic Nerve**.

The Phrenic Nerve descends inferiorly from the cervical vertebrae and innervates(provides nervous stimulation to) the **Diaphragm**.

The Brachial Plexus emerges from the spinal cord at **C5-T1**. As the name suggests, the nerves of the Brachial Plexus move distally, controlling the muscles of the **upper limb**. There are five primary nerves of the Brachial Plexus:

- Radial
- Musculocutaneous
- Axillary
- Median
- Ulnar

The **Radial Nerve** is located on the posterior arm and forearm, and innervates the Triceps Brachii, Anconeus, Brachioradialis, and Wrist Extensors.

The **Musculocutaneous Nerve** is located in the anterior arm, and innervates the Biceps Brachii, Brachialis, and Coracobrachialis.

The **Axillary Nerve** is primarily located in the armpit, and innervates the Teres Minor and Deltoid.

The **Median Nerve** is located in the anterior arm, forearm, and hand, and innervates the Wrist Flexors, and most muscles on the lateral side of the hand.

The **Ulnar Nerve** is located on the anterior arm, medial forearm, and medial hand, and innervates the Wrist Flexors and most muscles on the medial side of the hand.

The Lumbosacral Plexus, as the name suggests, emerges from the **entire span** of the Lumbar and Sacral vertebrae. The major nerves of the Lumbosacral Plexus include:

- Sciatic
- Femoral
- Obturator
- Tibial
- Common Peroneal
- Deep Peroneal
- Superficial Peroneal

The **Sciatic Nerve** is a large nerve located on the posterior thigh. The Sciatic Nerve is actually both the Tibial Nerve and the Common Peroneal Nerve bundled together. Once the Sciatic Nerve reaches the back of the knee, it branches off into two separate nerves. The Sciatic Nerve innervates the Hamstring muscle group.

The **Femoral Nerve** is located on the anterior thigh, and innervates the Quadriceps muscle group, Iliacus, Sartorius, and Pectineus.

The **Obturator Nerve** is located on the medial portion of the thigh, and innervates the Adductor muscle group.

The **Tibial Nerve**, after branching off the Sciatic nerve, runs down the posterior leg, and innervates the Gastrocnemius, Soleus, Tibialis Posterior, and Plantaris.

The **Common Peroneal Nerve**, after branching off the Sciatic Nerve, actually branches off into two other nerves of its own: The Deep Peroneal and Superficial Peroneal Nerves.

The **Deep Peroneal Nerve** is located on the anterior leg, and innervates the Tibialis Anterior.

The **Superficial Peroneal Nerve** is located on the lateral portion of the leg, running along the fibula, and innervates the Peroneus Longus and Peroneus Brevis.

The Cranial Nerves

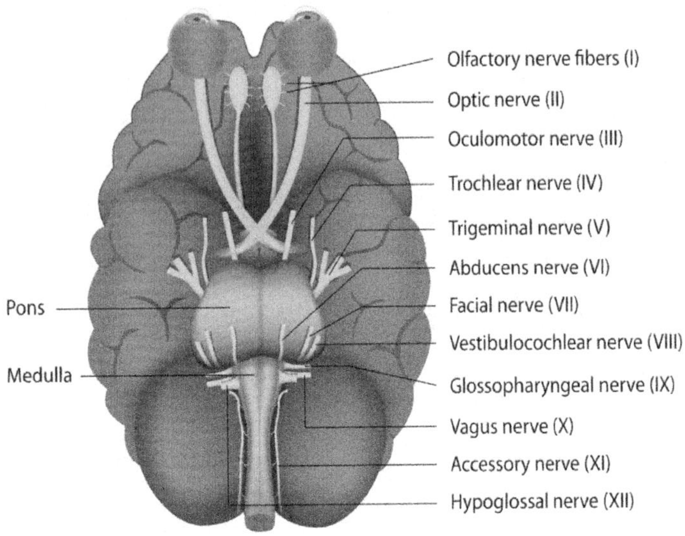


The Cervical Plexus

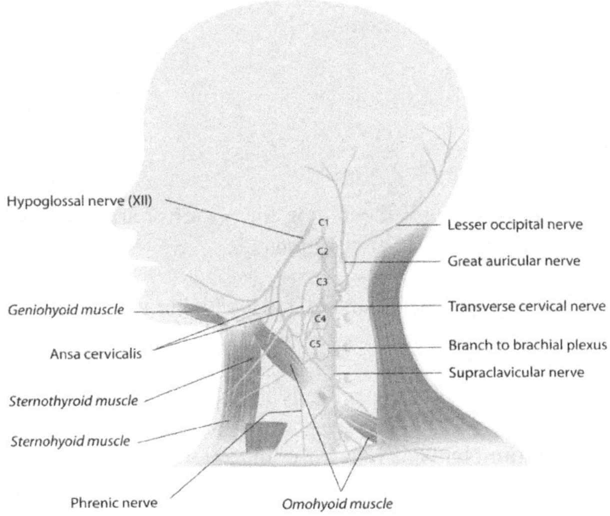


The Brachial Plexus

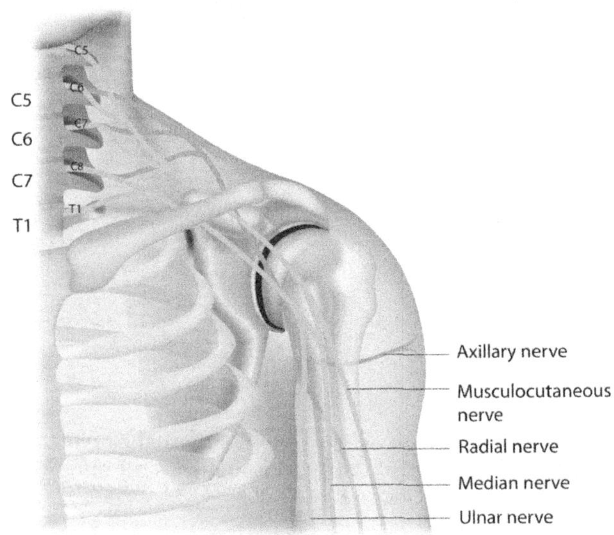


The Lumbar Plexus

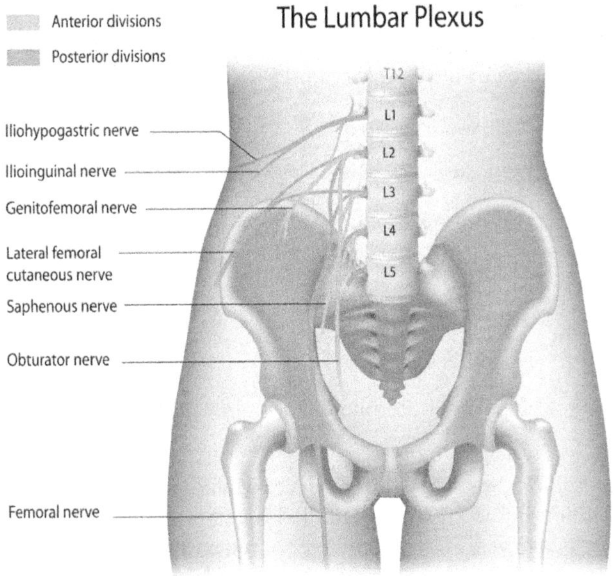

### Autonomic Nervous System

The autonomic nervous system helps to regulate **homeostasis** by release of hormones, controlling heart rate, breathing rate, and other bodily functions. There are two divisions of the autonomic nervous system: the **Sympathetic Response**, and the **Parasympathetic Response**.

The sympathetic response is also known as "**fight-or-flight**". When the body is in a state of **stress**, the sympathetic response helps the body respond by releasing **norepinephrine** into the blood stream, which increases heart rate and blood sugar. The digestive organs will also shut down, and blood will be pulled from these organs and supplied to the muscles for use.

The parasympathetic response is also known as "**rest-and-digest**". When the body is in a state of **relaxation**, the parasympathetic response helps the body to calm itself. It decreases the body's heart rate, and increases blood flow to the digestive organs to increase **peristalsis**. The parasympathetic response, decreasing heart rate, and peristalsis are all controlled by Cranial Nerve X, the **Vagus Nerve**.

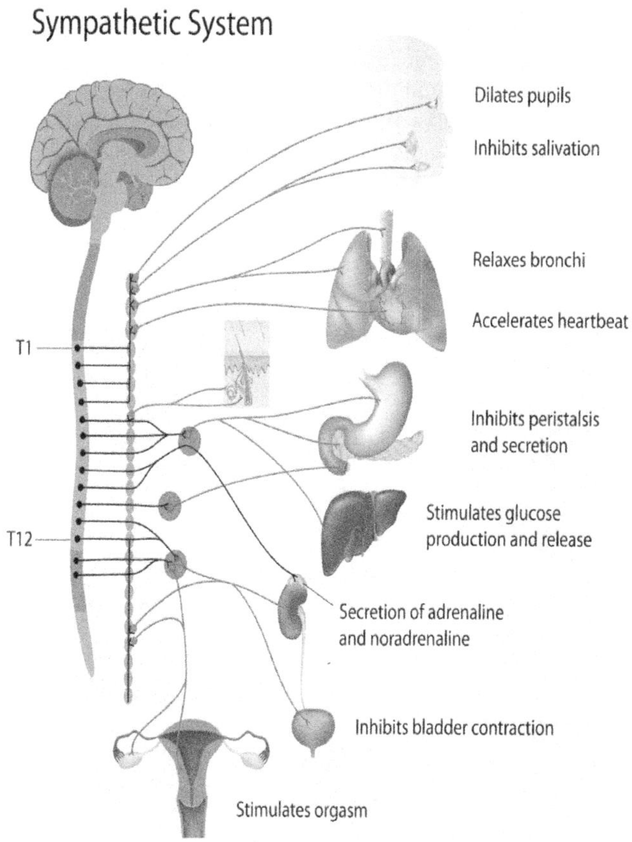


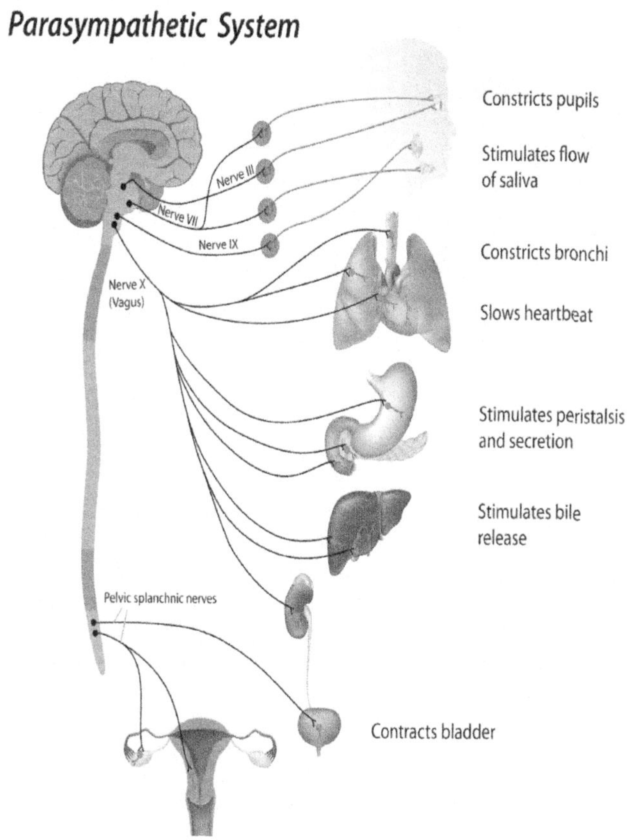

**Medical Tests and Equipment**

**Computerized Axial Tomography(CT/CAT Scan):** Computerized Axial Tomography, also known as CT or CAT Scan, is an imaging technique in which a snapshot is taken of a part of the body on a given body plane. This allows viewing of structures in the body from differing points of view. CT is extremely similar to MRI, but uses X-ray to produce images instead of magnetic fields.

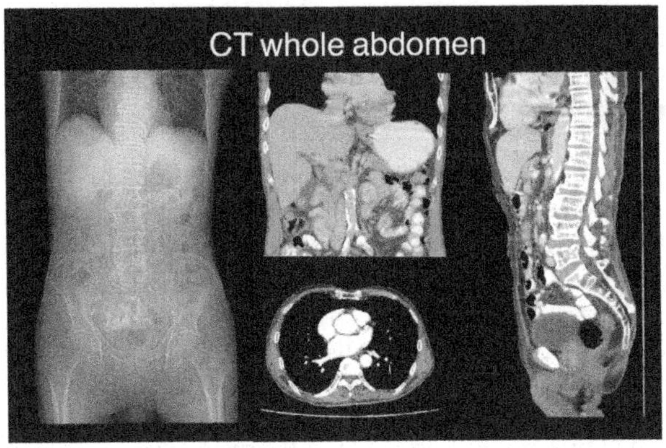


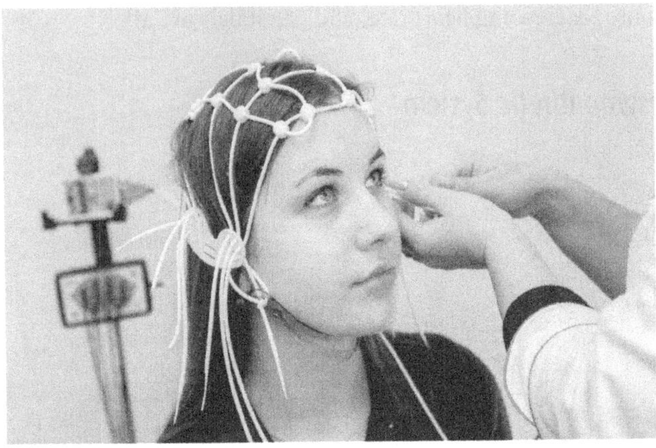

**Electroencephalogram(EEG)**: An electroencephalogram is a test used to detect the electrical activity of the brain. It uses electrodes placed around the head that attach directly to the scalp to detect electric activity. Electroencephalograms are performed to help diagnose brain disorders, such as encephalitis, tumors, epilepsy, and damage to the brain from concussions.

**Myelogram**: A myelogram is an imaging procedure used to view problems that may be occurring in the spinal canal. Special dyes are injected into the spinal column, and the patient is given X-rays, which allow the structures inside the spinal canal to be properly viewed. Myelograms are used to examine conditions such as herniated discs, infections such as meningitis, and tumors in the brain or spinal cord.

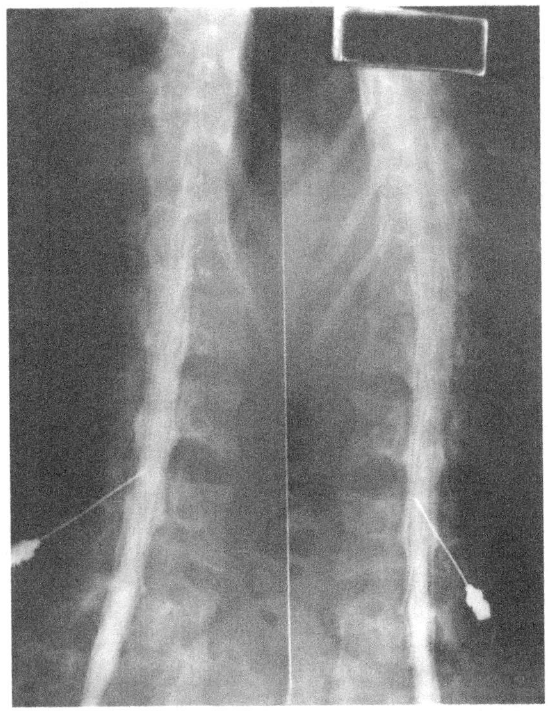

# Nervous System Pathologies

## Alzheimer's Disease

Alzheimer's Disease, the most common form of dementia, is an overarching term for **memory loss**, **confusion**, and a **general loss** of **intellectual abilities**. Alzheimer's is a result of brain tissue gradually dying over time. Increased age is a risk factor of developing Alzheimer's, and becomes much more common after the age of 65 in those affected.

### *Causes*

While the exact cause of Alzheimer's is unknown, environmental factors are the most likely culprit. Few people with Alzheimer's disease develop the disease due to genetic factors.

Two factors strongly contribute to the death of nervous tissue: plaque and tangles. Plaque is the formation of deposits of a protein known as beta-amyloid, which develops in the space between nerves, restricting communication between nerve cells. Tangles are the development of another protein known as tau inside the nerve cells, which can cut off the natural flow of nutrients through cells.

### *Symptoms*

Symptoms begin with difficulty remembering information, such as locations of items or things just learned. As the condition progresses, more brain tissue is lost, and a person may have difficulty making decisions, identifying people or places, and become more irritable or aggressive. Later stages of Alzheimer's may see the loss of the ability to read, write, dance, sing, and other activities learned early in life.

### *Treatments*

There is no cure for Alzheimer's, but there are treatments available that can help manage the condition. Medications may be prescribed that can help with memory loss and other cognitive symptoms. In later stages, other medications may be prescribed that can help with memory, speech, and the ability to perform simpler tasks.

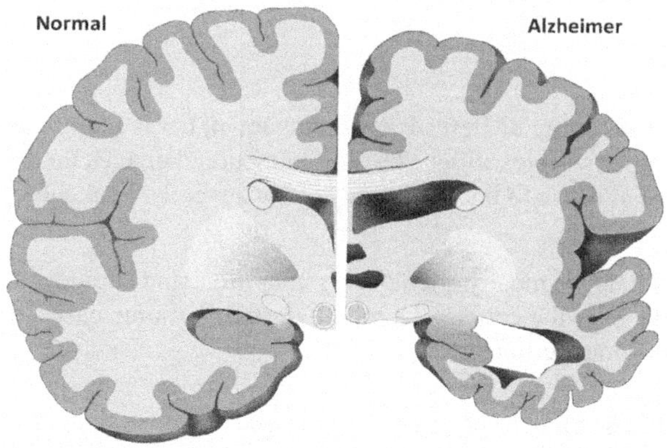


### *Contraindications*

Alzheimer's Disease is not contraindicated, although precautions may be taken in advanced stages of the disease. A person the client knows and is familiar with may stay in the room to assist with the client if the client becomes forgetful regarding their location.

## Amyotrophic Lateral Sclerosis

*(a-: without; my/o-: muscle; -trophic: nourishment)*

Amyotrophic Lateral Sclerosis(ALS) is a **degenerative** disorder affecting **motor neurons**, which control muscles. The nerve degeneration causes **loss** of **voluntary muscle control**, and can eventually lead to death within five years of diagnosis due to respiratory failure. A small percentage of people diagnosed with ALS survive longer than five years.

Amyotrophic Lateral Sclerosis is also known as **Lou Gehrig's Disease**, named for the baseball player who was diagnosed with the condition in 1939.

### *Causes*

The precise cause of ALS is unknown. Genetics seem to play a factor. Men are more likely to develop the condition than women, and it is much more common in people over the age of 50.

## Amyotrophic Lateral Sclerosis (ALS)

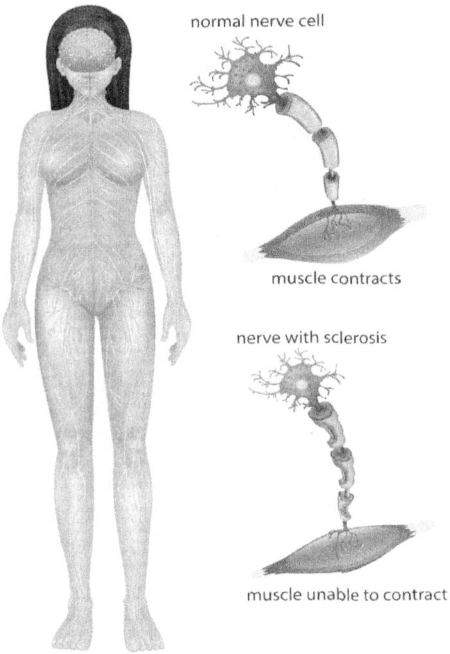


***Symptoms***

Symptoms of ALS begin subtly and may not be noticeable until they become more advanced. A person may experience muscle cramping and twitching, weakness in the muscles of the arms, legs, and neck, trouble chewing and swallowing, and slurred speech as the muscles responsible for vocalization are affected. As the disease progresses, muscle atrophy sets in and the person loses the ability to stand or walk.

***Treatments***

There is no cure for ALS, but treatment options may include medication to assist with muscle pain and cramping, physical therapy and speech therapy, and the use of ventilators as natural breathing support fails.

***Contraindications***

Massage is indicated for Amyotrophic Lateral Sclerosis. In advanced stages, the therapist may need to assist the client on and off the table. Because the muscles have atrophied, lighter pressure should be performed to avoid damaging tissue.

## Bell's Palsy

*(palsy: paralysis)*

Bell's Palsy is a condition affecting the **facial nerve**, causing **paralysis** on **one side of the face**.

***Causes***

The exact cause of Bell's Palsy is unknown, but is likely the result of an attack to the facial nerve(cranial nerve VII) by the herpes simplex virus. The inflammation damages the nerve, causing the muscles of the side of the face controlled by the facial nerve to become paralyzed or severely weakened. The side of the face affected may also become numb.

Bell's Palsy is mostly a temporary condition, and should resolve over the course of a month or two. In some cases, it can become permanent.

***Symptoms***

Symptoms, which are usually only present on one side of the face, include the inability to close the eye, difficulty chewing, twitching of muscles in the face, and watery eyes. These symptoms typically resolve within three weeks at the earliest, but may persist for several months, or even become permanent.

***Treatments***

A person with Bell's Palsy may take corticosteroids to help treat the muscle weakness. Self care, including facial exercises, are recommended.

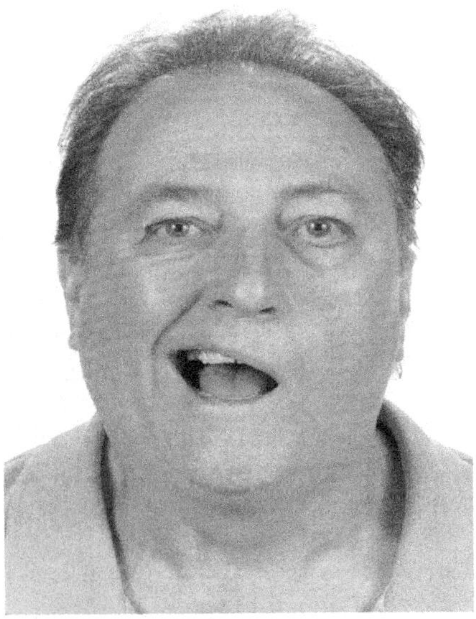

Bell's palsy presenting with paralysis of the left side of the patient's face

***Contraindications***

Bell's Palsy is indicated for massage. The side of the face that is paralyzed should be massaged lightly to avoid damaging any tissue. The client may not be able to tell the therapist if the massage is too deep around facial structures, so lighter massage on the affected area should be performed.

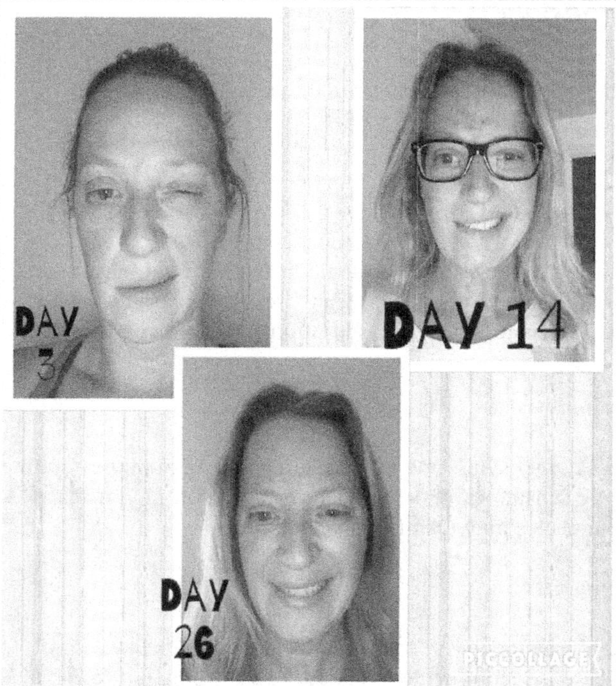


**Melissa, Bell's Palsy**

Tell me about the time you first noticed the effects of Bell's Palsy.

*Aug 30, 2016 I went to a concert. I was having pain in my jaw(the right side) - like a wisdom tooth growing in. And my right eye was so dry. I frequently get earaches so the ear pain (right side) didn't phase me. Aug 31, 2016 I was sitting outside having coffee and reading. The coffee kept dribbling down my face and my eye was so irritated. I tried winking and blinking to help with the irritation but I noticed I couldn't. When I looked in the mirror, my mouth was starting to droop and my eye couldn't close all the way.*

Did you experience any other symptoms?

*Because Bell's Palsy doesn't have any warning signs, the aches, pains, and irritation didn't mean anything. Just a bad day. Prior to BP, I had experienced heachache, neck pain (stiffness), tooth pain, eye irritation, ear ache. And the stress! The stress of everything and not knowing how to deal with certain issues. My anxiety and panic were combined with stress. The doctor thought that was why I got it as intense as I did. The first week of BP my face got worse. The pain in my neck was brutal. I was incredibly fatigued. Most days it took me two hours to get up the energy to drive eight minutes away to pick up my niece.*

Were you prescribed any medications? Or given any exercises to do?

*Yes. An antiviral and a steroid.*

Did these medications help?

*Yes and no. They worked on repairing the nerve, but they also cause other problems - not roid rage, more like roid annoyance which brought on headaches and made my neck a lot tighter.*

How is the Bell's Palsy now? Do you still experience symptoms, or has it resolved?

*From a support group I've learned BP never fully goes away. Meaning lasting effects from it - I am sensitive to light and sound. I get instant headaches when I walk into an office building because of the lighting. My ear will ache in weather changes. I can hear things really sharply but I can't always hear people talking to me. My face is mostly normal, I can tell Idon't smile evenly and my eyes are not the same. I had it for about six weeks before going back to mostly normal.*

Have you received massage therapy on the face since it appeared?

*I was told to get on medication within 72 hours for best results. Most people think they are having a stroke because of the droopiness of the face. I found facial exercises to do and massaged my face & neck 4-6x a day. I did the massage myself since I knew what was causing pain. Emu oil as lotion and a drop of peppermint oil to help with energy. Heating pads were a huge help. A big problem for me was that all food tasted like cardboard. I had that happen a few days before it hit.*

If you were to receive a massage from another person, what would you tell them in regards to the treatment and how to proceed?

*Very gentle on the face, but dig your elbow into my neck.*

## Carpal Tunnel Syndrome

Carpal Tunnel Syndrome is a condition caused by compression of the **median nerve** between the carpals and the **transverse carpal ligament**.

***Causes***

Several factors may contribute to the development of carpal tunnel syndrome, although the most common cause is **repetitive movements**. These repetitive movements can cause straining of the tendons that run through the carpal canal, which can place pressure on the median nerve. If the transverse carpal ligament tightens, it can also place pressure on the median nerve. When pressure is placed on the median nerve, numbness, pain, or tingling sensations may be experienced in the thumb, index, ring, and lateral side of the ring finger.

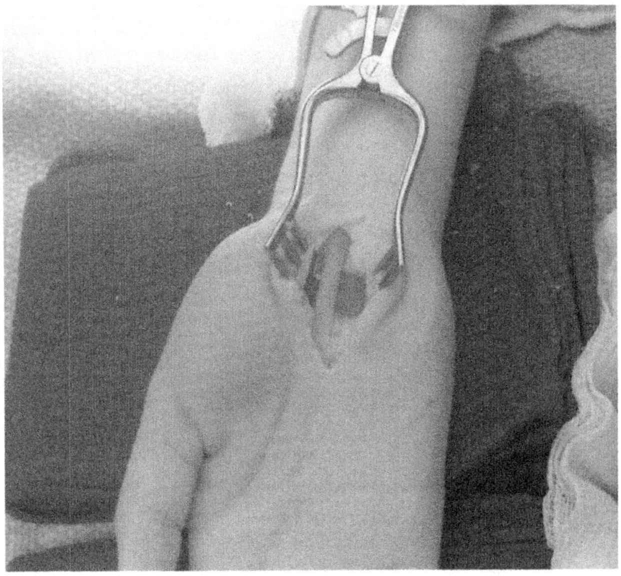

Median nerve, seen above during carpal tunnel release surgery

***Symptoms***

Carpal tunnel syndrome often results in pain, numbness, and tingling sensations in the hand and wrist. Atrophy of the hand muscles may result due to lack of use.

***Treatments***

Several treatments are available for carpal tunnel syndrome. Self-care is recommended, including stretching the forearm and wrist flexors, massaging the transverse carpal ligament and hand muscles, and icing the area. Because carpal tunnel syndrome is often caused by repetitive actions, ceasing these actions is recommended. Non-steroidal anti-inflammatory medications may be prescribed. Surgery to remove the transverse carpal ligament may also be an option if the condition is severe.

***Contraindications***

Massage is indicated for carpal tunnel syndrome. Cross-fiber and circular friction on the transverse carpal ligament should be performed to help loosen adhesions in the area. Application of heat can help soften the ligament, and allow more space in the carpal canal.

## Cerebral Palsy

*(cerebral: brain; palsy: paralysis)*

Cerebral Palsy is a disorder of the **brain**, causing difficulty with **movement** and **muscle tone**. Cerebral palsy is typically caused by **damage** to the **brain** that occurs during development. The most common time damage to the brain causes cerebral palsy is before birth.

As the condition progresses, symptoms appear that may affect posture and the proper development of muscle. This can cause problems with walking, standing, and swallowing, amongst other actions.

The condition affects each person differently, depending on the amount of brain damage suffered. Some people may have mild symptoms, while others may have much more severe symptoms.

***Causes***

Causes of cerebral palsy include infections during pregnancy(such as rubella, chickenpox, herpes, and toxoplasmosis), restricted blood flow to the brain during instances such as pregnancy(such as if the umbilical cord wraps around the baby's neck), infections the fetus may acquire that can damage the brain, or even injury to the head that may occur with falls.

***Symptoms***

Symptoms of cerebral palsy vary with severity. Symptoms involving the muscular aspect of the body may include difficulty walking due to poor muscle development or coordination, difficulty eating or swallowing, problems developing proper speech, especially stiff muscles, tremors, and differing muscle tone throughout the body.

Symptoms involving the brain due to damage may include seizures, difficulty perceiving pain, problems with vision and/or hearing, and difficulty learning. In addition, psychiatric conditions may also be present, such as ADHD.

***Treatments***

There is no cure for cerebral palsy. A person with cerebral palsy will likely need specialist care throughout life. Care is dependent on the symptoms present. If a person has problem with speech, a speech pathologist would be recommended. Physical therapists can help with muscle function. If mental disorders are present, a mental health specialist or psychologist may help. A neurologist may help with any function affected by specific brain damage.

***Contraindications***

Massage is indicated for clients with cerebral palsy. Depending on severity, the therapist may need to help the client on and off the table.

## Concussion

A concussion is an **injury** to the **brain**, usually caused by a **blow to the head**, that may impair brain function temporarily. Loss of consciousness and tremors may result, although they aren't common.

***Causes***

A concussion is caused by trauma to the head, which causes the brain to violently collide with the inner lining of the skull, damaging it. Common causes of concussions are automobile accidents and contact sports such as football, hockey, or mixed martial arts. Having a prior concussion may make concussions easier to occur with subsequent head trauma.

***Symptoms***

Acute symptoms of a concussion may include dizziness, nausea and vomiting, headache, loss of consciousness, confusion, ringing ears, and loss of short term memory around the time of the concussion.

A person may experience prolonged headaches, dizziness, and difficulty processing information for days after experiencing a concussion. Long-term, if a person has suffered multiple concussions throughout life, they may be at risk of developing permanent brain damage, a condition known as Chronic Traumatic Encephalopathy, or CTE. This can cause symptoms similar to Alzheimer's Disease, such as loss of memory, confusion, depression, and more.

***Treatments***

After suffering a concussion, a person should rest and avoid any activity that may over-stimulate the brain, such as reading, writing, watching television, or playing video games. A person should wait until receiving medical clearance before returning to sports. Headaches resulting from concussion may be treated with pain relievers such as acetaminophen, but blood thinners such as aspirin should be avoided due to risk of bleeding in the brain.

***Contraindications***

In the acute stage immediately following a concussion, massage is considered an absolute contraindication. After a few days and clearance from a doctor, massage may be performed. People who have suffered from a concussion should avoid any activity that may excessively stimulate the brain, and massage may be one of those.

## Encephalitis

*(encephal-: brain; -itis: inflammation)*

Encephalitis is primarily a **viral** infection that results in **inflammation** of the **brain**.

***Causes***

Causes of encephalitis vary, but may include mosquito-borne viruses, such as West Nile, the herpes simplex virus, and the rabies virus. Symptoms of encephalitis are usually mild, with the infected person suffering no more than flu-like symptoms, but severe cases may result in brain damage or death.

***Symptoms***

Symptoms of encephalitis vary depending on severity. Mild cases result in flu-like symptoms, such as fever, headache, general body ache, and fatigue. More severe cases may result in unconsciousness, seizures, weakness, and difficulty speaking or hearing.

***Treatments***

Because most cases of encephalitis are mild, treatment often consists of bed rest, and letting the virus work through its course. Antiviral medications may also be administered via an IV if the infection is more severe.

***Contraindications***

Because encephalitis is contagious and a serious medical condition, it is an absolute contraindication. Massage may be performed after the condition has completely resolved.

## Epilepsy

*(epi-: above; -lepsy: seizure)*

Epilepsy is a nervous disorder usually caused by **over-stimulation** of the **brain**, which may produce **seizures**. Seizure severity varies, and a person may not be diagnosed with epilepsy unless they have experienced two or more seizures with unknown causes.

A seizure that occurs in only one specific region of the brain is called a focal seizure. A seizure that occurs in every part of the brain is known as a generalized seizure.

***Causes***

In roughly half of people who have been diagnosed with epilepsy, there is no known cause. Trauma to the head or damage to the brain, such as strokes, may cause epilepsy. Genetics may play a role in epilepsy. Infections such as meningitis or encephalitis may also lead to epilepsy.

***Symptoms***

While symptoms vary, common symptoms include seizures, loss of consciousness, and staring blankly for a few moments. Epilepsy commonly stops occurring on its own.

***Treatments***

Anti-epileptic medications are the most common form of treatment for people with chronic epilepsy. If seizures persist, surgery may be performed in which the part of the brain suffering from seizures is removed, as long as that part of the brain is not responsible for vital functions of the body.

***Contraindications***

Massage on a client with epilepsy is indicated, however, precautions should be taken. If a trigger is known, it should be avoided. If a client has a seizure while receiving massage, the therapist should not attempt to put fingers in the client's mouth to prevent choking on the tongue, or catch the client if they fall off the table. The therapist should stay with the client and time the seizure. If the seizure lasts for five minutes or longer, or another seizure occurs quickly after the initial seizure, medical treatment should be sought immediately.

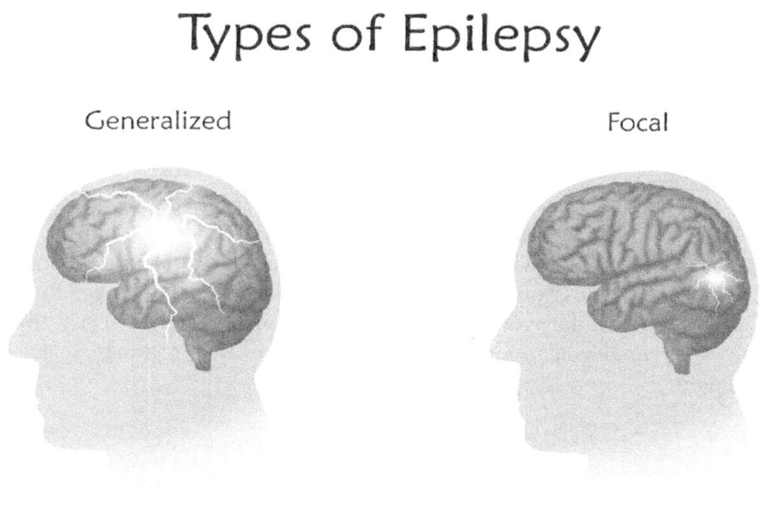


## Meningitis

*(mening-: meninges; -itis: inflammation)*

Meningitis is **inflammation** of the **meninges**, protective connective tissue surrounding the brain and spinal cord. In the US, meningitis is most commonly caused by **viral infection**. However, certain **bacterial** and **fungal infections** may also cause meningitis. Bacterial meningitis is the most severe form of meningitis, usually preceded by a sinus or ear infection.

### *Causes*

Being exposed to a pathogen, such as streptococci bacterium, or West Nile virus, are the causes of meningitis. Exposure to these may differ, and contracting them does not necessarily mean a person will develop meningitis. West Nile virus, which also may cause encephalitis, is often transmitted by mosquitoes.

Rarely, meningitis may be caused by things that are not infectious, such as medications or allergies to certain chemicals.

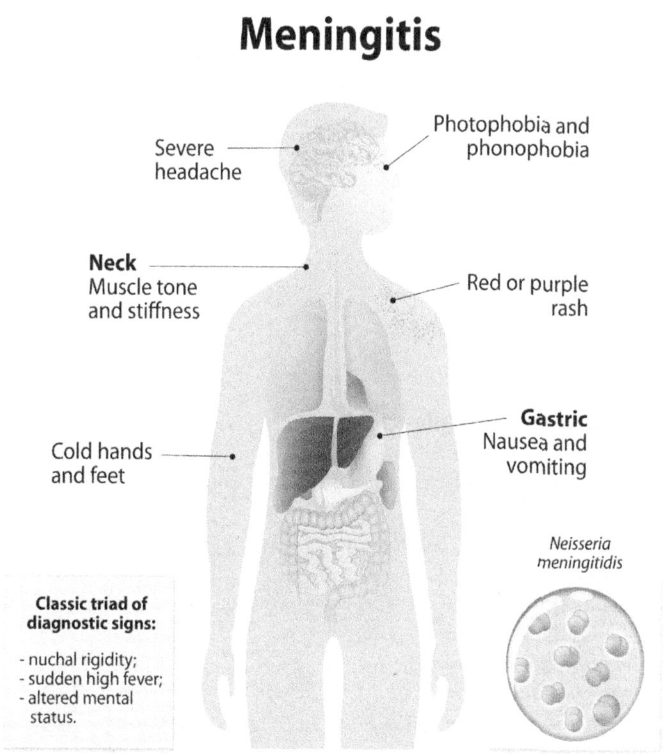


### *Symptoms*

Symptoms vary depending on the underlying cause. Viral meningitis may present with symptoms extremely similar to influenza, and will likely clear up on their own within a couple weeks. Fever, headache, nausea, vomiting, and an unusually stiff neck are symptoms to watch for. Meningitis is considered a medical emergency, and a person with suspected meningitis should be seen by a medical professional right away.

### *Treatments*

Bacterial meningitis is treated with intravenous antibiotics to combat the infection, and a course of corticosteroids to prevent inflammation in the brain. Draining the infection from the sinuses may be helpful. Viral meningitis, however, is far less serious, and often clears up after a couple weeks. Treatment for viral meningitis is simply rest and increasing fluid intake. Pain relievers may also help if a person has general body aches or is suffering from mild fever.

***Contraindications***

Because meningitis is a contagious condition, it is an absolute contraindication to massage. Massage may be performed after the condition has completely resolved.

## Multiple Sclerosis

*(scler-: hard; -osis: condition)*

Multiple Sclerosis is an **autoimmune** disorder, affecting the **myelin sheaths** that protect the axons of the Nervous System.

***Causes***

The cause of Multiple Sclerosis is unknown, but may be hereditary, and even environmental factors have been linked to the development of the disease. The disease begins with the body's immune system attacking the myelin sheaths, the protective fatty layers surrounding axons. These sheaths help to insulate the axons and prevent damage to the axons. When the myelin sheath is attacked and destroyed, it exposes the axons, which can have many different effects. Impulses traveling along an axon may terminate at the site of myelin degeneration, which may cause loss of functions. Scar tissue may form over the axons, which leads to extreme pain.

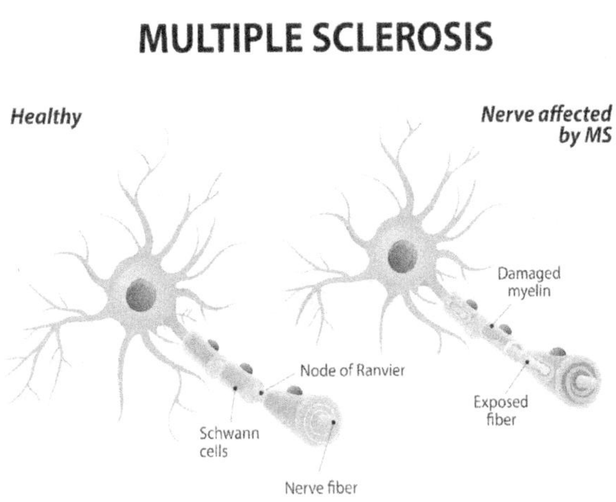


***Symptoms***

Symptoms of Multiple Sclerosis in acute stages include pain, weakness, fatigue, numbness(usually in the face), tingling sensation, blurry vision, and difficulty walking.

***Treatments***

There is no cure for Multiple Sclerosis. People may be prescribed disease-altering drugs that may suppress the functions of the immune system. People may seek other means of managing Multiple Sclerosis and the accompanying pain and fatigue, including massage therapy, yoga, and meditation.

***Contraindications***

Massage in the acute stage of Multiple Sclerosis may be performed, but it is highly unlikely a client will seek massage because of the pain involved. Modalities that do not involve touching, such as Reiki, may be recommended and performed in these instances. In the post-acute stage, massage may be performed.

**Rhiannon, Multiple Sclerosis**

How long has it been since you were diagnosed with Multiple Sclerosis?

*I was diagnosed in February of 2014.*

What symptoms were you experiencing that led you to seeing a doctor?

*Well, it started back in November of 2013, I woke up and my middle through pinky fingers on my left hand were numb and tingly. Then by the time I was admitted in the hospital it had kind of slowly progressed to being the entire right side of my body from the top of my head to the tips of my toes. The first time I went to the doctor was in January, and I tried three separate times at three separate urgent cares and doctors offices before I finally went to the emergency room. By the time I ended up in the ER not only was I half numb and tingly, but my dexterity and vision were off, I had major anxiety, my speech and dexterity were off, and the whole left side of my body was puffy.*

*When I was admitted they said my white blood cell count was also off. Both the nurses and I were in the belief that I would be diagnosed with leukemia of some kind.*

What led the doctors to come to the conclusion it was MS and not leukemia?

*Ultimately it was when I had my spinal tap. The MRI's were showing that it was likely, but the spinal tap definitively showed it was MS.*

What does a spinal tap show that indicates MS?

*To be honest with you I'm not totally sure. Something to do with the way the fluid separates, and if certain things grow or don't grow inside of it. I think they send it to a lab to sit and be tested for 24-48 hours.*

What was your initial reaction after receiving the diagnosis?

*The very first thought I had was "Oh my God, Montel Williams!" And then I looked at my mom, who is the toughest lady I know, and she started to cry. Then I completely lost it and cried super hard off and on for the rest of the week I was in the hospital. Then I had a honeymoon period where I would joke and laugh about it. About six weeks after my diagnosis the other shoe dropped and I was in a really heavy depression for about 3 or 4 months. And then something just kind of clicked inside of me and I refused to let it rule my life.*

Did you know what MS was before the diagnosis?

*Yes, sort of. I remember coming home from high school and turning on the TV and listening to the Montel Williams talk show, and I remembered when he retired and announced his MS diagnosis and I thought "Wow, his career is over." So that was my first thought when I was diagnosed, "Oh no, my life is over." What I did NOT know, is that there are four different types of MS, and that every person affected has a different path with the disease. And the science of treating MS has really come along extensively in the last 20 years. Managing the disease is much more achievable than it used to be.*

How has MS impacted your every-day life?

*Well, for the first year I wasn't on any medication, and every day was like a roll of the dice. Some mornings I would wake up feeling fine and be fine all day. Some days I would wake up and be super tingly and numb, with heavy brain fog and slurred speech. Some days I'd start fine and end terrible, or vice versa. Once I started my medication Gilenya, it's been mostly smooth sailing. Once in a blue moon I'll get a little tingly or wobbly, or my speech will be funny, but usually it only happens if I'm absolutely exhausted, and once I get a really good night's sleep and take it easy for a few days it goes away. The only symptom I deal with on a regular basis is heat intolerance. Many people with MS have the same issue, our bodies just do not regulate temperature very well. The summertime can feel terrible, it's like I'm walking through cement waste deep inside a volcano. It's miserable. But I've gotten pretty savvy with avoiding too much heat.*

So you experience periods of remission and exacerbation. How long do these periods typically last, or is it pretty varied?

*When I was med free I had about 6 or 7 mini relapse/exacerbations, being on medication the things I experience are just little micro flares, really. I haven't had a full relapse since being diagnosed, thankfully. I feel very fortunate to have a handle on it now.*

How much pain does the MS cause when you experience a flare-up?

*Med free- anywhere from minor to excruciating. On Med- discomfort to medium level pain. Once in a super super blue moon I'll get what's called an MS hug, and that is excruciating. It's like someone squeezing the life out of your torso, it's hard to breathe or move.*

Have you received massage therapy since your diagnosis?

*Not professionally, no. I feel like it would be super helpful with fatigue though.*

In the acute stage, do you think you would want to receive a massage?

*Yes.*

## Myasthenia Gravis

*(my-: muscle; asthenia: weak; gravis: grave)*

Myasthenia Gravis is a condition that affects the ability to use muscles usually under **voluntary control**. Myasthenia gravis is an **autoimmune** disorder, in which the immune system attacks **acetylcholine receptor sites** in the muscles, which prevent proper communication between nerves and muscles to take place. This can cause the muscles to become weak and atrophy as a result.

***Causes***

The exact cause of myasthenia gravis is unknown, but it is thought that the thymus gland produces antibodies directly responsible for reducing nerve transmission to muscles. There may be a connection to abnormally large thymus glands or tumors in the thymus and the development of myasthenia gravis.

***Symptoms***

People with myasthenia gravis experience muscle weakness, usually in the eyes, face, throat, neck, arms, and legs. In regards to the eyes, it can cause the eyelids to droop. Trouble speaking or swallowing may occur, and it may also affect facial expressions.

***Treatments***

Because myasthenia gravis is an autoimmune disorder, immunosuppressants are often used to combat the condition. Other medications, such as pyridostigmine, allow better communication between muscles and nerves, and may be prescribed. If a tumor is present in the thymus, surgery to remove it may be performed.

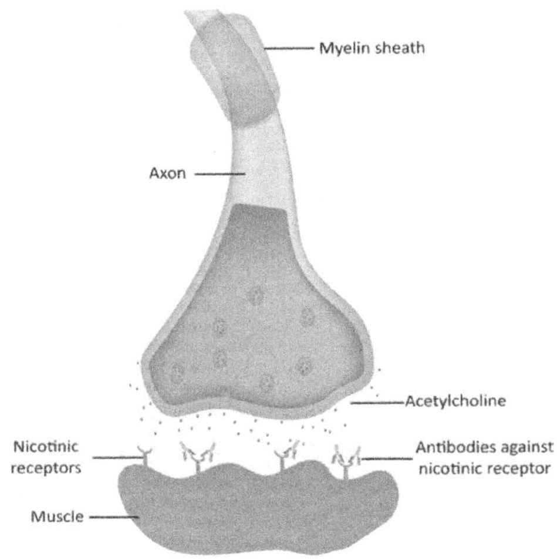


***Contraindications***

Massage may be performed on a client with myasthenia gravis. If a tumor is present on the thymus, the area should be avoided.

## Paralysis

*(paraleyin: disable)*

Paralysis is a **loss of function** of a part of the body. This condition can affect a small area, or a large portion of the body.

***Causes***

Paralysis is caused by **damage** to a nerve that innervates a muscle or muscles. When a nerve is damaged, it can cause weakness(partial paralysis) in a muscle, making it extremely difficult to use, or even result in complete loss of function. The three main types of paralysis that result in complete loss of function are paraplegia, quadriplegia, and hemiplegia.

Paraplegia is paralysis affecting the lower limbs. This is typically caused by an injury to the spinal cord, but may also be caused by conditions such as spina bifida.

Quadriplegia(also known as tetraplegia) is paralysis affecting all four limbs and the trunk. This is typically caused by an injury to the spinal cord around the C4 vertebrae, which eliminates nerve supply to the limbs.

Hemiplegia is paralysis that affects one side(hemisphere) of the body. This is typically caused by a stroke, transient ischemic attack, or even multiple sclerosis.

***Symptoms***

Primarily, paralysis results in loss of sensation. Depending on which type of paralysis, different parts of the body may lose sensation. In the initial acute stage of paralysis, a person may experience weakness, extreme pain in the back, head, or neck, difficulty walking or standing, difficulty breathing, and loss of control over the bladder or bowels. In the acute stage, a person needs medical attention immediately.

***Treatments***

Treatment for paralysis may be helpful in cases of partial paralysis, where there is still some function. Physical and occupational therapy may also help the nervous tissue regenerate.

***Contraindications***

Massage may be performed on an area that is paralyzed. Because the muscles involved will be atrophied, massage should be light to avoid damaging underlying tissue. Stretching and range-of-motion exercises may be performed to help with muscle elasticity.

## Parkinson's Disease

Parkinson's Disease is a motor disease that results in **trembling** due to a loss of the neurotransmitter **dopamine**.

***Causes***

There is no known cause of Parkinson's Disease. Neurons in the brain that produce dopamine are gradually destroyed. Dopamine is the neurotransmitter that stabilizes the body during motor movements, especially fine movements like writing. When dopamine levels in the body drop, trembling and shaking increases. Over time, as dopamine levels drop, the trembling increases. As dopamine continues to drop, larger movements become affected, like walking and talking.

***Symptoms***

Symptoms of Parkinson's Disease include tremors, which usually begin in the hands and fingers and advance to larger body areas, difficulty writing, slower movement, difficulty in speech, and the loss of movements such as blinking.

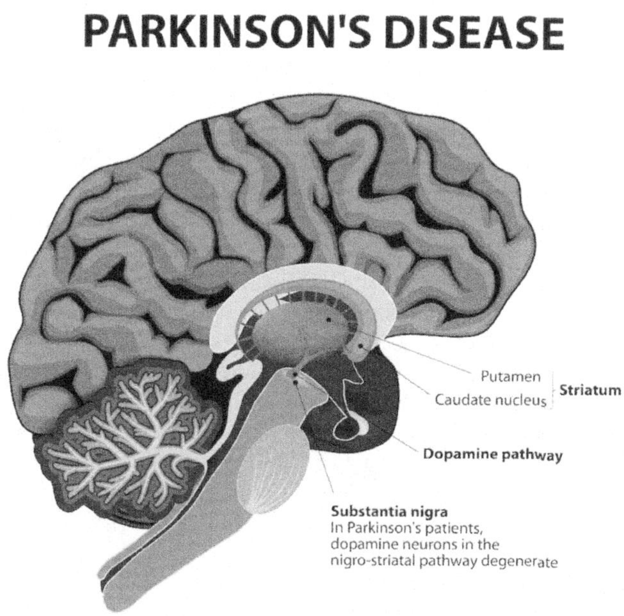


***Treatments***

While there is no cure for Parkinson's Disease, treatments are available to help manage the condition, including dopamine replacement medications.

***Contraindications***

Massage is indicated for clients with Parkinson's Disease. In advanced stages, when a client is unable to lie on a table without the entire body trembling, a doctor's note may be requested. In these advanced stages, the therapist may need to help the client on and off the table.

## Sciatica

Sciatica is a condition causing pain radiating down the buttocks, posterior thigh, and leg.

***Causes***

Sciatica is most commonly caused by a **herniated disc** in the lumbar vertebrae, which puts compression on the nerves that comprise the **sciatic nerve**. Bone spurs may also place pressure on the nerves.

Piriformis Syndrome is often confused with sciatica. Piriformis syndrome is caused by tightness in the piriformis muscle, which may place substantial pressure on the sciatic nerve.

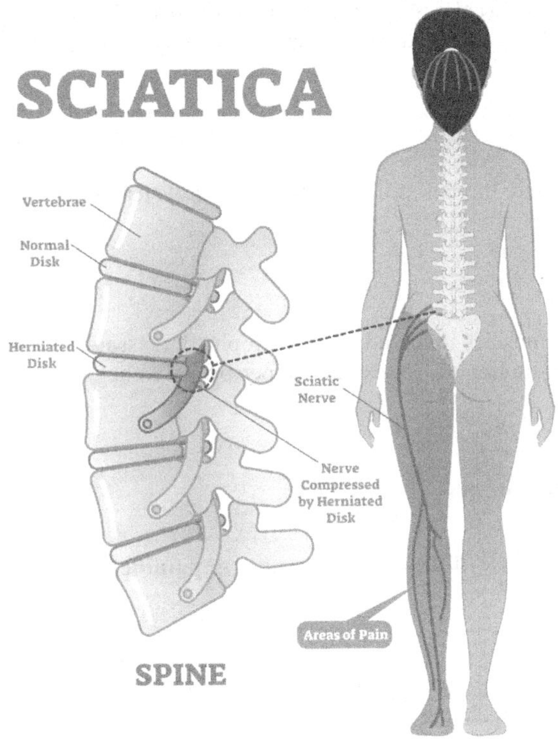


***Symptoms***

The primary symptom of sciatica is pain in the posterior leg, thigh, and glutes, usually only on one side of the body. There may also be numbness and tingling in the affected area.

***Treatments***

Treatment for sciatica may include physical therapy, anti-inflammatory medications, or surgery if the condition is severe enough.

***Contraindications***

Massage is indicated for sciatica. However, if sciatica is the result of a herniated disc, the site of disc herniation should be considered a local contraindication. Stretching techniques, especially in the glutes, may help ease some pain associated with sciatica.

## Spina Bifida

*(spina: spine; bifida: split)*

Spina Bifida is a **congenital** condition, caused by the **spinal cord** and **vertebrae not forming properly**. During development, the neural tube(which forms into the brain and spinal cord and associated structures) fails to close properly in one portion. This can cause problems in the development of the spinal cord and vertebral column. A portion of the spinal cord and nerves may protrude from their usual location into the back.

There are three types of spina bifida: Spina Bifida Occulta, Meningocele, and Myelomeningocele. Spina bifida occulta is the least severe, and people who have it may not even know it. Only a small portion of the vertebral column doesn't form properly. In meningocele, the meninges protrude through the opening created by the portion of the vertebrae not formed properly. The protrusion creates a fluid-filled sac, which does not contain any portion of the spinal cord. Myelomeningocele, the most severe form of spina bifida, is caused by numerous openings in the vertebral column in the lower back, causing the spinal cord and protective membranes to protrude through them. This can result in a visual sac in the lower back.

***Causes***

There is no known cause of spina bifida, although genetics may play a factor. Other factors that may contribute include a lack of vitamin B-9(folate) during pregnancy, certain medications such as anti-seizure medications, and obesity.

***Symptoms***

Symptoms of spina bifida vary based on severity and type of spina bifida. Spina bifida occulta and meningocele often present with no symptoms. Myelomeningocele may make a person more susceptible to serious infection, as the sac may be visible through the skin, and isn't given an extra layer of protection provided by the skin.

People with spina bifida may have difficulty walking and problems with waste elimination, amongst other less severe symptoms.

***Treatments***

Treatment may not be required for spina bifida occulta. Other times, treatment is required. If a doctor detects the presence of spina bifida before birth during an ultrasound, pre-birth surgery may be performed before the 26th week to repair the defect. Meningocele requires surgery to place the meninges back into the vertebral column and repair the opening, and is performed after birth. Surgery for myelomeningocele is also performed after birth, and much like surgery for meningocele, places the nerves and tissues back into the vertebral column, and the openings are repaired.

***Contraindications***

Spina bifida is considered a local contraindication and the area should be avoided.

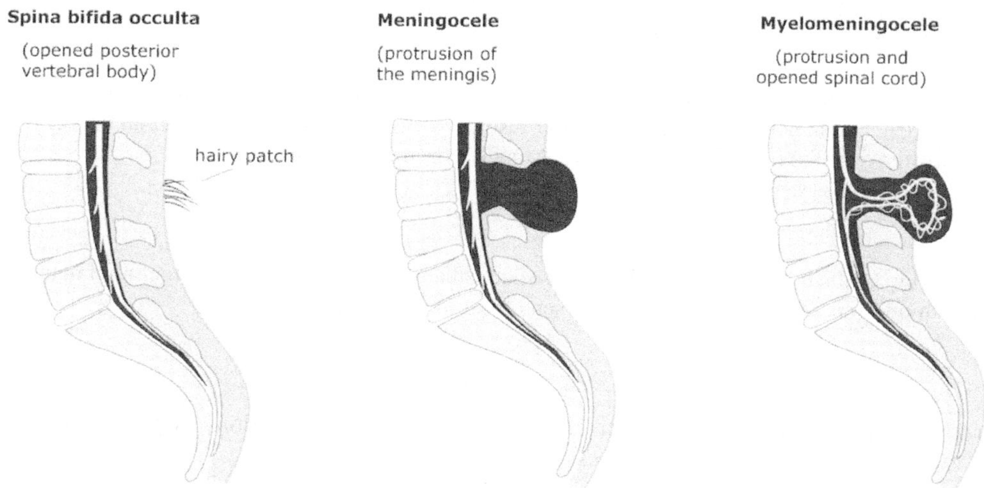


## Thoracic Outlet Syndrome

Thoracic Outlet Syndrome is a condition caused by **compression** of **nerves** and **blood vessels** passing through the **thoracic outlet**.

***Causes***

Thoracic outlet syndrome may be caused by tight muscles, including **pectoralis minor** and **scalenes**, obesity, and tumors in the neck, such as those seen in Non-Hodgkin's Lymphoma.

***Symptoms***

Pressure placed on the nerves and blood vessels may cause pain, numbness, and weakness in the upper limb. If a blood vessel is compressed, it may cause the hand to turn a bluish color due to lack of circulation, cause pain and fatigue in the arm, and coldness in the hands and fingers. If a nerve is compressed, numbness in the limb and atrophy of the muscles innervated by the nerve may result.

***Treatments***

Treatments primarily consist of stretching of the tight muscles to release pressure on the nerves and blood vessels. In the case of a tumor, surgery to remove the tumor may be required.

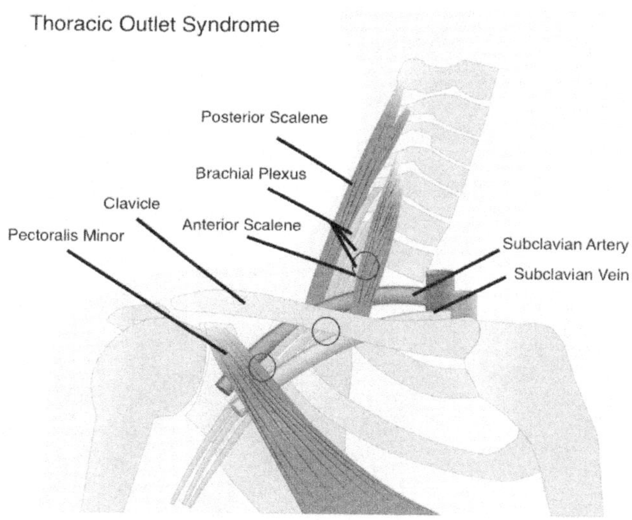

*Contraindications*

Massage is generally indicated for thoracic outlet syndrome. Massaging the scalenes and pectoralis minor may assist in releasing pressure on the area, returning sufficient blood supply to the area. Sensation may return to the upper limb as a result. If thoracic outlet syndrome is the result of tumors, the area should be avoided, and massage would be a local contraindication.

## Trigeminal Neuralgia

*(neur-: nerve; -algia: pain)*

Trigeminal Neuralgia is a chronic condition causing **extreme pain** in the **face**.

*Causes*

The **trigeminal nerve**(cranial nerve V) sends sensory information from the face to the brain. When a blood vessel comes into contact with the trigeminal nerve at the brain stem, it results in dysfunction of the trigeminal nerve. This dysfunction results in hyper-sensitivity of the face, making even light touch extremely painful.

*Symptoms*

Extreme pain in the face, which may last from days to weeks, is the primary symptom of trigeminal neuralgia. This pain is typically only felt in one side of the face, but may worsen over time.

*Treatments*

Treatments for trigeminal neuralgia include medications to reduce pain, botox injections, or possible surgery to reduce pressure on the trigeminal nerve caused by blood vessels.

*Contraindications*

Massage for trigeminal neuralgia is generally not contraindicated, but everything is dependent on the severity of pain experienced by the client. If pain is severe, massage may be considered a local contraindication, or the client may not want to be massaged at all and the appointment would need to be rescheduled. If massage is able to be performed, the therapist should not use a face rest, instead opting to use a pillow for the client to rest their head upon while prone.

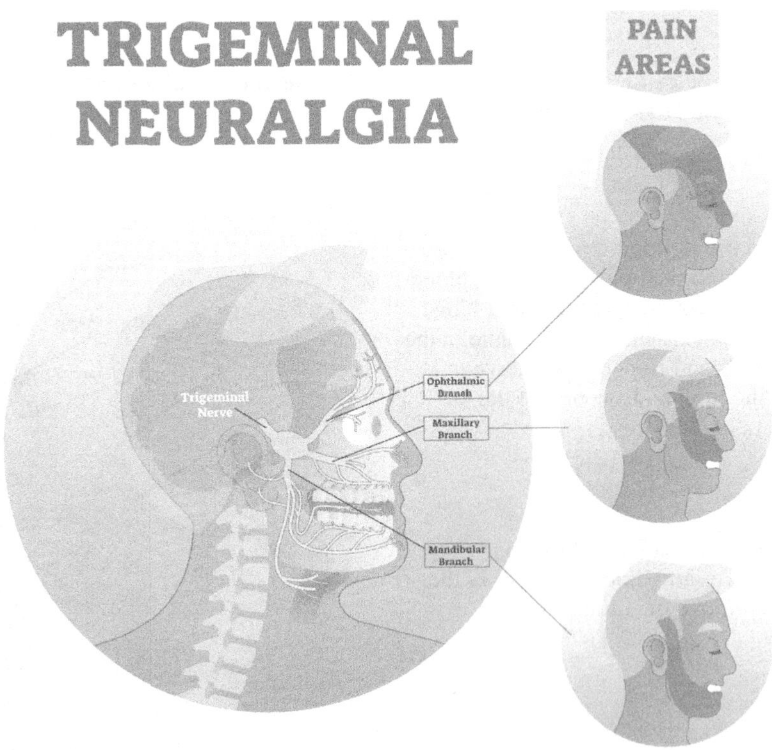

# Nervous Pathologies

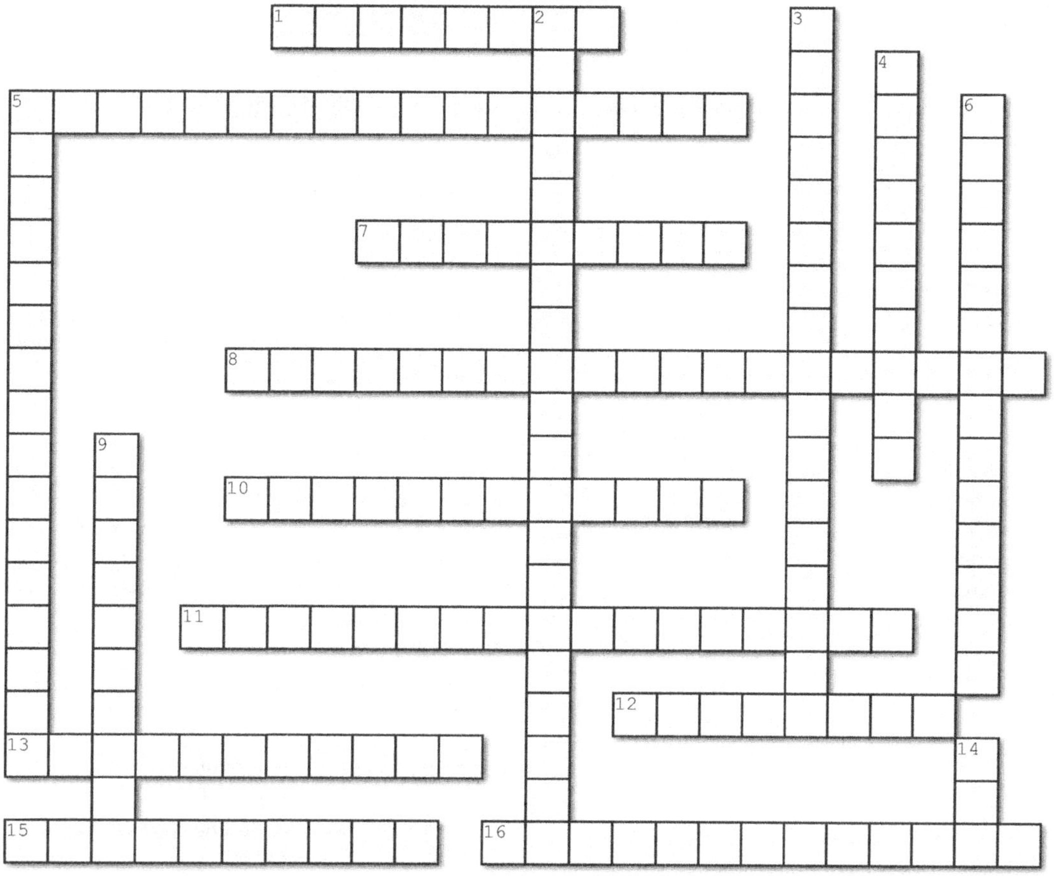


## Across

**1.** Compression of the sciatic nerve, most commonly the result of a herniated disc in the lumbar region
**5.** Degeneration of myelin sheaths in the central nervous system
**7.** Loss of function of part of the body
**8.** Hyper-sensitivity of the face due to irritation of cranial nerve V
**10.** Inflammation of the brain resulting from a viral infection
**11.** Reduction of neurotransmitter dopamine, results in trembling or shaking
**12.** Over-stimulation of the brain, which may result in seizures
**13.** Failure of the neural tube to form properly, which may cause part of the spinal cord to protrude from the vertebral column
**15.** Inflammation of the meninges, most commonly caused by a viral infection
**16.** Damage to the brain during brain development, causing difficulty with movement and muscle tone

## Down

**2.** Compression of the median nerve by the transverse carpal ligament
**3.** The most common form of dementia
**4.** Paralysis of one side of the face, caused by irritation of the facial nerve
**5.** Autoimmune disorder that attacks the acetylcholine receptor sites in muscles, affecting voluntary movements
**6.** Compression of nerves and blood vessels going into the arm by tight muscles in and near the neck
**9.** An injury to the brain resulting from a blow to the head
**14.** Abbreviation, degenerative disorder affecting motor neurons that causes a loss of voluntary muscle control over time

Answer Key on Page 287

# Nervous Quiz

1. The sympathetic nervous system is also referred to as
A. Housekeeping
B. Rest and digest
C. Fight or flight
D. Central

2. Dopamine is an example of a
A. Neurotransmitter
B. Synapse
C. Neuron
D. Dendrite

3. Autoimmune disorder affecting myelin sheaths in the central nervous system
A. Multiple sclerosis
B. Myasthenia gravis
C. Parkinson's disease
D. Alzheimer's disease

4. There are how many pairs of spinal nerves in the peripheral nervous system
A. 24
B. 12
C. 18
D. 31

5. Motor axons carry nerve impulses
A. Towards the cerebellum
B. Towards the brain
C. Away from the brain
D. Away from muscle

6. Cranial nerve VII is involved in
A. Bell's palsy
B. Cerebral palsy
C. Trigeminal neuralgia
D. Hemotaxis

7. Compression of the following nerve by the transverse carpal ligament results in carpal tunnel syndrome
A. Median
B. Ulnar
C. Radial
D. Musculocutaneous

8. Multiple sclerosis is what type of disorder
A. Bacterial
B. Autoimmune
C. Viral
D. Ulcerative

9. A person trembling during fine motor movements is a sign of
A. Alzheimer's disease
B. Parkinson's disease
C. Anemia
D. Bell's palsy

10. Infection caused by bacteria or virus that causes inflammation of the meninges, resulting in vomiting, headache, and fever
A. Osteomyelitis
B. Meningitis
C. Impetigo
D. Encephalitis

11. Paralysis of one half of the face, caused by stimulation of the Herpes Simplex virus, which affects the Facial nerve
A. Graves' disease
B. Cerebral palsy
C. Trigeminal neuralgia
D. Bell's palsy

12. If a client presents with trigeminal neuralgia, the best modification to the massage table would be
A. Remove the head rest and have client lay with their head turned to the side, or supine
B. Elevate the right hip with bolsters
C. Only position the client in a semi-reclined position
D. Have the client place both arms across the chest to relax the platysma

13. Congenital condition in which the spine and vertebrae do not form properly, causing the spinal cord to protrude through the defective portion of the spine
A. Myasthenia gravis
B. Spina bifida
C. Amyotrophic lateral sclerosis
D. Trigeminal neuralgia

14. Over-stimulation of the brain, which may cause seizures
A. Sciatica
B. Encephalitis
C. Meningitis
D. Epilepsy

15. Viral infection commonly spread by mosquitoes that causes inflammation of the brain
A. Meningitis
B. Alzheimer's disease
C. Encephalitis
D. Bell's palsy

Answer Key on Page 289

# Reproductive System and Pathologies

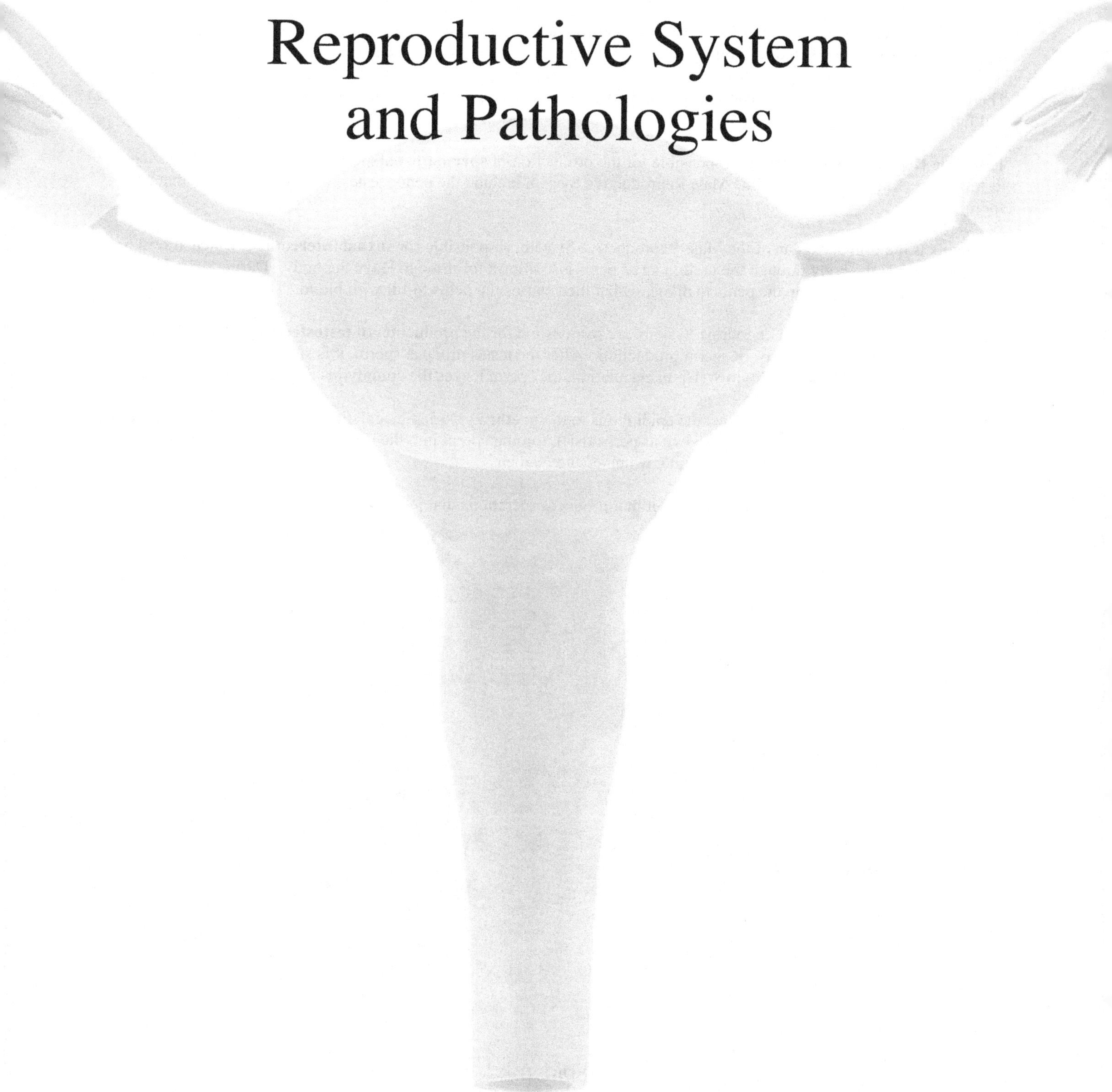

# Reproductive System

The Reproductive System is responsible for **reproduction,** or the creation of offspring. Many organs and structures in the reproductive system are shared with other body systems, such as the urethra, testes, and ovaries.

There are two subcategories: the **Male Reproductive System** and **Female Reproductive System**. Each vary in structures and function.

The **Male Reproductive System** is responsible for the production of **spermatozoa**(sperm) and male hormones, such as testosterone. Major structures of the Male Reproductive System include the penis, testes, scrotum, and ducts that carry sperm.

The **penis** is the primary organ of the Male Reproductive System, responsible for **sexual intercourse**, which allows passage of sperm outside the body through the urethra. The penis also allows for urine to leave the body. During sexual arousal, nerves cause blood vessels in the penis to dilate, which then causes the penis to fill with blood. This results in an erection.

The **testes**, as discussed in the Endocrine System, are responsible for the production of **testosterone**. They are also responsible for **spermatogenesis**, or sperm production. After the testes produce sperm, it is stored in a tube located atop each testicle, known as the **epididymis**. Upon ejaculation, the sperm leaves the epididymis and enters the vas deferens.

The **vas deferens** are tubes that connect the epididymis to the **urethra**. During ejaculation, smooth muscle in the walls of the vas deferens contract rhythmically(known as peristalsis), forcing sperm into the urethra. The sperm mixes with secretions from structures such as the prostate, which creates semen.

The **prostate** is a gland located near the bladder that produces secretions that join with sperm to create **semen**.

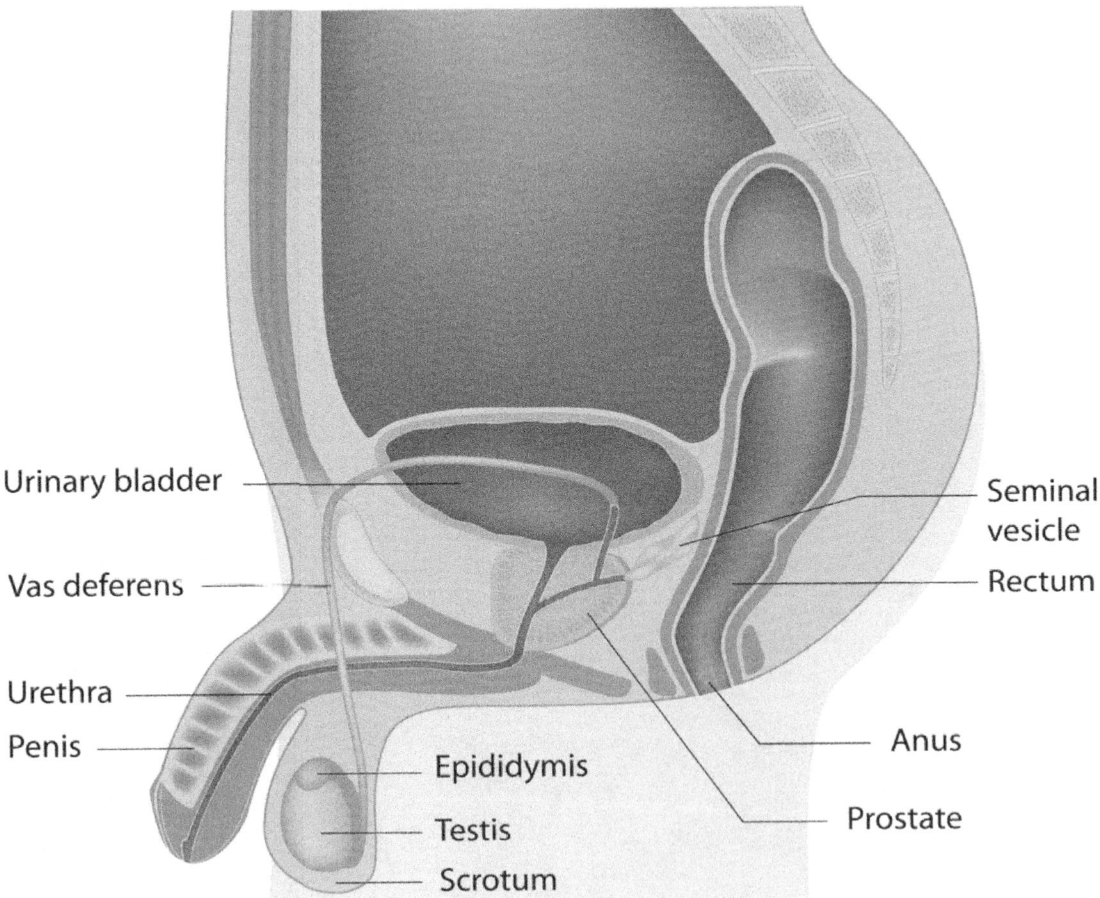

The **Female Reproductive System** is responsible for the production of **egg cells**, estrogen, progesterone, and **fetal development**. Major structures of the Female Reproductive System include the vagina, ovaries, fallopian tubes, uterus, and cervix.

The **vagina** is the **passageway** located between the cervix and the opening to the outside of the body. The vagina is often confused with the outer, visible portion, known as the vulva. The vagina allows a passageway for the penis during sexual intercourse.

The **ovaries**, as discussed in the endocrine system, are responsible for the production of estrogen and progesterone. The ovaries are also the structures that produce and release **egg cells(oocytes)** in women. Eggs are typically released once a month from one ovary.

The **fallopian tubes** allow **passage** of oocytes from the ovaries to the uterus. Fertilization most commonly occurs in the fallopian tubes.

The **uterus** is an inverted pear-shaped organ responsible for the **development of a fetus**. Upon fertilization, the embryo attaches to the wall of the uterus. The placenta develops, which connects to the embryo, providing it with blood flow and nutrients to help it grow. During childbirth, the placenta detaches from the uterus and exits through the cervix and vagina.

The **cervix** is a narrow, circular passage that connects the **vagina to the uterus**. During pregnancy, the cervix is closed by a thick layer of mucous. During childbirth, the cervix dilates widely, which allows a passage for the child to pass through.

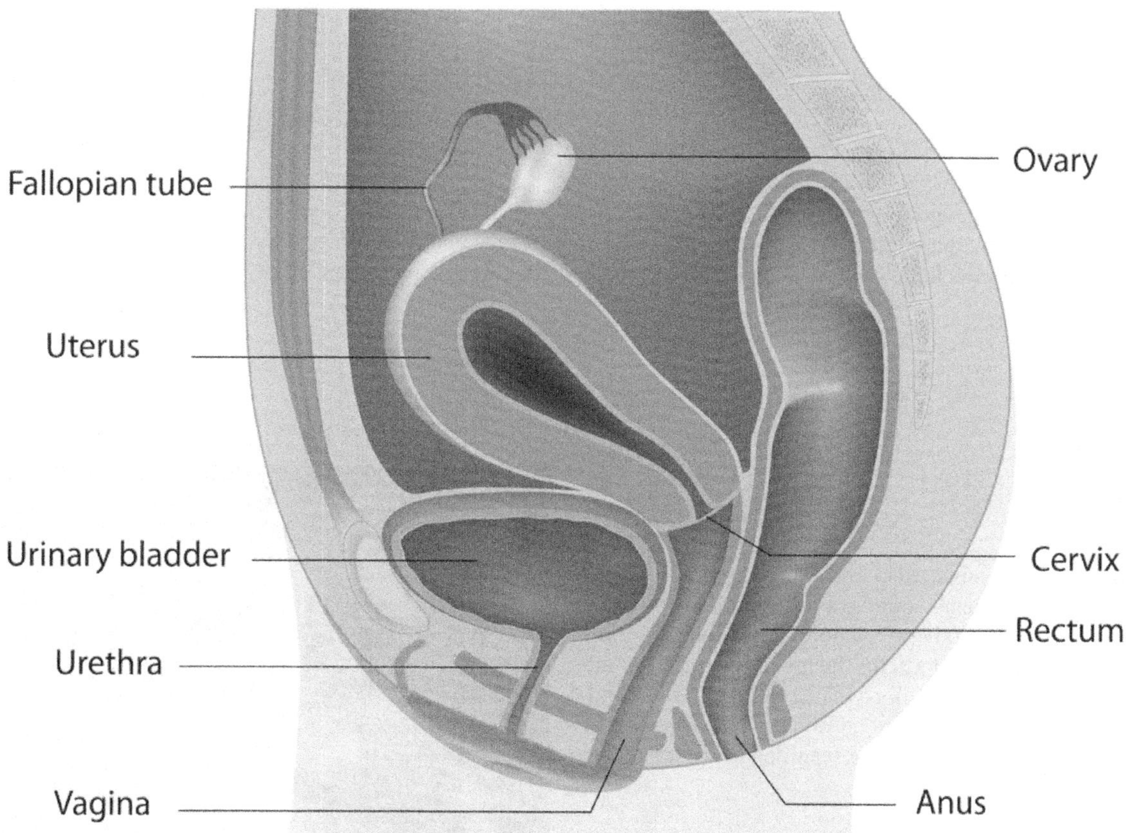

**Medical Tests and Equipment**

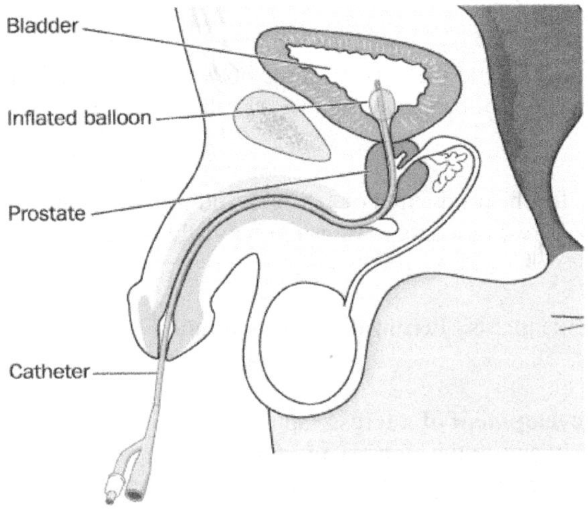


**Catheter**: A catheter is a small tube inserted into a part of the body to help fluid drain. The most common form is a urinary catheter. These are inserted into the urethra and into the urinary bladder. From there, fluid is able to drain freely from the bladder.

**Epidural:** An epidural is a medical procedure used to block pain and sensation in the lower body. It is performed by injecting analgesics and anesthetics around the spinal cord in the lumbar region. The medications are delivered via a catheter inserted into the site of injection. Epidurals are commonly used during labor to eliminate pain associated with child birth.

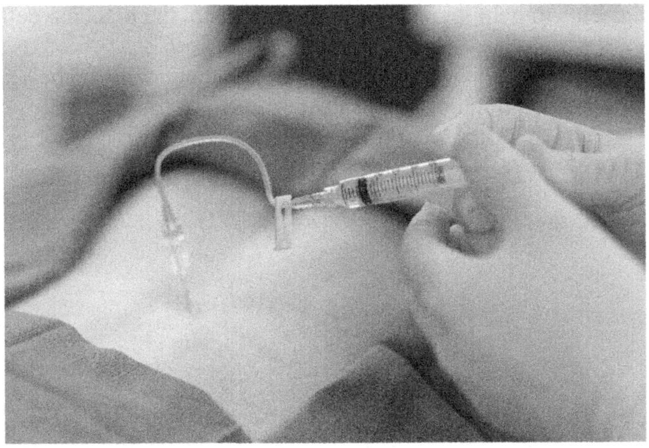

**Mammogram**: A mammogram is a procedure used to detect breast cancer in patients who are not showing any symptoms. It uses an X-ray to view the internal breast tissue. A mammogram is typically performed by placing the breast between two glass plates that compress the tissue. Compressing the tissue allows the X-ray to view all of the breast without missing anything.

**Ultrasound**: An ultrasound, also known as sonography, is an imaging technique utilizing sound waves to produce pictures of structures inside the body. Commonly, ultrasound is used to view the development of a fetus during pregnancy, but may also be used to examine infections inside the body, liver and gallbladder function, and heart conditions. The part of the machine that is used to perform the scanning is known as the transducer.

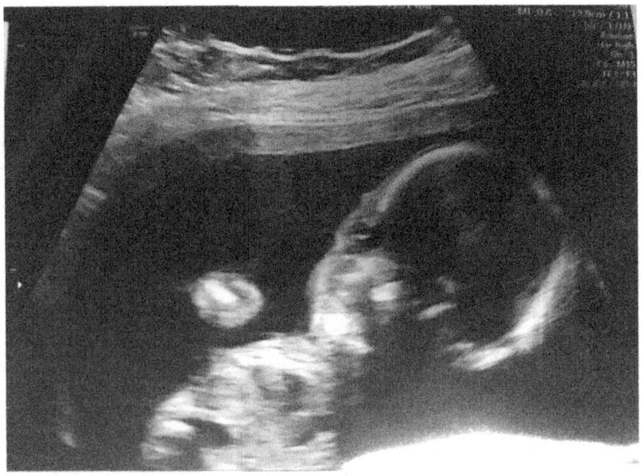

# Reproductive System Pathologies

## Amenorrhea

*(a-: without; men-: menstruation; -rrhea: discharge)*

Amenorrhea is a **lack of menstruation** that takes place **over three menstrual cycles**. This most commonly occurs with pregnancy, although hormones and issues with reproductive organs may also contribute.

***Causes***

The main cause of amenorrhea is pregnancy. As a woman ages and experiences menopause, amenorrhea will also occur. Birth control may also stop menstruation, along with other medications such as antidepressants.

Problems with hormone production, such as if a woman has polycystic ovarian syndrome(PCOS), may also prevent menstruation. Stress may also lead to hormonal imbalance.

***Symptoms***

A lack of menstruation is the main symptom of amenorrhea. Other symptoms may include headaches, change in vision, production of acne, and loss of hair.

***Treatments***

Treatment depends on the root cause. If pregnancy is the cause, normal menstruation should return after pregnancy. Stopping birth control will return menstruation. Medications to treat hormonal imbalances may be prescribed. In cases such as PCOS, surgery may be performed to remove the cyst or cysts causing problems, or remove the ovary completely. Reducing stress may also help reestablish menstruation.

***Contraindications***

Massage is generally not contraindicated for amenorrhea.

## Chlamydia

Chlamydia is a **bacterial infection** of the reproductive system, known as a sexually transmitted infection. It occurs most commonly in sexually active women, but anyone may contract it via sexual or oral intercourse.

***Causes***

Direct contact to the bacteria during vaginal, anal, or oral intercourse may result in contraction of chlamydia. Despite contracting the bacteria, a person may not know they have it, as symptoms do not always appear.

***Symptoms***

Discharge from the penis or vagina, painful urination, and pain in the abdomen are common symptoms of chlamydia, although as previously stated, symptoms don't always appear. If symptoms do occur, they usually appear a couple weeks after contracting the bacteria.

***Treatments***

If any symptom is seen, a person should see a doctor to get diagnosed. If diagnosed with chlamydia, antibiotics are prescribed to kill the bacteria, and the infection is usually resolved within a couple weeks after starting medication.

***Contraindications***

Because massage is not generally performed on the genital area, massage is indicated for a client with chlamydia. If massage is performed on the genital region, gloves should be worn and properly disposed of after the massage.

## Dysmenorrhea

*(dys-: difficult; men-: menstruation; -rrhea: discharge)*

Dysmenorrhea, known as **menstrual cramps**, is pain experienced during menstruation, typically at the beginning of menstruation. The pain usually goes away after a few days. Pain may be experienced in the lower abdomen and lower back, and may be either dull or more intense and interfere with daily life.

Sometimes, dysmenorrhea may be the result of more serious problems, such as endometriosis.

***Causes***

During menstruation, the uterus sloughs off its inner lining by contracting. The release of substances such as prostaglandins, which are associated with pain and inflammation, cause the uterus to contract, and pain results.

***Symptoms***

Symptoms include a dull ache in the lower abdomen or back, potential nausea, and headaches.

***Treatments***

Usually, over-the-counter pain relievers such as ibuprofen are taken to assist with the management of pain. If dysmenorrhea is the result of another more serious condition, surgery to correct the issue may be performed, such as removing fibroids from the uterus.

***Contraindications***

Massage for dysmenorrhea is dependent on the symptoms being experienced. Generally, it is not contraindicated. If a client is experiencing pain and cramping, massage of the abdomen and/or lower back may need to be avoided depending on the client's pain. If the client is nauseated, the massage may need to be rescheduled.

## Endometriosis

*(endo-: inside; metri-: uterus; -osis: condition)*

Endometriosis is an **abnormal growth** of **uterine lining**, known as the **endometrium, outside the uterus**. The lining often grows on the ovaries and fallopian tubes. The tissue still behaves like normal uterine lining, breaking down and bleeding during each menstrual period. The tissue stays inside the body, whereas during a normal menstrual period, the uterine lining is expelled from the body. Scar tissue and cysts may form, especially involving the ovaries, and pain may be present.

***Causes***

There is no exact cause that has been determined. Some theories include menstrual blood flowing backwards through the fallopian tubes and out to the pelvic cavity, possible complications from surgeries such as C Section, or even problems with the immune system that make it difficult to break down the growth of tissue.

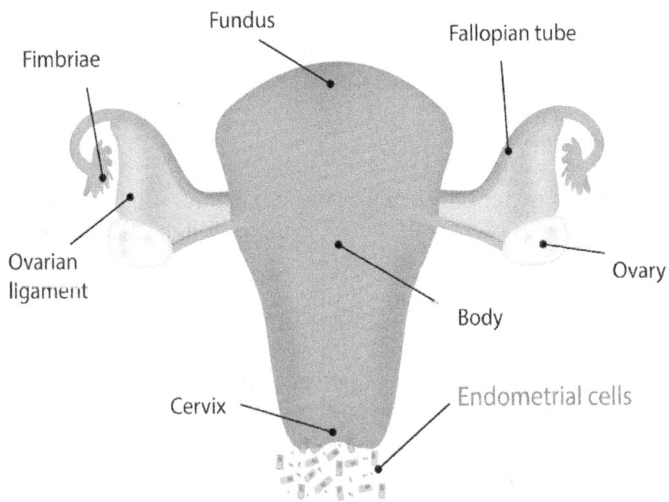


***Symptoms***

Painful menstruation, sometimes severe, may occur. Excessive bleeding and infertility may also occur as a result due to blockage of the fallopian tubes by endometrial tissue.

***Treatments***

There are many treatments available. Pain medication may be prescribed to manage pain, while birth control may be administered to help regulate hormones responsible for building up uterine lining. Surgery is an option to remove endometrial tissue. If other treatments are not helpful, a hysterectomy may be performed to completely remove the uterus.

***Contraindications***

Massage of a client with endometriosis is generally not contraindicated. However, if a client is experiencing severe pain as a result, massage should not be performed and should be rescheduled.

## Genital Herpes

Genital Herpes is a **viral infection** of the **genitals**, caused by contact with the **Herpes Simplex 2 Virus**. Herpes Simplex 1 may also cause genital herpes, but is usually only transmitted during oral sex, and is much less common than Herpes Simplex 2. The virus is primarily transmitted sexually, and a person who has contracted it may not know they have it due to symptoms not being present immediately after infection.

***Causes***

Exposure to the herpes simplex virus through sexual contact is the cause of genital herpes.

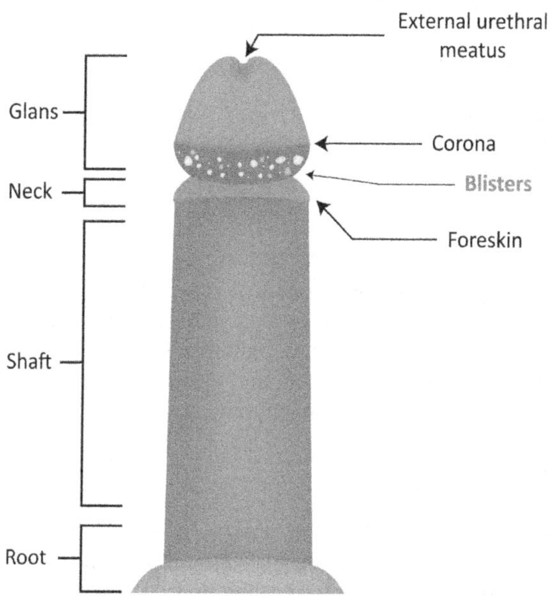


***Symptoms***

Symptoms are often recurring, and a person may experience them several times a year. Symptoms include pain, itching, ulceration, skin that forms a crust that scabs, and the development of red bumps or white blisters that contain fluid.

***Treatments***

There is no cure for genital herpes. Antiviral medications may be prescribed to help slow the progression of symptoms.

***Contraindications***

Because massage is not generally performed on the genital area, massage is indicated for a client with genital herpes. If massage is performed on the genital region, gloves should be worn and properly disposed of after the massage to avoid contracting the virus.

## Genital Warts

Genital Warts is the development of **warts** in the **genital region**. Genital warts is one of the most common sexually transmitted infections. Genital warts are caused by coming into contact with the **human papilloma virus(HPV)**, the same virus that causes cervical cancer(page 260).

***Causes***

Genital warts are caused by the human papilloma virus. Not every strain of HPV causes genital warts, and the virus is generally destroyed by the body before warts can develop.

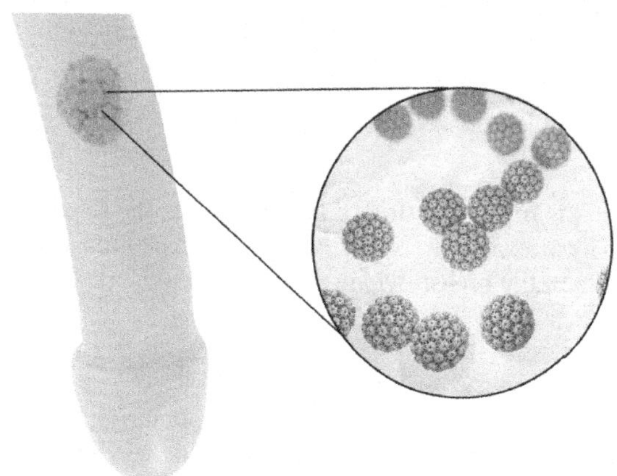

***Symptoms***

Warts form around the genitals. The warts may itch or cause discomfort. Like other warts, genital warts may go away on their own and return later.

*Treatments*

Most common treatment is application of topical creams that either boost the immune system to destroy the warts, or creams that destroy the wart tissue. Surgical removal may be performed if warts are larger or are unresponsive to topical creams.

*Contraindications*

Because massage is not generally performed on the genital area, massage is indicated for a client with genital warts. If massage is performed on the genital region, gloves should be worn and properly disposed of after the massage to avoid contracting the virus.

## Gonorrhea

*(gono-: semen, seed; -rrhea: discharge)*

Gonorrhea is a **bacterial infection** of the genital region. The infection results from sexual contact with the **Neisseria bacterium**. Although gonorrhea most commonly affects the genitals, it can also infect the mouth, throat, eyes, and rectum.

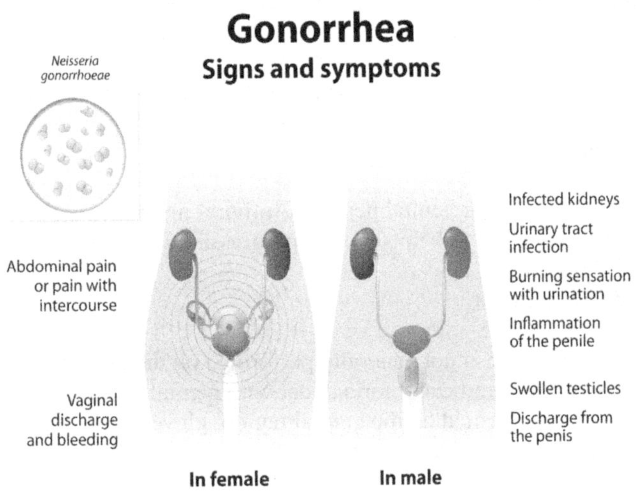


*Causes*

Sexual contact is the most common cause of bacteria transmission in gonorrhea.

*Symptoms*

Commonly, symptoms of gonorrhea never appear, and a person may not know that they have been infected. When symptoms do appear, they include discharge from the penis or vagina, pain during urination, and bleeding from the vagina between menstrual periods in women.

*Treatments*

People with gonorrhea are treated with antibiotics to kill the bacteria. A course of antibiotics should be completed, even if symptoms have disappeared in the middle of the prescribed dose.

*Contraindications*

Because massage is not generally performed on the genital area, massage is indicated for a client with gonorrhea. If massage is performed on the genital region, gloves should be worn and properly disposed of after the massage.

## Mastitis

*(mast-: breast; -itis: inflammation)*

Mastitis is **inflammation** of **breast tissue**, the result of a **bacterial infection**. Mastitis most commonly occurs after pregnancy as a result of breast feeding. The breast may become red and tender. If not properly treated, an abscess may develop in the breast, which would need to be drained surgically.

*Causes*

Bacteria is a common cause of mastitis, entering the breast while breast feeding. Not properly draining the breast after bacteria has entered the breast can provide a suitable environment for the bacteria to reproduce.

A blockage in a milk duct may also produce mastitis, causing bacteria to become trapped, leading to infection. Breasts should be sufficiently drained to prevent blockages.

*Symptoms*

Breasts may become red and swollen, a fever may present, and the breasts may be more tender than normal.

*Treatments*

Antibiotics are useful in treating mastitis caused by bacterial infection. Again, if an abscess is present, it may need to be surgically drained. Over-the-counter pain relievers may help with general aches associated with breast inflammation.

*Contraindications*

Mastitis is a local contraindication for massage. If a client presents with mastitis, the client may need to be placed into side-lying position to reduce pressure on the breasts. Massage of the breasts should be avoided. If fever is present, massage should not be performed.

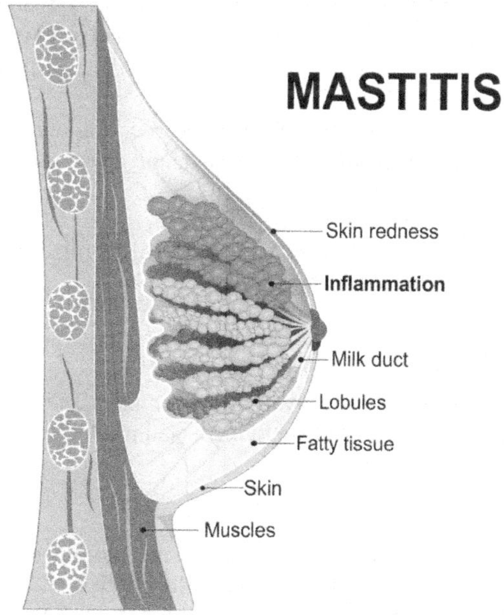


## Menopause

Menopause is the **permanent cessation of menstrual cycles**. As a woman ages, her body naturally produces less estrogen and progesterone, two hormones vital in regulating menstruation. The average age of a woman to reach menopause is 51, at which point the ovaries no longer release eggs, and menstruation stops. Osteoporosis(page 237) is a common side effect of menopause.

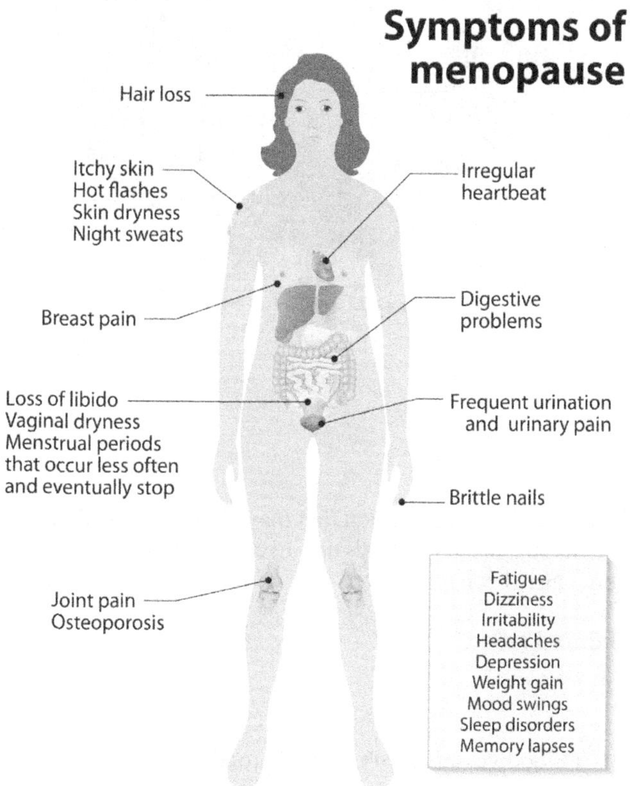


*Causes*

Most commonly, menopause is a result of natural aging. Less commonly, it is associated with other medical procedures, such as hysterectomy(surgical removal of the uterus), problems arising from the ovaries, or even temporary menopause seen with chemotherapy or radiation treatments stemming from cancer.

*Symptoms*

There are numerous symptoms associated with menopause, depending on the stage of menopause a person is in. Hot flashes and changes in mood are common. Hair may become thin and brittle. A person may see increased weight gain, and experience problems sleeping.

*Treatments*

There are no treatments to prevent menopause from occurring. Treatments are available that may help with some symptoms associated with menopause. Hormone replacement therapy can help maintain estrogen levels in the body, which may assist with hot flashes and reduce the chances of developing osteoporosis.

*Contraindications*

Massage is indicated for clients with menopause. If a client is experiencing hot flashes, anything that produces heat, such as heat pads, should not be used. Cold packs may be used to help with hot flashes.

## Polycystic Ovarian Syndrome

*(poly-: many; cyst-: bladder)*

Polycystic Ovarian Syndrome(PCOS) is a disorder marked by the development of small **fluid-filled sacs** in an **ovary**, which may prevent eggs from being released, and cause problems with estrogen and progesterone release. It is more commonly seen in obese women.

Polycystic Ovarian Syndrome may lead to infertility, miscarriage, the development of gestational and/or Type 2 Diabetes, and hypertension during pregnancy.

***Causes***

The precise cause of Polycystic Ovarian Syndrome is unclear, but factors that may contribute include excessive amounts of insulin in the blood, which can lead to increased production of male specific hormones, and genetic factors.

***Symptoms***

Common symptoms include a lack of regular menstrual cycle, cysts that develop in an ovary(which may affect both ovaries), increased amounts of facial hair, and increased acne due to excessive amounts of male hormones.

***Treatments***

Because Polycystic Ovarian Syndrome occurs more commonly in obese women, weight loss is recommended to combat the condition. Certain medications may be prescribed to help regulate estrogen and progesterone levels in the body, reducing the effects of male hormones.

To help with ovulation, medications such as Metformin may be prescribed.

If the cysts in the ovary are too large, surgery to remove the ovary completely may be performed.

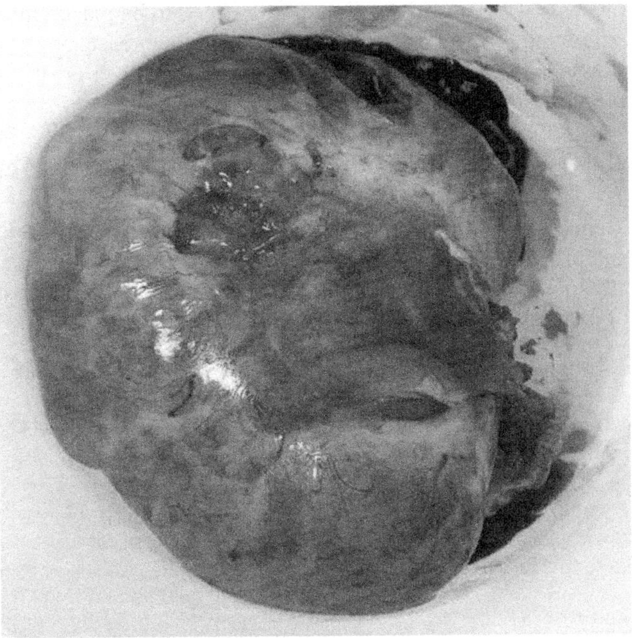

Ovary containing cysts, roughly the size of a grapefruit

***Contraindications***

Massage is generally indicated for a client with Polycystic Ovarian Syndrome.

## Preeclampsia

*(pre-: before; -eclampsia: a convulsive state)*

Preeclampsia is a potential complication of pregnancy, and is considered a serious condition that may potentially lead to death if left untreated. Preeclampsia may be a sign of damage to organs such as the kidneys and liver. It is marked by **high blood pressure** and **increased protein** in the **urine** where there hasn't been any before.

Because preeclampsia is a serious condition, it may lead to **early induced labor**.

***Causes***

Causes of preeclampsia often involve blood vessels in the placenta. If blood vessels aren't formed properly and are unable to effectively deliver blood to the fetus, it can result in preeclampsia. Other disorders, such as gestational hypertension, may result in preeclampsia.

***Symptoms***

Although preeclampsia may be asymptomatic, common symptoms include hypertension, an abnormally large amount of protein in the urine, nausea, headaches, and abdominal pain. The amount of urine being produced may decrease, as well as the levels of thrombocytes in the blood.

***Treatments***

Treatments before delivery are available, but the only way to completely rid the body of preeclampsia is to deliver the child. Severe complications may arise until then, including stroke and seizures. Medications include corticosteroids to improve thrombocyte levels in the blood, and antihypertensives to lower blood pressure.

***Contraindications***

Massage of a client with preeclampsia should generally be avoided until after the child has been delivered and the condition resolves.

## Premenstrual Syndrome

Premenstrual Syndrome is the predictable occurrence of a series of symptoms around the time a woman leading up to menstruation.

***Causes***

Hormonal changes are thought to be a major contributing factor to the development of premenstrual syndrome. During menstruation, **hormone levels change** dramatically, and this can cause changes in behavior and thought processes.

***Symptoms***

Symptoms are extremely varied, and no one person experiences exactly the same symptoms as another. Common symptoms include depression, mood swings, changes in appetite, fatigue, headache, bloating, feeling anxious, fluid retention, and tenderness in the breasts.

***Treatments***

Despite changes in lifestyle being the preferred treatment, a doctor may prescribe medications if symptoms are more severe. Diuretics help with excessive fluid accumulation, and antidepressants may help with hormone regulation associated with mood swings. Lifestyle changes may include increasing exercise and incorporating massage therapy or yoga to promote relaxation and reducing stress.

***Contraindications***

Massage is indicated for premenstrual syndrome.

## Prostatitis

*(prostat-: prostate; -itis: inflammation)*

Prostatitis is **inflammation** of the **prostate**, a small gland located beneath the bladder in males. Prostatitis commonly affects men over the age of 50, but can occur at any age.

The prostate produces fluids that mix with sperm to create semen, connecting with the urinary tract. **Bacteria** may enter into the prostate through the urine, resulting in acute prostatitis.

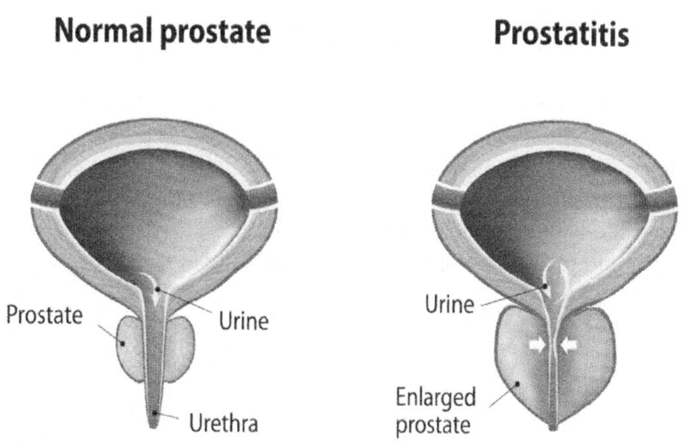


***Causes***

The most common cause of prostatitis is a bacterial infection. Damage to the nerves that control urination may also lead to the development of prostatitis.

### *Symptoms*

Difficulty urinating is a common symptom of prostatitis. Painful urination may present, along with the need to frequently urinate at night. A person may experience pain in the abdomen and pelvis, and the urine may look cloudy.

### *Treatments*

Most commonly, prostatitis is treated with antibiotics. Non-steroidal anti-inflammatory drugs may also help alleviate inflammation of the prostate, but will not fix the underlying cause of the condition.

### *Contraindications*

Massage is indicated for a client with prostatitis.

## Syphilis

Syphilis is a **bacterial infection** of the genitals, most commonly spread by **sexual intercourse**. Syphilis is easily treatable, but may lie dormant in the body for years before becoming activated. Advanced stages of a syphilis infection can cause bra in or heart damage, and can be fatal.

### *Causes*

Direct sexual contact with a person infected by syphilis transmits the bacteria. Although less common, the bacteria may be transmitted during childbirth(known as congenital syphilis), or through direct contact to syphilis lesions during activities such as kissing.

### *Symptoms*

There are several different stages of a syphilis infection. The first stage is known as primary syphilis, and presents with a small sore that is usually painless on the area where infection occurred. Secondary syphilis presents with a widespread rash that usually starts on the torso, then spreads over the entire body. Latent syphilis occurs when there are no symptoms, but a person is still infected by the bacteria. Tertiary syphilis, which develops in the late stages of a syphilis infection, may cause damage to the brain, heart, liver, or eyes. The amount of damage caused could lead to stroke, dementia, and the development of aneurysms.

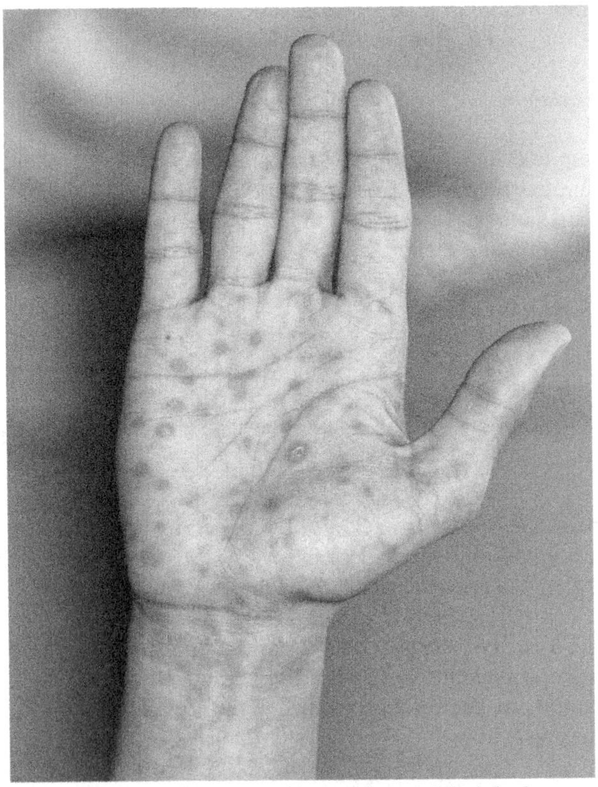

Widespread rash seen with secondary syphilis infection

### *Treatments*

Because syphilis is caused by bacteria, antibiotics are prescribed to destroy the infection. Early stage syphilis is easily treatable.

### *Contraindications*

Because massage is not generally performed on the genital area, massage is indicated for a client with syphilis. If massage is performed on the genital region, gloves should be worn and properly disposed of after the massage.

# Reproductive Pathologies

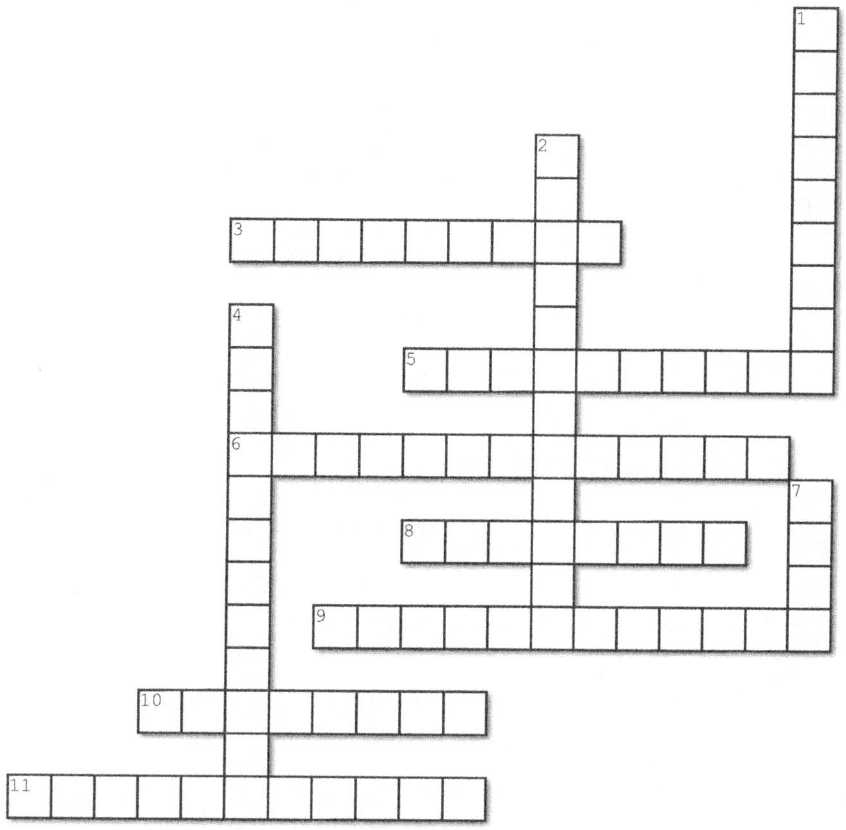


**Across**

**3.** Permanent cessation of menstrual cycles

**5.** Lack of menstruation that takes place over three menstrual cycles

**6.** Abnormal growth of uterine lining outside the uterus

**8.** Bacterial infection that, if left untreated, causes a widespread rash and damages the brain and liver

**9.** The development of raised thick patches of keratin in the genital region, caused by exposure to the human papilloma virus

**10.** Inflammation of breast tissue, most commonly caused by bacterial infection

**11.** Inflammation of the prostate

**Down**

**1.** Bacterial infection of the genitals caused by exposure to Neisseria bacteria

**2.** Cramping experienced during menstruation

**4.** Serious condition seen during pregnancy marked by increased protein in urine and high blood pressure

**7.** Abbreviation, the development of fluid-filled sacs in an ovary

Answer Key on Page 287

# Reproductive Quiz

1. The vas deferens connect which structures
A. Epididymis to the prostate
B. Urethra to the urinary bladder
C. Seminal vesicle to the prostate
D. Urethra to the epididymis

2. Chlamydia and gonorrhea are both
A. Bacterial infections
B. Fungal infections
C. Viral infection
D. Parasitic infections

3. Permanent cessation of menstrual cycles, a natural result of aging
A. Dysmenorrhea
B. Premenstrual syndrome
C. Menopause
D. Amenorrhea

4. In addition to egg cells, the ovaries produce
A. Epinephrine
B. Progesterone
C. Growth hormone
D. Follicle-stimulating hormone

5. Endometriosis
A. Abnormal growth of the uterine lining that takes place outside the uterus
B. Development of cysts in the ovaries
C. Lack of menstrual cycle for three or more consecutive months
D. High blood pressure and increased protein in urine due to organ damage

6. Bacterial infection that presents with a widespread rash in the secondary stage of infection
A. Gonorrhea
B. Chlamydia
C. Mastitis
D. Syphilis

7. The testes are responsible for the production of which hormone
A. Estrogen
B. Growth hormone
C. Testosterone
D. Adrenaline

8. The fallopian tubes create a passageway for
A. The penis during intercourse
B. Egg cells during ovulation
C. Estrogen and progesterone to enter the blood stream
D. The fetus to exit the uterus

9. Inflammation of the breast, commonly caused by a bacterial infection
A. Mastitis
B. Endometriosis
C. Amenorrhea
D. Gonorrhea

10. Genital warts and genital herpes are caused by
A. Viral infections
B. Bacterial infections
C. Fungal infections
D. Parasitic infections

11. The development of fluid-filled sacs in an ovary that may prevent egg cells from being released
A. Menopause
B. Dysmenorrhea
C. PCOS
D. Prostatitis

12. Cramping during menstruation which may last for a few days
A. Amenorrhea
B. Dysmenorrhea
C. Mastitis
D. PCOS

13. Organ responsible for growing and developing a fetus
A. Ovary
B. Vagina
C. Uterus
D. Fallopian tubes

14. Spermatogenesis takes place
A. In the testes
B. In the prostate
C. In the epididymis
D. In the penis

15. Inflammation of the prostate caused by bacterial infection
A. Prostatitis
B. Syphilis
C. Gonorrhea
D. Chlamydia

Answer Key on Page 289

# Respiratory System and Pathologies

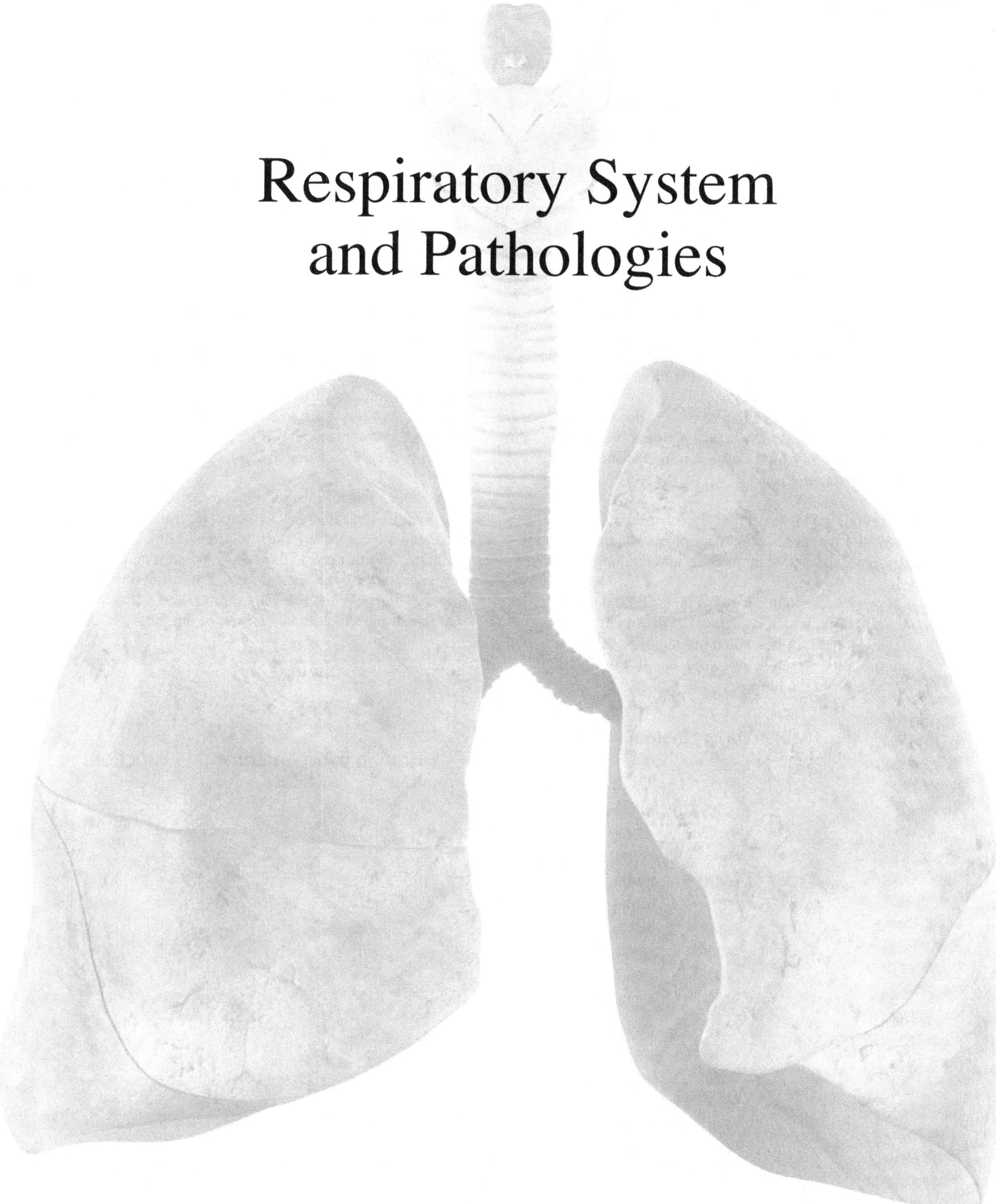

# Respiratory System

The Respiratory System has one essential function: to bring **oxygen** into the body, and eliminate wastes such as **carbon dioxide** from the body. The main organs of the Respiratory System are the **lungs**. The left lung has two lobes and is smaller than the right lung, which has three lobes. This is due to the presence of the heart on the left side of the chest.

Conduction of air is controlled by the **nose**. Air enters the body through the nose, and is filtered by **hair** and **mucous**. The nose also warms the air as it enters the body.

The **larynx**, also known as the voice box, is a short tube located inferior to the pharynx. As air passes over the vocal cords in the larynx, the vocal cords vibrate, which produces **sound**. This, along with the tongue, produces speech.

Sitting atop the larynx is a flap of tissue known as the **epiglottis**. Upon swallowing, the epiglottis lies on top of the larynx, blocking any food or fluid from entering the larynx, which **prevents choking**.

Connecting to the larynx inferiorly is a tube of cartilage known as the **trachea**, or the wind pipe. The trachea is the primary passageway for air to enter into the lungs.

Once air enters the lungs, it goes into each lung through **bronchial tubes**, which branch off of the trachea. These tubes branch into smaller tubes called bronchioles. Bronchial tubes secrete **mucous**, which helps to trap any dirt or debris that have made it into the lungs.

At the end of the bronchioles are tiny **air sacs**, known as **alveoli**. The alveoli resemble a cluster of grapes. Capillaries attach to the alveoli and move blood across the surface of the alveoli. This allows carbon dioxide to detach from the erythrocytes and exit the blood stream, and also allows oxygen to enter the blood stream and attach to erythrocytes. Alveoli are where **gas exchange** occurs in the Respiratory System.

Respiration is accomplished by contraction of the **diaphragm**, a large muscle connected to the rib cage that separates the chest from the abdomen. The diaphragm creates a **vacuum** inside the chest. When it contracts, it descends, pulling the chest down. This allows air to enter into the lungs. When the diaphragm relaxes, it ascends up into the chest, which forces air out of the lungs.

The Respiratory System

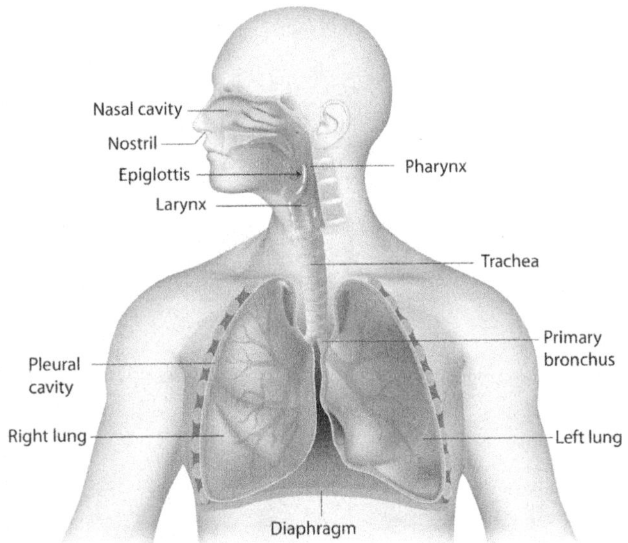


Human Lung Anatomy and Function

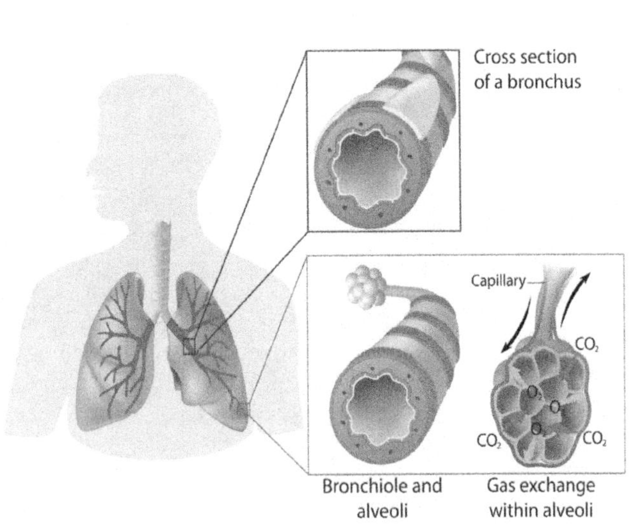

**Medical Tests and Equipment**

**Nebulizer**: A nebulizer is a form of an inhaler that turns liquid medication into a mist. Nebulizers are often used during asthma attacks, as the medication in mist form is easier to inhale than a regular inhaler which requires the patient to take a deep breath.

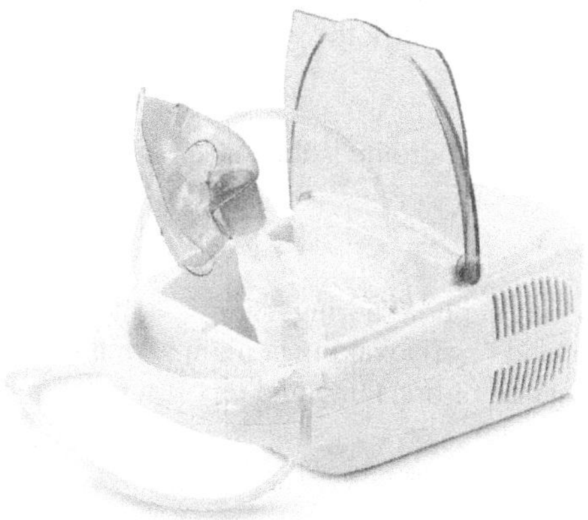

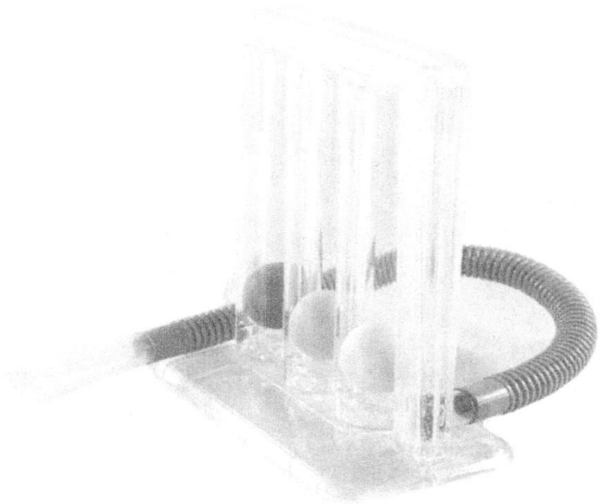

**Spirometer**: A spirometer is a device used to measure the volume of air being inhaled and exhaled by the lungs. This is used to determine if there are any obstructive or restrictive abnormalities in a person's breathing. A spirometer is mainly used to help diagnose or measure conditions such as asthma, bronchitis, and emphysema.

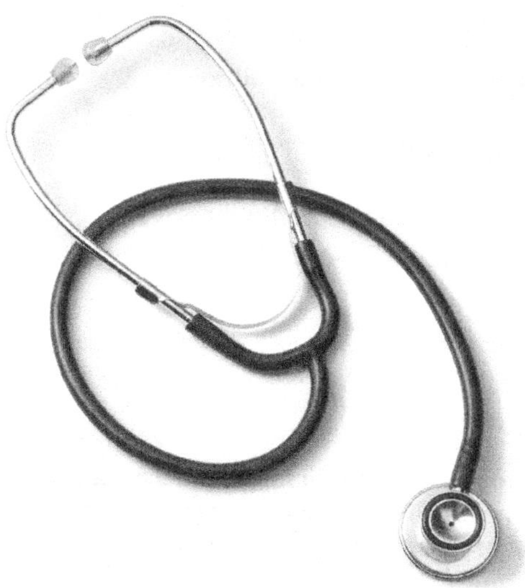

**Stethoscope**: A stethoscope is an auditory instrument used to listen to the internal body, most commonly the heart and lungs. It consists of two ear plugs connected to metal tubes, which then connect to rubber tubing. At the end of the tubing are two structures, the diaphragm and the bell. The diaphragm transmits higher frequency sounds to the ears, while the bell transmits low frequency sounds.

## Respiratory System Pathologies

### Apnea

*(a-: without; -pnea: breathing)*

Apnea, commonly referred to as sleep apnea, is a **temporary cessation of breathing** during sleep. Apnea may be a serious condition, depending on the patient. There are three types of sleep apnea: central sleep apnea, obstructive sleep apnea, and complex sleep apnea syndrome.

People who are overweight have a much higher rate of occurrence than others. Advanced age and being male are also common demographics for the development of sleep apnea.

***Causes***

Central sleep apnea is the result of the brain not stimulating muscles responsible for breathing. A patient may experience shortness of breath due to lack of oxygen intake. This form of sleep apnea is not common.

Obstructive sleep apnea is the result of throat muscles relaxing, which causes the air passages to narrow or completely close upon inhalation. This reduces the amount of oxygen getting into the body. As a result, the brain may force the patient awake momentarily to unblock the airways. People with obstructive sleep apnea often snore, and may even sound as if they are choking.

Complex sleep apnea syndrome is diagnosed when a person experiences both common and obstructive sleep apnea.

***Symptoms***

Symptoms of apnea include snoring, shortness of breath upon waking, fatigue, and briefly waking at night. Another person may see the cessation of breathing and report it to the patient.

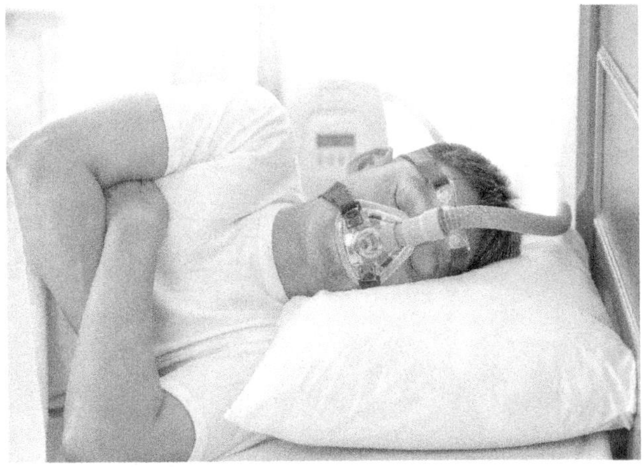

Utilization of CPAP to assist in breathing support

***Treatments***

Less severe forms of apnea may require less drastic forms of treatment, such as losing weight. In more severe forms, a person may be instructed to wear a CPAP(continuous positive airway pressure) machine during sleep, which increases air pressure in the airway, keeping the airways open enough for adequate oxygen intake to occur.

If other treatments are ineffective, surgery may be performed to remove tissue in and around the airway, which can increase the passageway for air to travel through.

***Contraindications***

Apnea is not contraindicated for massage.

## Asthma

Asthma is a chronic respiratory disease that causes **constriction** of the **airways**, restricting oxygen intake.

***Causes***

Asthma affects the **smooth muscle** in the **walls** of the **bronchial tubes**. Typically, when a person inhales an irritant(such as dust or smoke), the smooth muscle spasms and constricts in an effort to reduce the irritant moving further into the lungs. The bronchi will also produce an excessive amount of **mucous**, which further restricts the flow of oxygen into the lungs.

***Symptoms***

Symptoms include wheezing, chest tightness, and shortness of breath. Treatment varies depending on the severity in acute stages. If it is mild, medication may not be required. If symptoms are more severe, bronchodilators may be required to calm and open the airways. In extreme cases, where regular bronchodilators do not work, medical attention should be sought. A nebulizer, with inhalable steroids, should be used with asthma attacks.

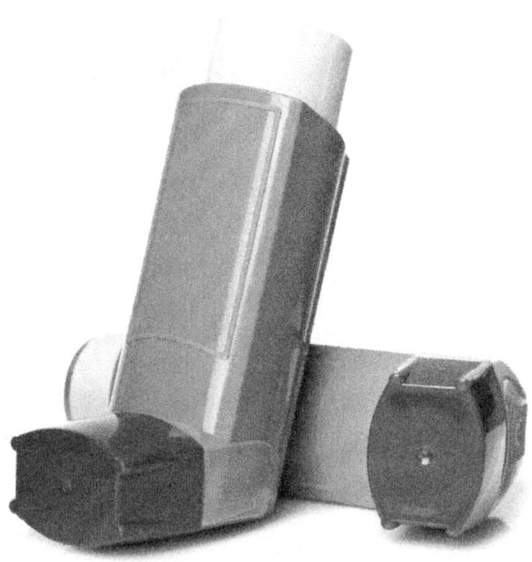

Asthma usually begins in childhood, but may disappear with age. Other times, it remains a chronic condition. Other factors such as smoking or obesity may lead to the development of asthma.

***Treatments***

Treatment for asthma primarily consists of the use of steroids and bronchodilators administered directly to the lungs via inhalers. If a person suffers from an asthma attack or has more severe forms of asthma, a nebulizer(which turns medication into a mist) may be required. Corticosteroids may also be used to lessen the chances of having an asthma attack.

***Contraindications***

In the acute stage, asthma is considered an absolute contraindication. Once breathing has returned to normal, massage may be performed. Tapotement may be performed on the back and chest to help loosen any excess phlegm that may be present.

Pathology of Asthma

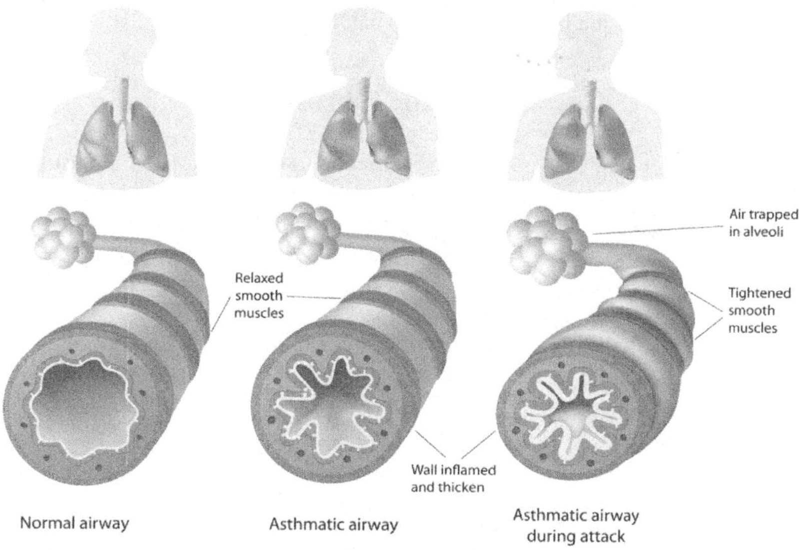


## Bronchitis

*(bronch-: bronchi; -itis: inflammation)*

Bronchitis is an inflammatory disease of the Respiratory System, restricting oxygen intake.

***Causes***

There are two different types of bronchitis: acute bronchitis and chronic bronchitis. **Acute bronchitis** is the result of a **primary** infection of the Respiratory System, such as influenza or pneumonia. These diseases affect the bronchial tubes, causing them to become irritated and inflamed. When these diseases resolve, the bronchitis will also resolve. **Chronic bronchitis** is the result of **constant irritation** to the bronchial tubes, caused by things such as **cigarette smoking** or exposure to things like **dust**. When exposure to the irritant ceases, the bronchitis will also cease.

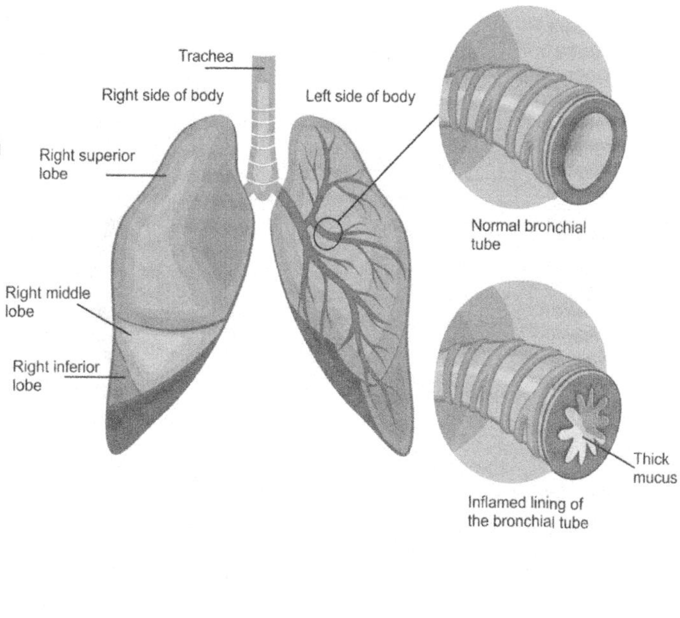


***Symptoms***

With both forms of bronchitis, there is an increased amount of mucous produced in the lungs, which makes breathing difficult. Increased coughing may be a side effect of the increase in mucous.

***Treatments***

Treatments vary depending on which type of bronchitis is involved. Acute bronchitis may require nothing more than a bronchodilator or cough suppressant. Because acute bronchitis is usually caused by a viral infection, antivirals may be prescribed to stop the advancement of the virus. Chronic bronchitis often requires the use of a bronchodilator, but not much else.

***Contraindications***

Acute bronchitis is considered an absolute contraindication, because it only appears as a secondary condition with another infection that is an absolute contraindication, such as influenza or pneumonia. Once these conditions resolve, the bronchitis will also resolve, and massage may be performed. Chronic bronchitis is indicated for massage. Tapotement may help loosen any excess phlegm as a result of the bronchitis, which can help breathing.

## Cystic Fibrosis

Cystic Fibrosis is a **genetic disorder** that causes **excessive mucous** to be produced in the **lungs and digestive tract**. The mucous produced is much thicker than normal mucous, and is extremely hard to expel from the body. The mucous can make it difficult to breathe, or to get digestive enzymes into the digestive tract from the pancreas.

***Causes***

The cause of cystic fibrosis is a mutated gene responsible for chloride moving in and out of cells. When chloride is unable to move to the surface of cells, it is unable to attract water to the cells. This causes mucous in several organs to become thicker than normal.

***Symptoms***

Symptoms of cystic fibrosis in the respiratory system include wheezing, shortness of breath, a cough that produces abnormally thick mucous, and an increased susceptibility to lung infections. Symptoms involving the digestive system include constipation, greasy feces, and lack of weight gain or growth. A person with cystic fibrosis will often exhibit abnormally high levels of salt in their sweat.

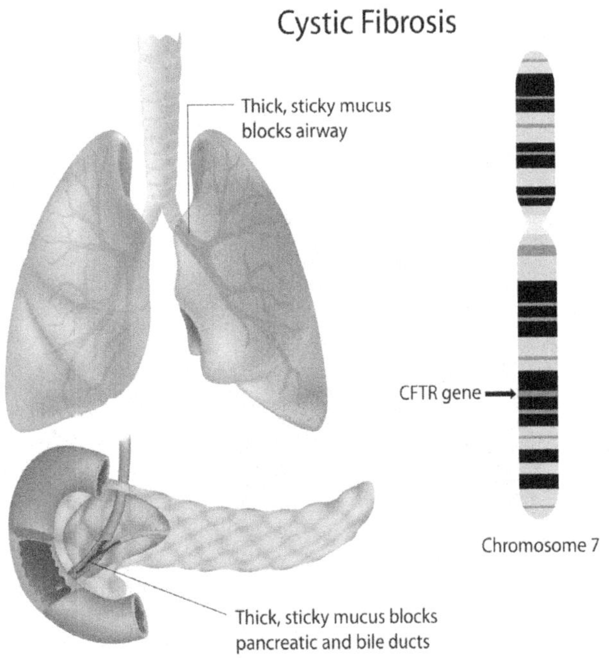


***Treatments***

Unfortunately, no cure exists for cystic fibrosis. Treatments are available to help manage the condition, however. These treatments include prescriptions designed to thin mucous, antibiotics to fight lung infections as they appear, bronchodilators to keep airways open, and pancreatic enzymes taken orally.

Physical therapy and massage therapy may be helpful in helping loosen phlegm in the respiratory tract. A patient with cystic fibrosis may use a vest that vibrates to help loosen phlegm.

***Contraindications***

Massage is indicated for cystic fibrosis. Tapotement may aid in loosening phlegm in the lungs.

## Emphysema

*(emphyso: inflate)*

Emphysema is a chronic condition of the lungs, resulting in difficulty bringing oxygen into the body and eliminating carbon dioxide from the body.

### *Causes*

Emphysema is caused by over-exposure to substances such as **cigarette smoke**. Constant irritation of the lungs by smoke can lead to degeneration of the **alveoli**, air sacs at the end of bronchial tubes where gas exchange takes place. When the alveoli degenerate, they lose surface area, which is what capillaries move across to eliminate carbon dioxide from the body and bring oxygen into the body. Lack of sufficient alveoli surface area makes gas exchange extremely difficult.

### *Symptoms*

Emphysema causes shortness of breath. A person with emphysema may be much more likely to develop a collapsed lung due to damage to the lungs.

### *Treatments*

Breathing exercises and oxygen supplementation may help control emphysema. If needed, bronchodilators can help relax the airways. If infections such as pneumonia occur, antibiotics may help.

### *Contraindications*

Massage is indicated for emphysema.

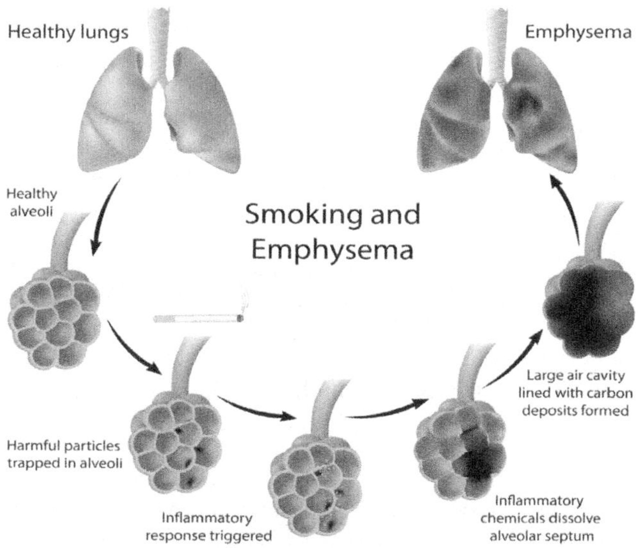


## Influenza

*(Italian "influenza": influence)*

Influenza is a highly contagious **viral** infection that primarily affects the **lungs**.

### *Causes*

There are many different strains of the flu virus. It is constantly mutating, so treatment can be difficult. **Vaccinations** are the primary form of prevention for influenza.

Influenza, during acute stages, results in fever, general malaise, body aches, runny nose, and cough. Symptoms generally last no more than a week. Depending on the person involved, it can be a moderate infection, or can be life-threatening. Children and the elderly are much more likely to have serious cases of influenza than the general population.

***Symptoms***

Influenza typically has a sudden onset of symptoms, including fever, body ache, fatigue, sore throat, nasal congestion, body chills, and sweating.

***Treatments***

Treatment for influenza is usually nothing more than rest and increased fluid intake. Antiviral medication may be prescribed, and may help reduce the length of the infection. Influenza usually clears up on its own.

***Contraindications***

Influenza is highly contagious, and is considered an absolute contraindication.

## Laryngitis

*(laryng-: larynx; -itis: inflammation)*

Laryngitis is **inflammation** of the **larynx**, also known as the voice box. Laryngitis may affect one's **ability to speak** due to the presence of the vocal cords inside the larynx.

***Causes***

There are many different causes of laryngitis. There are two main types of laryngitis: acute and chronic. **Acute laryngitis** is commonly the result of trauma to the larynx caused by yelling, or caused by an acute infection. Once the larynx has had time to heal, or the infection goes away, the inflammation should dissipate and the voice should return to normal. In **chronic laryngitis**, common causes include smoking and acid reflux.

***Symptoms***

Symptoms include difficulty speaking, pain in the throat, and dry coughing. In some cases, the voice may be completely lost, and in others, the voice is only hoarse.

***Treatments***

If laryngitis is not caused by an infection, resting the voice is extremely helpful. If bacterial infection is the cause, antibiotics may aid in destroying bacteria causing the inflammation. Most cases of infectious laryngitis are viral, however, and won't be helped by antibiotics.

Lozenges may aid in soothing the throat, as well as using humidifiers.

***Contraindications***

Massage on a client with laryngitis depends on the cause. If the cause of laryngitis is an infection, massage should be considered an absolute contraindication. If the cause of laryngitis is trauma, such as shouting, massage is indicated.

## Pleurisy

Pleurisy is **inflammation** of the **pleural membrane** surrounding the **lungs**. Pleurisy is commonly caused by another condition. Two types of pleurisy exist: **wet pleurisy** and **dry pleurisy**. Wet pleurisy occurs when there is an increased accumulation of fluids inside the membranes. Dry pleurisy occurs when the fluid between the membranes lessens.

***Causes***

Causes of pleurisy are varied, ranging from infections(such as influenza or pneumonia) to autoimmune disorders. A small number of medications may irritate the pleural membranes.

***Symptoms***

Shortness of breath and chest pain upon inhalation are two extremely common symptoms. Shortness of breath is caused by a conscious effort by the patient to not inhale, because inhalation causes pain.

***Treatments***

Treatment depends on the cause of pleurisy. A viral infection requires rest and proper hydration as the virus works its course through the body. A bacterial infection requires antibiotics to kill the bacteria.

***Contraindications***

Pleurisy is considered an absolute contraindication until the condition has completely resolved.

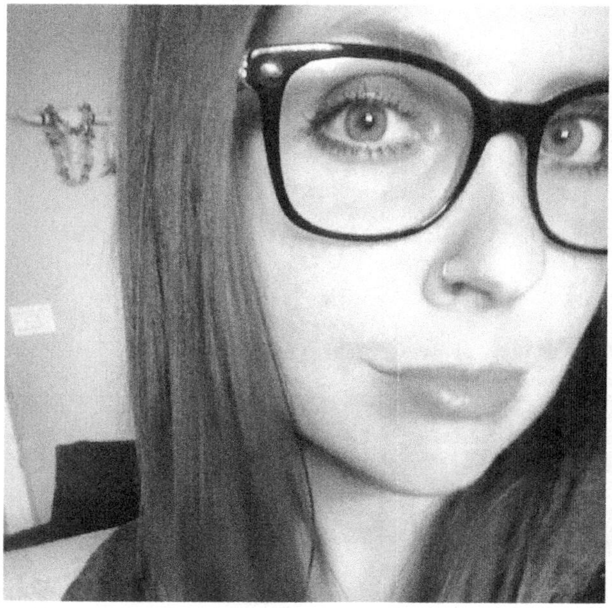

**Ashley, Pleurisy**

When were you diagnosed with pleurisy?

*The first time was like ten years ago.*

The first time?

*They told me I had it. Then I went to the ER several times and they told me that's what it was.*

What kind of symptoms were you experiencing ten years ago?

*Chest pain and tightness when breathing, shortness of breath and burning in my back.*

How long were you experiencing these symptoms before going to the ER?

*About a day or so. It progressively got worse as time went on. I was worried it was my heart.*

Had you had any heart issues up until that point?

*Yes, tachycardia uncontrolled by medication.*

How did the doctors conclude that you had pleurisy?

*X-ray and exam.*

What kind of exam?

*They took my vitals, listened to my heart and lungs.*

Do you know if you have wet pleurisy or dry pleurisy?

*Dry.*

After the diagnosis, what did they tell you to do to manage it?

*They said there's not much you can do for it.*

Did they tell you it would go away eventually?

*They said it could come and go.*

Did it go?

*Eventually I felt better, then it would come back.*

How often would it come back?

*I've had it about 6 times.*

How long does it usually last?

*Usually 2-3 weeks.*

Are the symptoms usually consistent every time?

*For the most part. Sometimes more intense than other times.*

When was the last time you've had it?

*Eight months ago.*

Have you ever been prescribed medication for it?

*Anti-inflammatories.*

Do they help?

*Not really.*

Typical Ashley luck.

*Absolutely.*

Are there any medications you've taken that make it worse?

*No, but I feel like Enbrel, because it's a biologic and it suppresses my immune system, it makes it more difficult to heal.*

Have you found anything that helps?

*No. Basically just trying to manage stress so I don't cause a flare up.*

So stress is one of the reasons you get pleurisy?

*Stress aggravates my lupus. The doctors think I have pleurisy because of lupus.*

Would you be looking to receive massage during a flare up of pleurisy?

*I would definitely be willing to try it!*

Does anything like aromatherapy or steam help?

*I've tried. It didn't.*

## Pneumonia

*(pneumo: lung)*

Pneumonia is a highly contagious infection of the lungs, resulting in a buildup of **fluid** in the **alveoli**.

***Causes***

The primary cause of pneumonia is **bacterial** infection(staphylococci), but may also be caused by a virus or fungi. The bacteria enters the body through breathing, which then infects the lungs.

***Symptoms***

Mild cases of pneumonia usually present with symptoms similar to those of influenza. Other symptoms may include pain in the chest upon breathing, coughing which may produce phlegm, fever, nausea, and shortness of breath. Symptoms can range for mild to severe, and even life threatening, based on the overall health and age of the person infected.

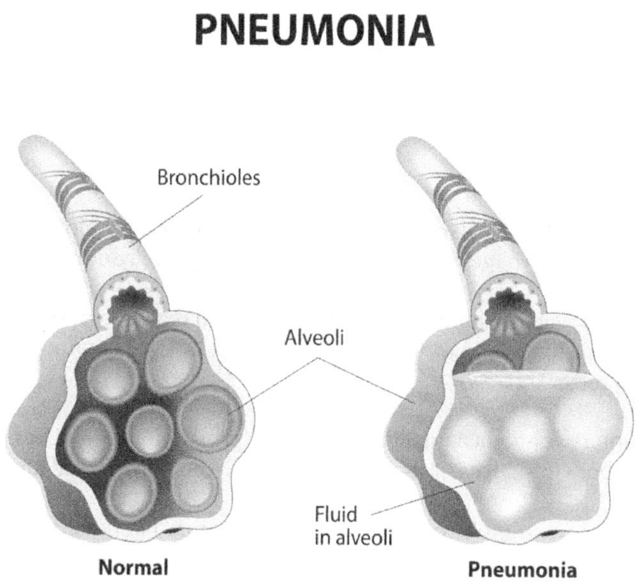


***Treatments***

Pneumonia is typically treated with antibiotics. Cough medicine and antipyretics may be prescribed to aid with coughing and to lower fever.

***Contraindications***

Pneumonia is a highly contagious condition, and is therefore an absolute contraindication.

## Pulmonary Edema

Pulmonary Edema is a potentially serious **collection of fluid** in the **alveoli**, which makes breathing extremely difficult.

***Causes***

The most common cause of pulmonary edema is a problem with the heart, such as difficulty regulating blood flow through the chambers due to damage to valves, or a build up of plaque in the coronary arteries. Other causes include infections such as pneumonia, pulmonary embolism, and even high altitudes when the body is not acclimated.

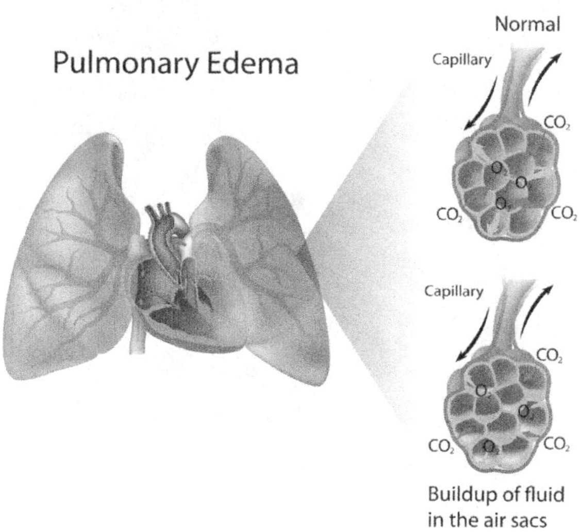


***Symptoms***

Symptoms vary from minor to severe. Shortness of breath, wheezing, coughing, chest pain, fatigue, and irregular heart beat are all common symptoms. Acute pulmonary edema should be seen by a doctor.

***Treatments***

Increasing oxygen intake is the first step in treatment, usually administered by an oxygen mask. To reduce the amount of fluid in the body, diuretics are prescribed. Other medications such as nitroglycerin and statins may be prescribed to help with reducing fluid from escaping the heart and entering into the alveoli.

### *Contraindications*

In the acute stage, pulmonary edema is an absolute contraindication, and massage should not be performed.

## Pulmonary Embolism

A Pulmonary Embolism occurs when a **blood clot** lodges into the **lung**, restricting blood flow vital to the lung. Pulmonary embolism is an extremely serious, life-threatening condition.

Clots form when there is damage to a tissue that has caused bleeding. If a clot dislodges from an artery or vein, it is then known as an embolus, and can freely travel through the cardiovascular system. If one of these clots gets stuck in an artery or vein, it can block blood from flowing further through that blood vessel, and may cause ischemia and necrosis, or may even lead to death.

### *Causes*

Pulmonary embolism is most commonly caused by a clot in the legs dislodging and getting stuck in the lung. Deep Vein Thrombosis(page 57) is one of the most common conditions that result in pulmonary embolism.

People who are immobile are more likely to develop blood clots than those who are not. When the legs move, the veins are able to stretch and move blood effectively, but when someone is immobile, blood may start to pool in the veins, and clots can form.

Surgery is another cause of blood clot formation in blood vessels. During surgery, tissue is cut open and sewn together, and the body produces clots in these vessels to help them heal and repair.

People who smoke or are overweight are more likely to develop pulmonary embolism than those that don't.

### *Symptoms*

Shortness of breath, coughing, and chest pain are three extremely common symptoms of pulmonary embolism. Pain in the legs may also be felt at the site of a blood clot. Irregular heart rhythm and dizziness may accompany a pulmonary embolism. If any of these are felt suddenly and are unexplained, a doctor should be seen immediately for treatment.

### *Treatments*

The acute stage of pulmonary embolism may require surgery to remove the clot, and a prescription of thrombolytics and anticoagulants to help break up the clot and prevent future clots from occurring.

Prevention of clot formation is important. When seated, getting up and moving can help get blood flowing again. Staying hydrated can help, as can wearing compression socks to assist circulation. After surgery, legs should be elevated to allow blood to efficiently flow towards the heart while under bed rest.

### *Contraindications*

In the acute stage, if pulmonary embolism is suspected, massage is contraindicated and the client should seek medical attention. If a client is taking blood thinners, lighter massage is indicated, as any damage to underlying tissue may cause significantly more bleeding than normal. If the site of a blood clot is known, that area is considered a local contraindication and should be avoided.

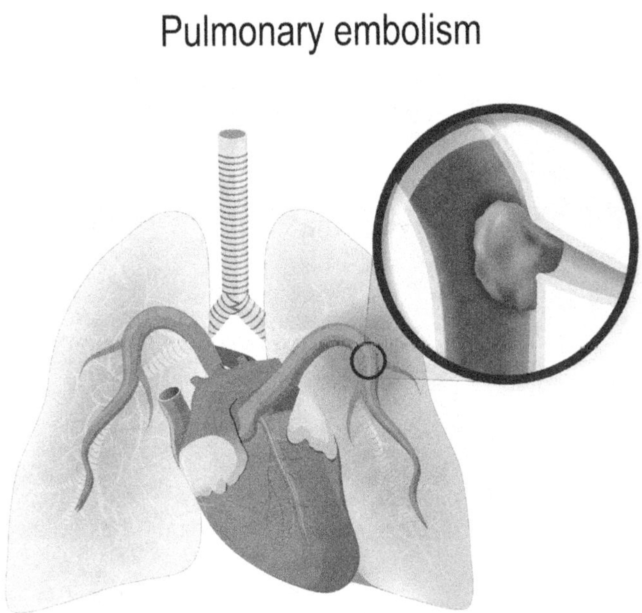

## Sinusitis

*(sinus: sinus; -itis: inflammation)*

Sinusitis is an acute condition causing **inflammation** and **swelling** in the **nasal sinuses**, which can result in **excessive mucous** production. It can also prevent mucous from properly draining from the sinuses, causing a person to feel a lot of pressure in the face around the nose and eyes. Bacterial infection may result, which can increase the amount of fluid present in the sinuses.

***Causes***

The most common cause of sinusitis is an acute viral infection, such as the common cold, which may in turn cause bacterial infection to take place.

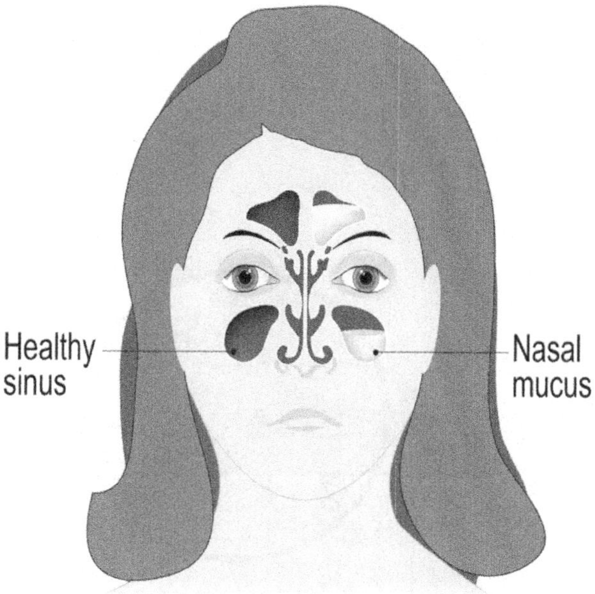


***Symptoms***

A person with sinusitis may experience pressure in the face around the nose, eyes, and ears, headache, a thick mucous produced by the nose usually presenting with a yellow or green color, and congestion in the nasal cavity.

***Treatments***

Decongestants are effective at helping to drain the nasal cavities, which can help ease pressure in the area. Nasal sprays can help alleviate inflammation and clean out the nasal cavity, further helping to reduce pressure. If bacterial infection is present, antibiotics may be prescribed.

***Contraindications***

During the acute stage, and due to being caused by a contagious viral infection, sinusitis is considered an absolute contraindication. Once the condition has resolved, a client may receive massage.

## Tuberculosis

Tuberculosis is a serious **bacterial infection** of the respiratory system, and is contagious. Exposure to tuberculosis may cause a person to acquire either **latent tuberculosis** or **active tuberculosis**. In latent tuberculosis, the bacteria enters the body but does not cause any problems or symptoms. This type is not contagious. However, if it becomes active tuberculosis, it becomes contagious. Active tuberculosis is when the bacteria is activated and symptoms of a tuberculosis infection are present.

***Causes***

Tuberculosis is contracted from another person through microscopic droplets spread through the air. This can be caused by actions such as coughing and sneezing.

Tuberculosis may have a better chance of becoming active in a person with HIV/AIDS, due to the compromised immune system.

***Symptoms***

Symptoms include chronic coughing, pain in the chest when breathing, fatigue, fever, and producing blood upon coughing. Night chills, sweating, and unexplained loss in weight may also be signs of an active tuberculosis infection. Tuberculosis may, in some instances, also affect structures and organs in the body such as the kidneys.

***Treatments***

The bacteria responsible for tuberculosis is extremely hard to destroy, so a person afflicted with the condition will need to take antibiotics for an extended period of time. This ensures the bacteria is completely destroyed and there is no chance of the bacteria becoming immune to the antibiotics being used.

***Contraindications***

Tuberculosis is a contagious condition, and is considered an absolute contraindication.

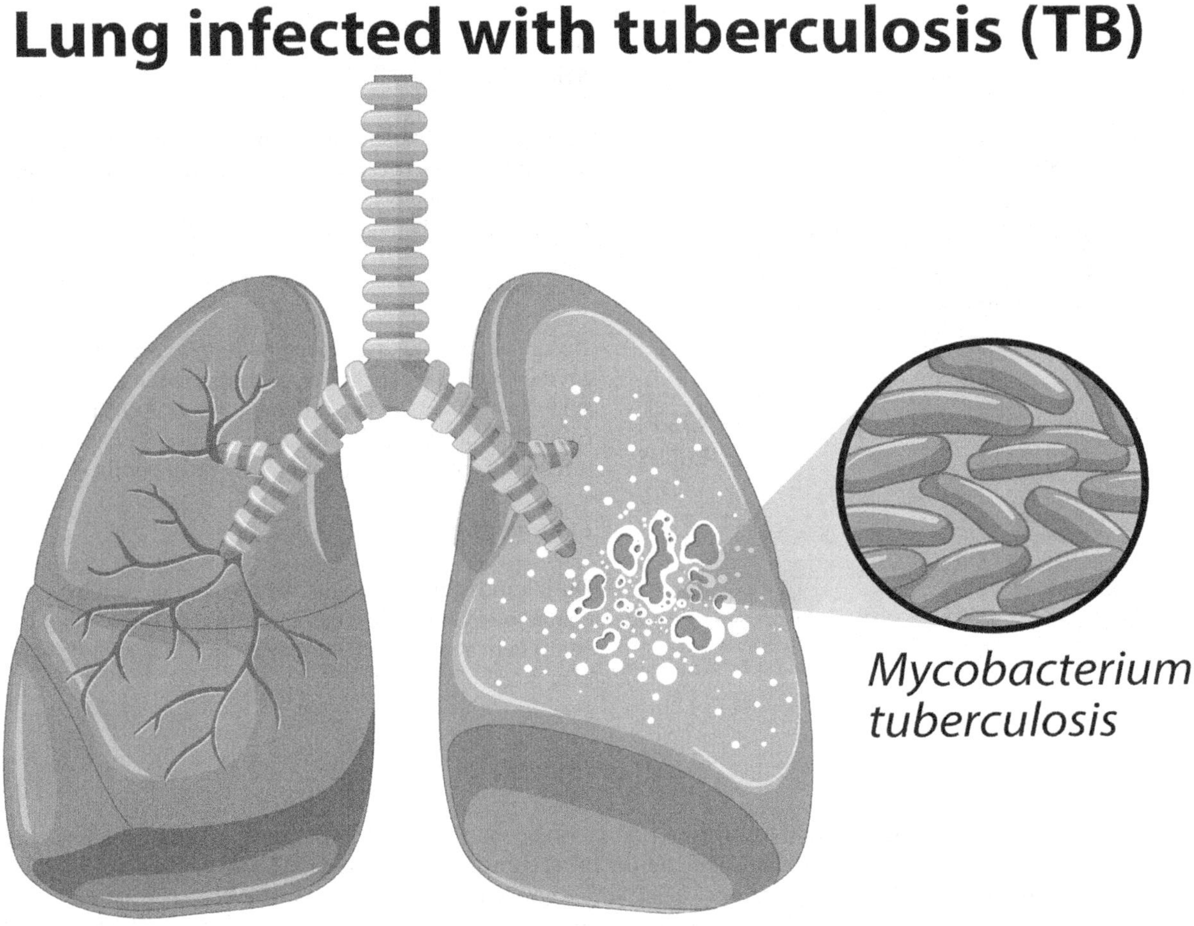

# Respiratory Pathologies

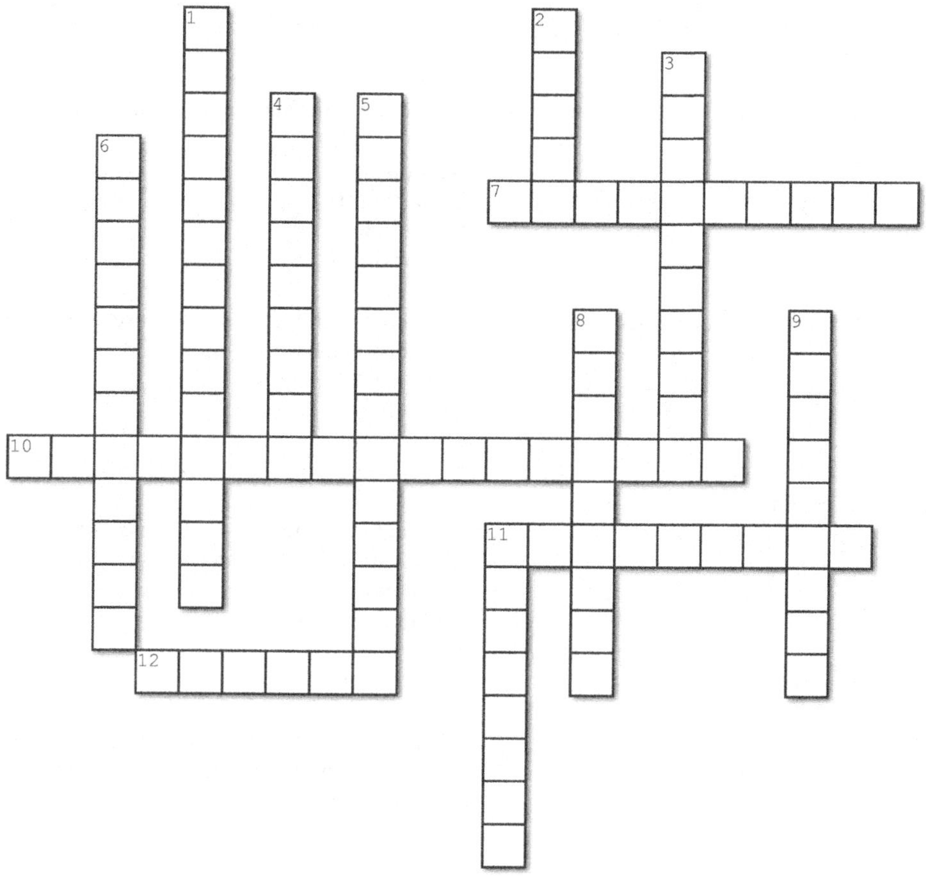


**Across**

**7.** Loss of voice due to inflammation of the voice box

**10.** A blood clot entering the lung that restricts blood flow to the lung

**11.** Highly contagious infection causing fluid to build up in the alveoli

**12.** Constriction of smooth muscle surrounding bronchial tubes, reducing oxygen intake

**Down**

**1.** Genetic disorder resulting in thick mucous being produced in the respiratory and digestive tracts

**2.** Temporary cessation of breathing during sleep

**3.** Inflammation of bronchial tubes, often caused by a primary infection or cigarette smoke

**4.** Destruction of alveoli, reducing alveoli surface area and oxygen intake

**5.** A collection of fluid in the alveoli most commonly caused by an issue with the heart

**6.** Bacterial infection of the lung spread through microscopic droplets of water in the air

**8.** Viral infection of the respiratory tract that may cause fever and nausea

**9.** Acute inflammation of the sinuses that causes an increased amount of mucous to be produced

**11.** Inflammation of the pleural membrane

Answer Key on Page 287

## Respiratory Quiz

1. Part of the respiratory passage that divides into the left and right bronchus
A. Larynx
B. Pharynx
C. Trachea
D. Epiglottis

2. Bronchial tubes branch out into smaller tubes called
A. Larynx
B. Alveoli
C. Trachea
D. Bronchioles

3. Drug used to treat acute asthma
A. Bronchodilator
B. Expectorant
C. Decongestant
D. Anticoagulant

4. Vibration of air produces speech, which is the responsibility of
A. Larynx
B. Pharynx
C. Trachea
D. Epiglottis

5. High altitudes can cause altitude sickness, a common form of
A. Hypoxia
B. Hypothermia
C. Hyperplasia
D. Frostbite

6. Apnea can be defined as
A. Lack of sufficient erythrocytes in the body
B. Temporary cessation of breathing, usually during sleep
C. Constriction of smooth muscle around bronchial tubes
D. Viral infection causing inflammation in the nasal cavity

7. Contagious bacterial infection typically spread through coughing or sneezing, which can cause pain upon breathing, chronic coughing, and bloody coughing
A. Strep throat
B. Tuberculosis
C. Influenza
D. Bronchitis

8. A collection of fluid in the lung alveoli, most commonly associated with a heart problem
A. Pulmonary edema
B. Asthma
C. Pneumonia
D. Tuberculosis

9. Acute inflammation of the sinuses, often the result of a viral infection
A. Sinusitis
B. Laryngitis
C. Bronchitis
D. Tonsillitis

10. Acute viral infection that results in general malaise, fever, and body aches
A. Pneumonia
B. Pleurisy
C. Tuberculosis
D. Influenza

11. Bacterial infection that causes fluid to build up in the alveoli, which can reduce oxygen intake
A. Pneumonia
B. Tuberculosis
C. Sinusitis
D. Influenza

12. Damage to the lungs that causes pain upon breathing and inflammation of the pleural membrane
A. Pulmonary edema
B. Pleurisy
C. Influenza
D. Pneumonia

13. Form of bronchitis caused by another condition or infection
A. Latent
B. Chronic
C. Active
D. Acute

14. Pulmonary embolism
A. Blood clot getting lodged in the lung
B. Build up of fluid in the alveoli
C. Excessive mucous production in the sinus
D. Constriction of bronchial tubes by smooth muscle

15. Genetic disorder that results in the body producing excessive amounts of mucous in the respiratory and digestive tracts
A. Emphysema
B. Asthma
C. Cystic fibrosis
D. Pleurisy

Answer Key on Page 289

# Skeletal System and Pathologies

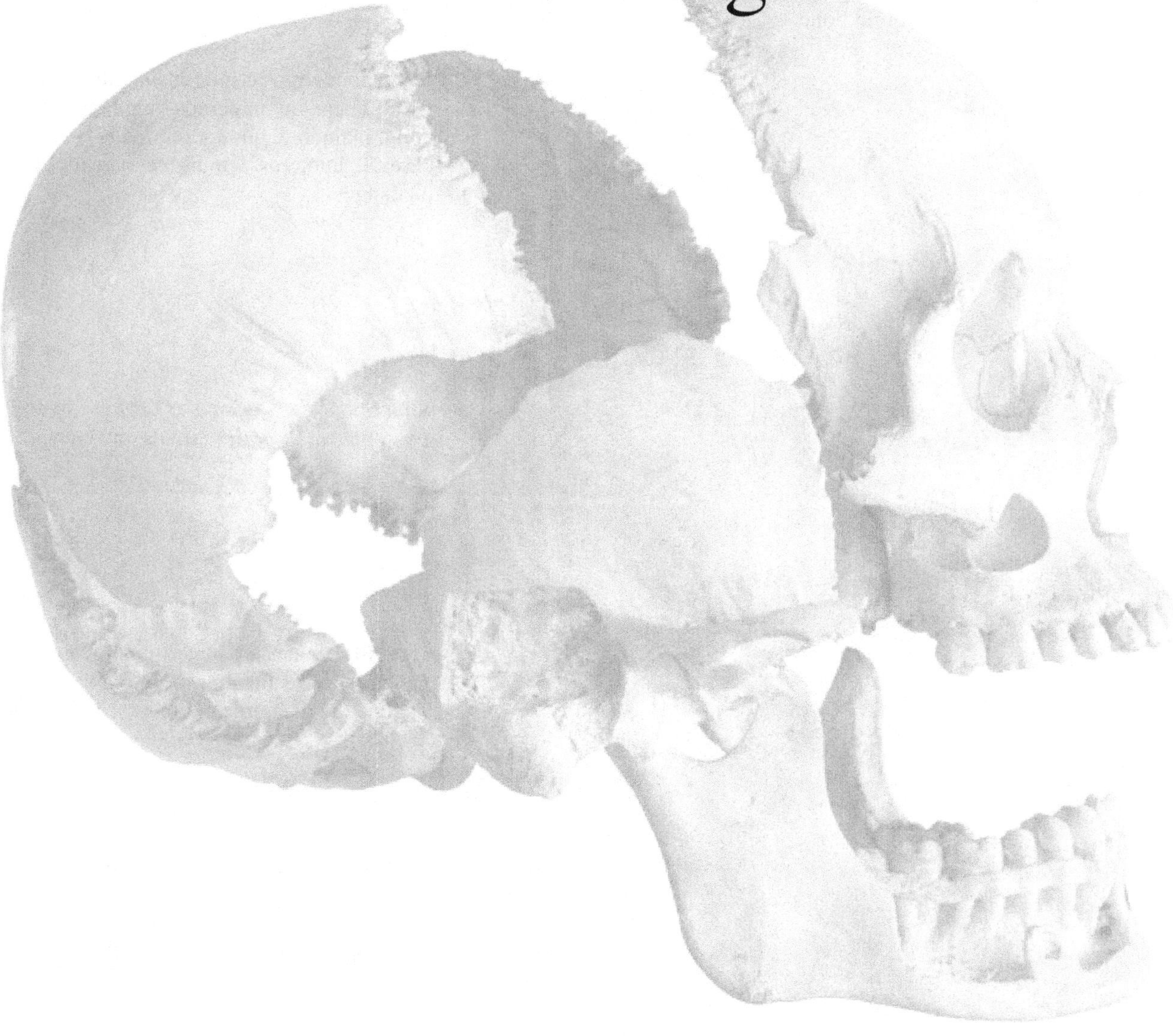

# Skeletal System

The Skeletal System is a vital component of movement. We wouldn't be able to move if we didn't have bones! Muscles attach to bones, and when a muscle contracts, it pulls on a bone(or bones), which performs an action. Bones also produce blood cells, provide stability for the body, and protect structures and organs in the body. Needless to say, bones are extremely important!

There are **206** bones in the human body. Each bone can be classified as one of the following: **Long** bone, **Short** bone, **Irregular** bone, **Flat** bone, **Sesamoid** bone.

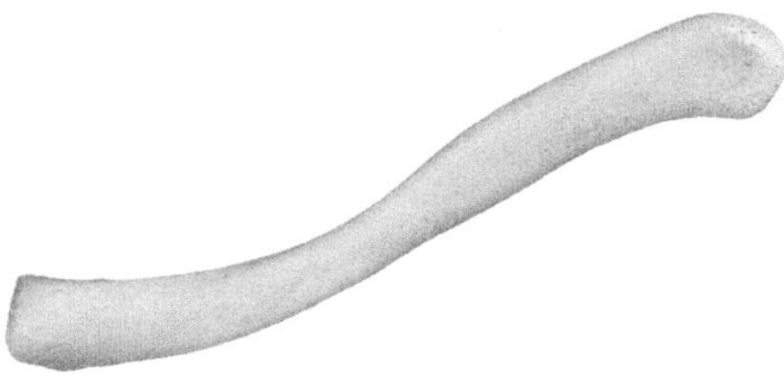

- **Long** bones appear **longer** than they are **wide**. There are numerous long bones in the body, including, but not limited to, the clavicle, humerus, femur, metatarsals, and phalanges.

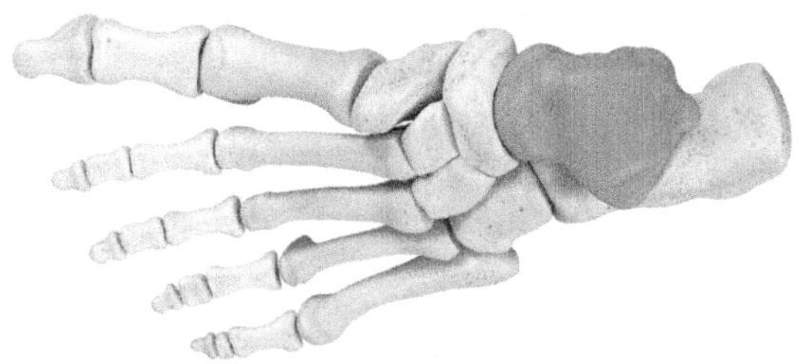

- **Short** bones are **as long** as they are **wide**. Examples include the carpals and tarsals.

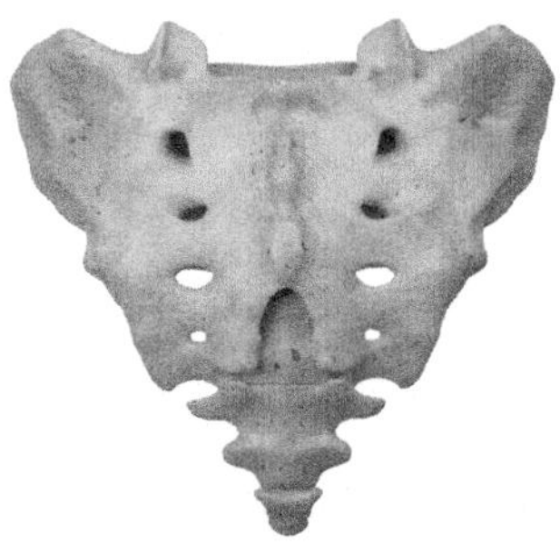

- **Irregular** bones are bones that have generally **unusual shapes**. Examples include the mandible, vertebrae, and pubis.

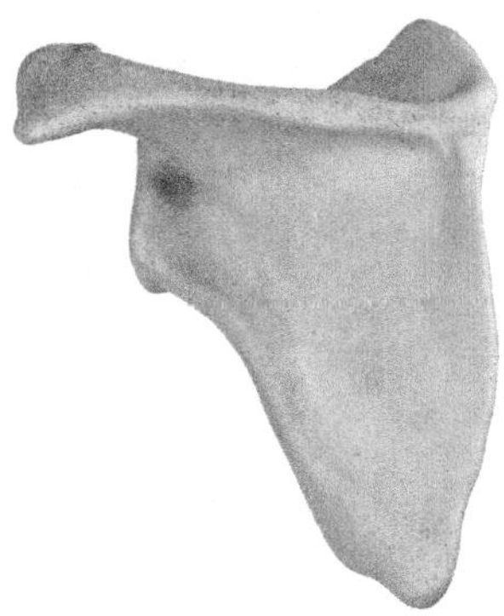

- **Flat** bones are named after how they look: **flat**. They are typically thin and flat. Examples include the scapula, ribs, and cranial bones.

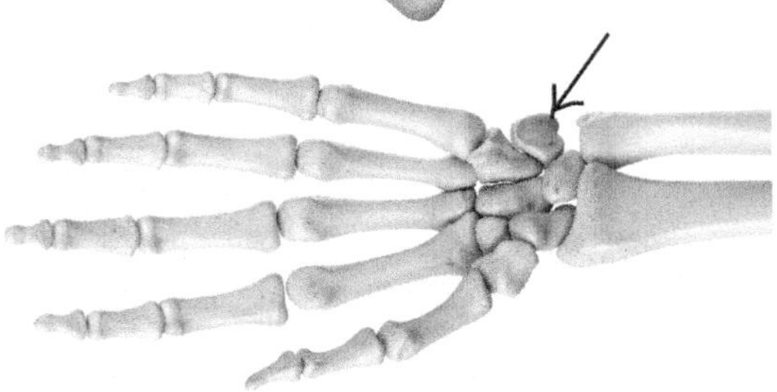

- **Sesamoid** bones are bones embedded **inside tendons**, and named after what they look like. They are rounded, and resemble **sesame seeds**. The primary examples are the patella and pisiform.

Long bones consist of three main parts: the **epiphyses**, the **metaphyses**, and the **diaphysis**. The epiphyses can be found on the **ends** of the long bone, where the bone articulates with other bones. The epiphyses are covered with cartilage to prevent friction between the articulating bone surfaces. The epiphyses are primarily made of spongy bone, which allows certain bones to withstand extreme pressure without fracturing.

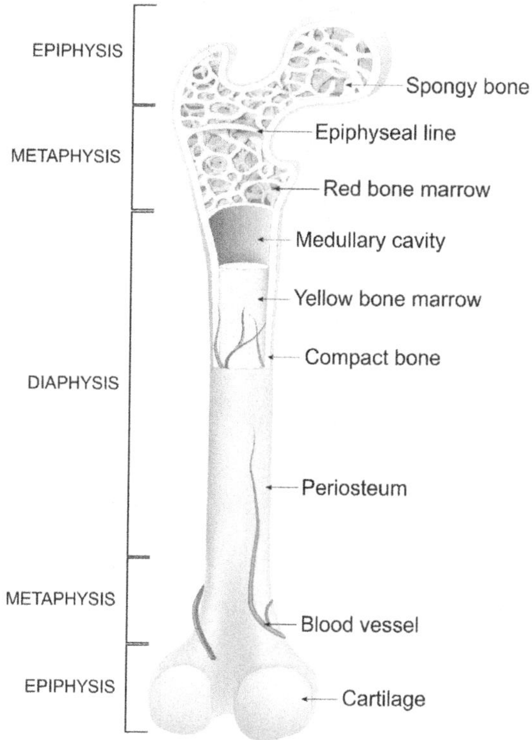


The **metaphyses** are the sections between the epiphyses and the diaphysis. Inside the metaphyses, there is a line of cartilage called the **epiphyseal plate/line**, and it is where **growth** in the bone takes place during childhood and adolescence. As a person grows, eventually the cartilage ossifies and becomes part of the bone, and growth in the bone no longer occurs.

The **diaphysis** is the **shaft** of the bone. Inside the shaft of the bone is the medullary cavity. The medullary cavity contains **red bone marrow** during childhood, which is the site of **red blood cell formation**. When the child ages, the red bone marrow is converted into yellow bone marrow, which is mainly just fat. The diaphysis is made of compact bone to provide as much strength as possible around the medullary cavity, while still giving enough space for the cavity itself to fill with marrow.

## Joints

Where bones come together is known as an **articulation**. Another name for articulation is "**joint**". Joints are where **movements** occur. We don't flex muscles, we flex joints!

All joints are classified as one of the following: **Synarthrotic**, **Amphiarthrotic**, or **Diarthrotic**. Synarthrotic joints are joints with little to **no movement** in them, such as the sutures in the skull. Amphiarthrotic joints are joints that are **slightly movable**, such as the intervertebral joints. Diarthrotic joints are **freely movable** joints, and have no real movement restrictions, such as in the shoulder or hip.

Joints have several structures that help create and support them. Between bones that articulate, on the **epiphyses**, there is **articular cartilage**. This type of cartilage is known as **hyaline** cartilage. It is a dense form of cartilage, very thick, and is a shock-absorber. Hyaline cartilage also **prevents friction** between the articulating bones, so bones don't rub against each other during movement.

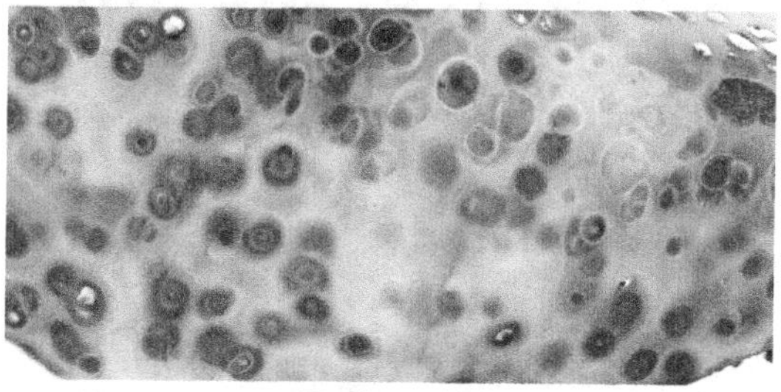

Hyaline cartilage

Certain joints have a specific type of cartilage in them known as a **labrum**. The labrum, found in the glenohumeral joint and iliofemoral joint, is used to **deepen** the joint, providing a deeper socket for these ball-and-socket joints. This provides more **strength** and **stability** for the joint.

Bones are held together by **ligaments**. Ligaments are avascular, meaning they are not supplied with blood by blood vessels. Ligaments are strong, but do not stretch very far before injury can occur. Tearing of ligaments such as the Anterior Cruciate Ligament is common in activities such as sports, or in car accidents.

Four of the most important joints joined together by ligaments are located in the skull, between the cranial bones. These synarthrotic joints are called **sutures**. The **sagittal** suture runs along a sagittal plane on the top of the head, connecting the two **parietal bones**. The **coronal** suture runs on a coronal plane, connecting the **frontal** bone to the **parietal** bones. The **squamous** suture runs on a sagittal plane, but is located on the side of the skull, connecting the **parietal** and **temporal** bones together. Finally, the **lambdoid** suture, named for its resemblance to the Greek letter "lambda", connects the **occipital** bone to the **parietal** bones.

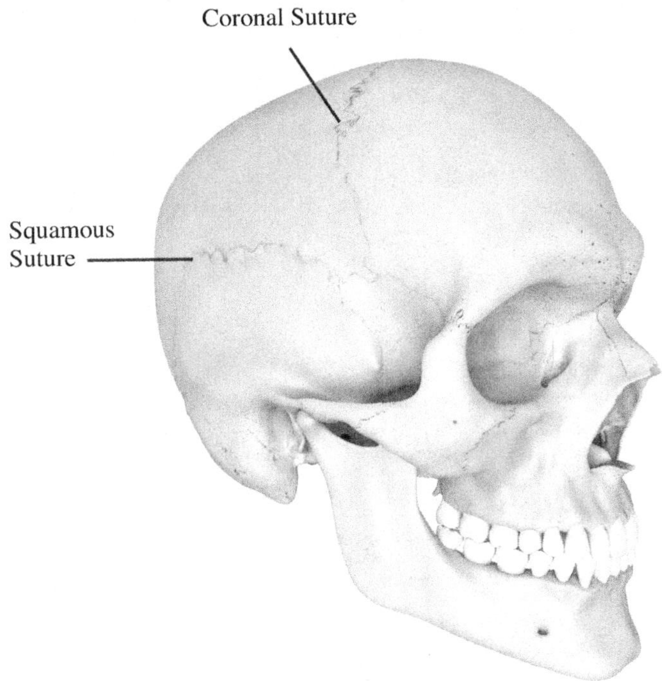


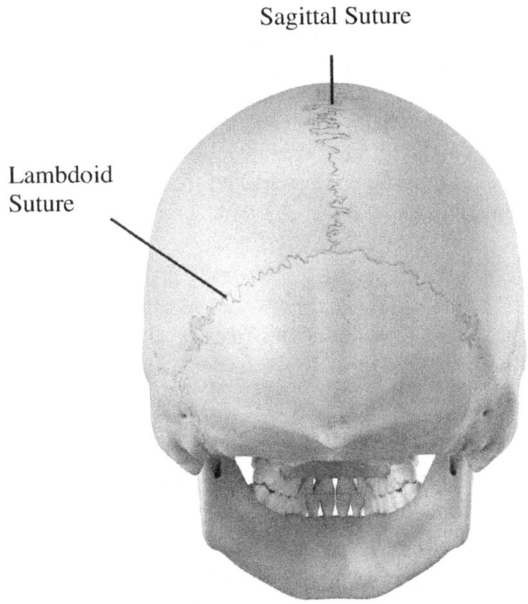


# Synovial joint of the knee

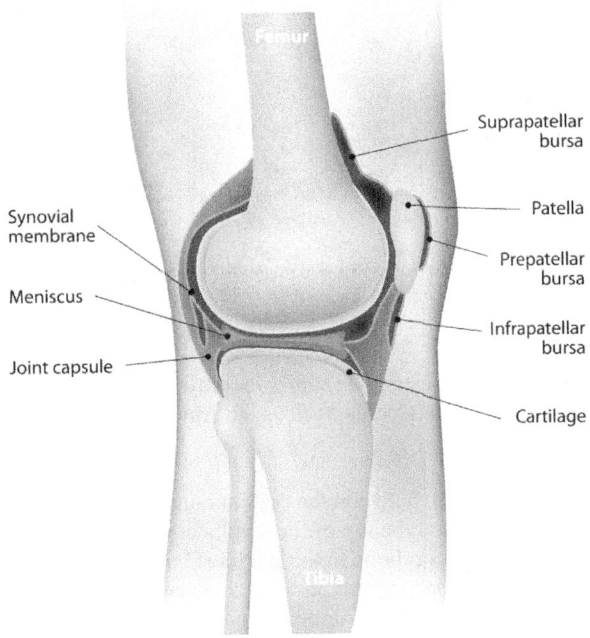


Inside the joint itself, a membrane is present, known as the **synovial membrane**. The synovial membrane produces a fluid that helps to lubricate the joint, known as the **synovial fluid**. Lubrication of the joint is key in keeping the joint functioning optimally. Surrounding the entire joint is thick, dense connective tissue known as the **joint capsule**. The joint capsule keeps everything inside the joint, such as the synovial fluid, and provides even more strength and support for the joint.

Muscles are held to bones via **tendons**. Tendons are similar to ligaments, but have a much more rich blood supply, and able to stretch further before injury occurs.

## Types of Diarthrotic Joints

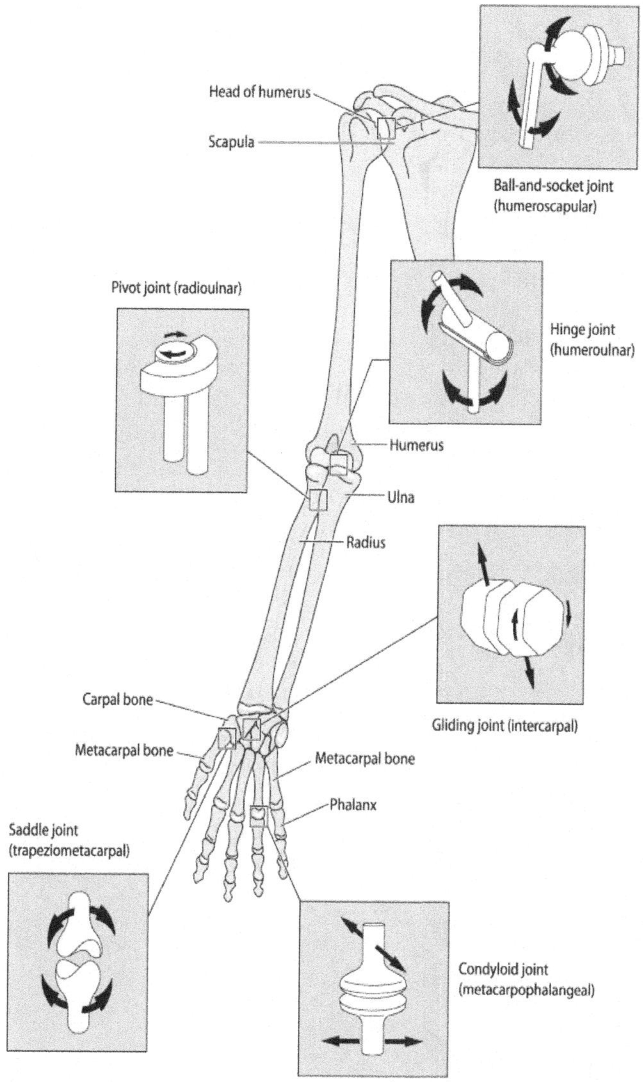


There are **six** different types of diarthrotic joints.

**Ball-and-Socket** joints feature one bone with a **ball** at the epiphysis, and another bone with a **socket**. The ball fits in the socket, creating a ball-and-socket joint. Examples include the shoulder and hip joints. Ball-and-socket joints have the most amount of movement, able to move the joint in really any direction.

**Hinge** joints act much like the hinge on a door, only opening and closing. Hinge joints only allow movement in **one plane**, allowing only **flexion** and **extension**. Examples include the elbow and knee joints.

**Pivot** joints allow only one type of movement: **rotation**. All they do is allow structures to turn. An example is the atlantoaxial joint, which lets us shake our head "no". This is rotation.

**Plane/gliding** joints are produced when the articulating bones have **flat** surfaces, and there is a **disc of cartilage** between the bones. This allows the joint to move, or glide, in any direction, although with slight movement. Examples include the joints between the carpals and tarsals.

**Saddle** joints are only located in one part of the body: the **carpometacarpal joint** of the **thumb**. Saddle joints are named after the appearance of the articulating bones. The articulating surfaces are both shaped like saddles. The two bones that create the saddle joint are the **first metacarpal** and the **trapezium**.

**Ellipsoid/condyloid** joints are extremely similar to ball-and-socket joints. On one bone, there is a **condyle**, which resembles a ball, but isn't as pronounced. This condyle fits into an **elliptical cavity** on another bone, which is similar to a socket, but not as deep. This allows movements such as flexion, extension, adduction, abduction, and circumduction. An example is the radiocarpal joint, created by the elliptical cavity of the radius meeting the condyle of the scaphoid.

## Skeleton Divisions

There are two divisions of the skeleton: the **Axial Skeleton** and the **Appendicular Skeleton**.

The Axial Skeleton contains all of the bones that do not correspond to any appendages: the **skull**, **vertebral column,** and **thoracic cage**. These bones make up the trunk.

The Appendicular Skeleton contains all of the bones that correspond to the appendages: the **humerus**, **radius**, **ulna**, **carpals**, **metacarpals**, **phalanges**, **femur**, **tibia**, **fibula**, **metatarsals**, **phalanges**, the **pectoral girdle**(clavicles and scapulae) and **pelvic girdle**(ilium, ischium, pubis, and sacrum).

## Bones of the Axial Skeleton

### Skull

The skull's primary function is to **protect the brain**. The bones that make up the skull are:

| | |
|---|---|
| Parietal | Mandible |
| Frontal | Vomer |
| Temporal | Ethmoid |
| Occipital | Sphenoid |
| Zygomatic | Nasal |
| Maxilla | Lacrimal |

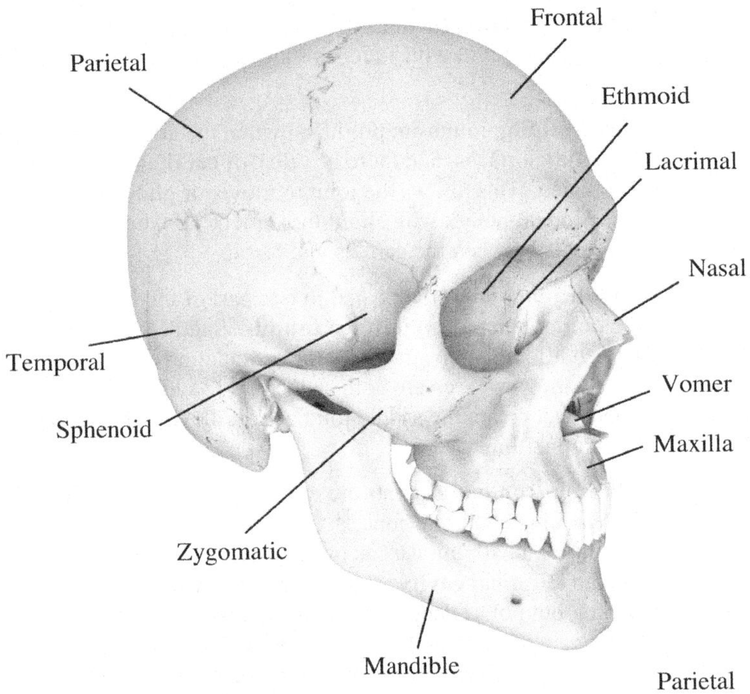


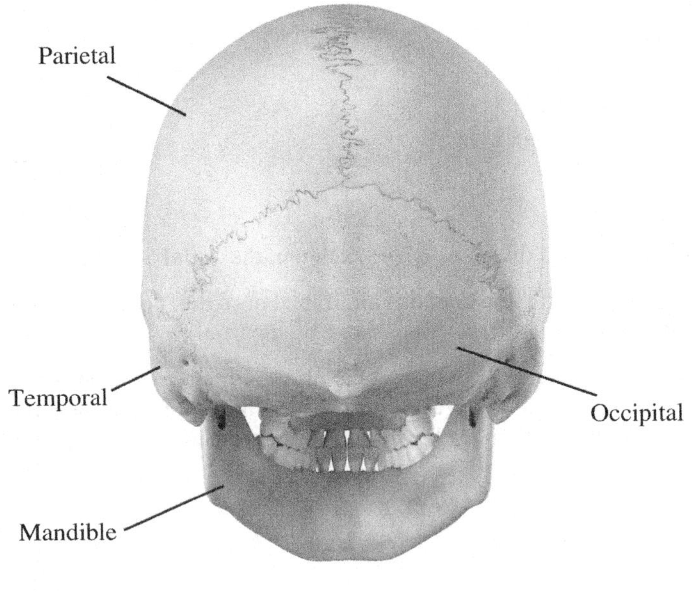

## Vertebral Column

The vertebral column consists of **26** individual bones. Its primary function is to **protect the spinal cord,** which runs through it. There are five different regions of the vertebral column. They are:

Cervical(7 vertebrae)
Thoracic(12 vertebrae)
Lumbar(5 vertebrae)
Sacral(1 vertebrae)
Coccygeal(1 vertebrae)

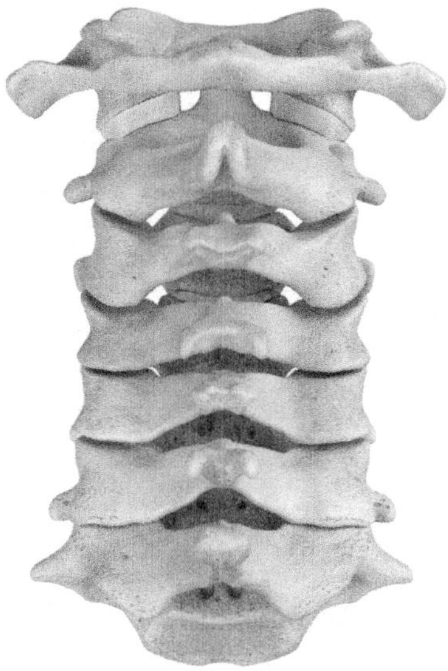

Cervical Vertebrae

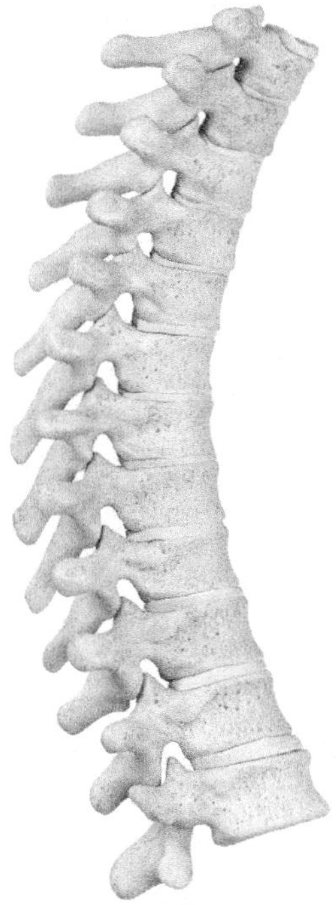

Thoracic Vertebrae

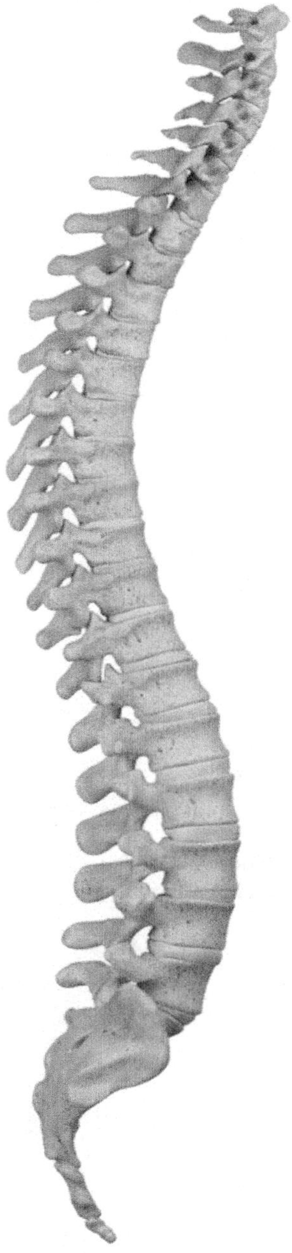

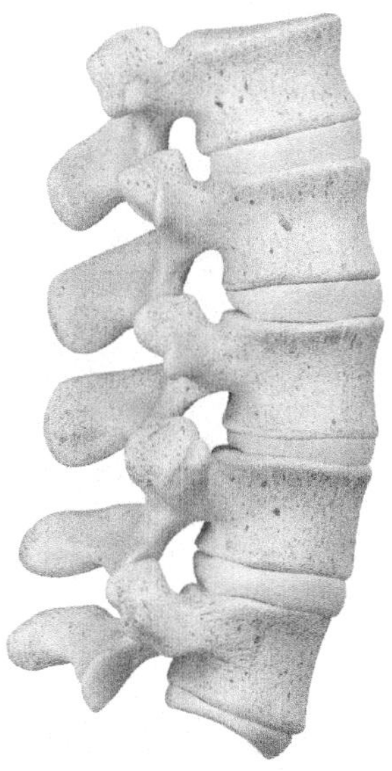

Lumbar Vertebrae

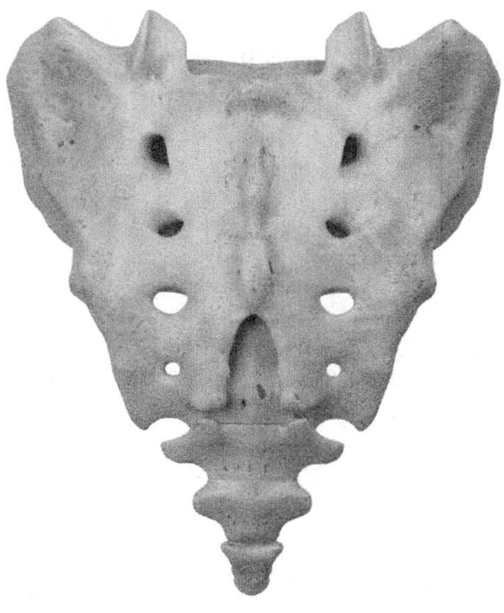

Sacrum and Coccyx

### Chest

The chest consists of the **rib cage**. The primary function of the rib cage is to **protect vital organs** inside the thorax, and assist in breathing by giving the diaphragm a place to attach. The rib cage consists of:

True ribs(superior seven ribs)
False ribs(inferior five ribs)
Floating ribs(ribs 11 and 12)

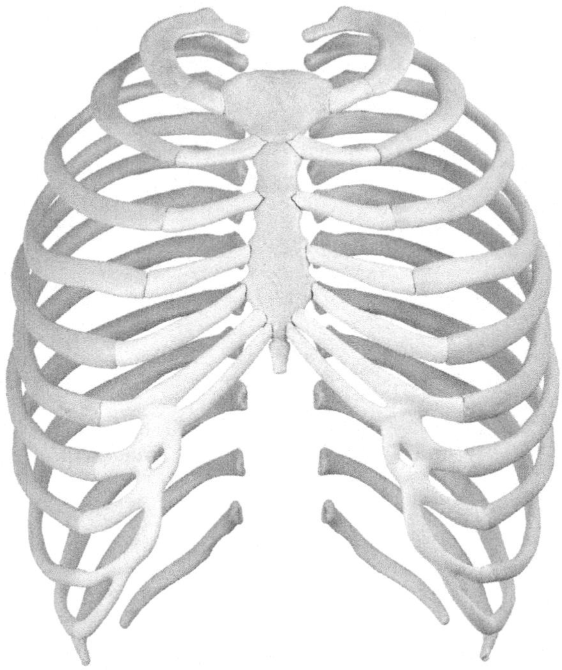

## Bones of the Appendicular Skeleton

### Pectoral Girdle

The pectoral girdle is responsible for holding the upper limbs to the body. The pectoral girdle consists of four bones:

Scapulae(two bones)
Clavicles(two bones)

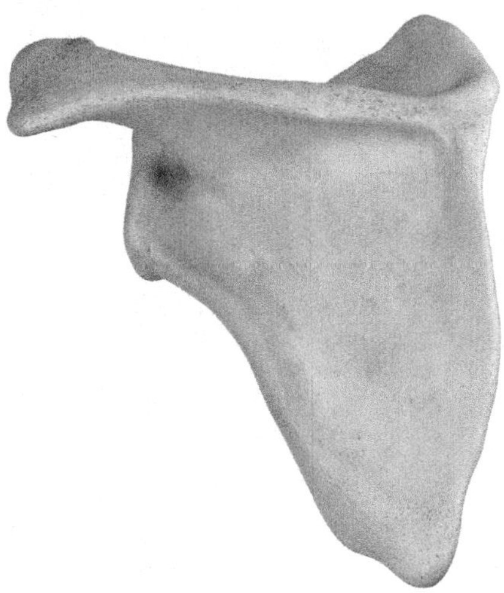

Scapula

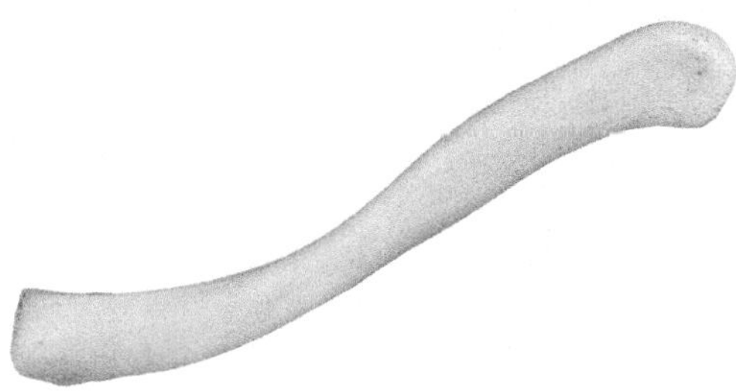

Clavicle

## Pelvic Girdle

The pelvic girdle is primarily responsible for holding the lower limbs to the body. The pelvic girdle contains:

Ilium(two bones)
Ischium(two bones)
Pubis(two bones)
Sacrum(one bone)

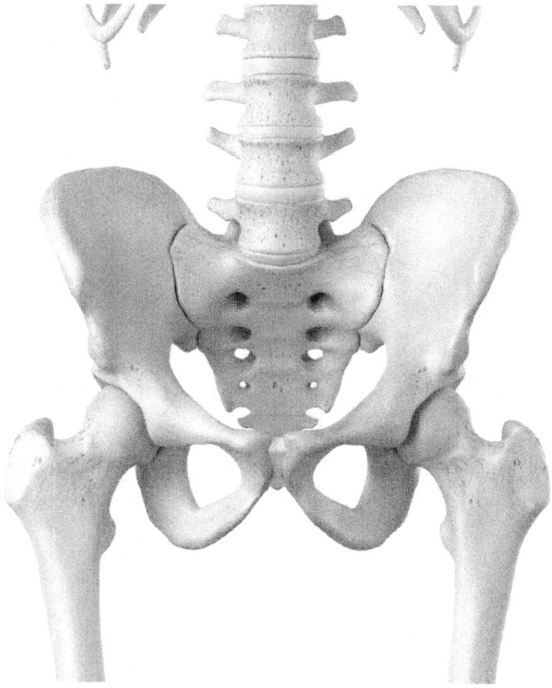

## Arm

The arm contains one bone:

Humerus

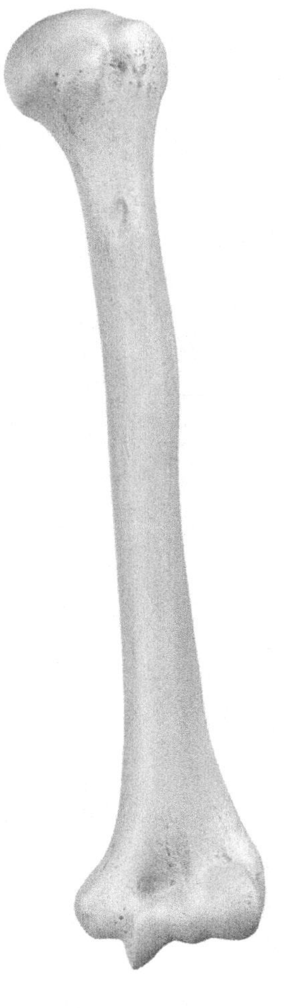

## Forearm

The forearm contains two bones:

Radius
Ulna

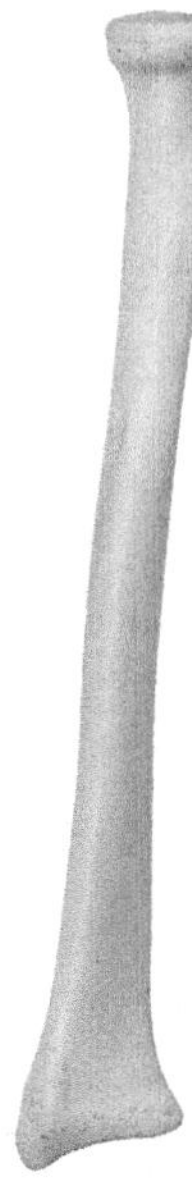

Radius

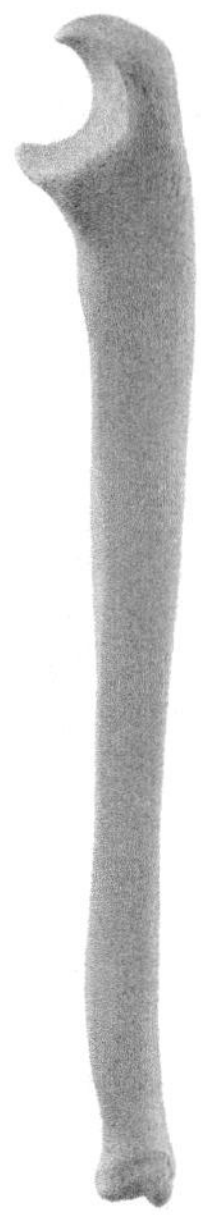

Ulna

## Wrist

The wrist is located distally to the forearm, and it contains the **carpal** bones. The carpal bones are divided into two separate lines, each containing four bones. The proximal line is listed first, then the distal line:

Proximal Line:
Scaphoid
Lunate
Triquetrum
Pisiform

Distal Line:
Trapezium
Trapezoid
Capitate
Hamate

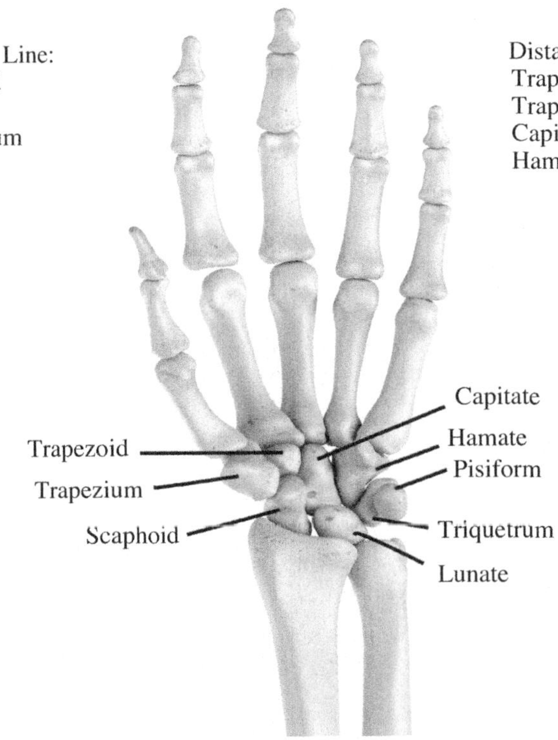

## Hand

The hand contains **19 bones** in each hand:

Metacarpals(5 bones)
Phalanges(14 bones)

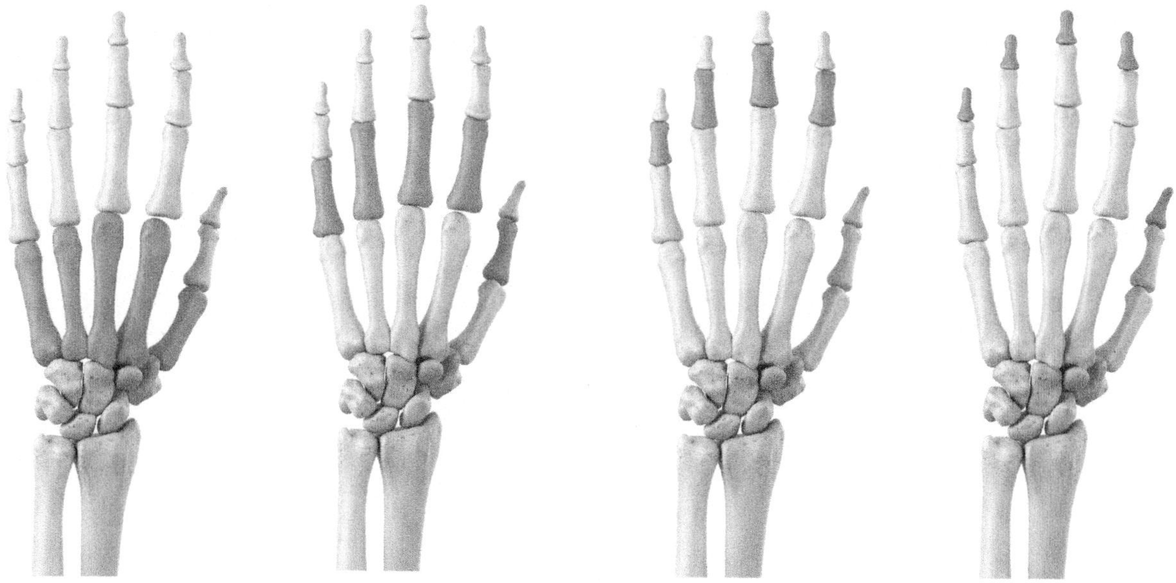

Metacarpals Proximal Phalanges Middle Phalanges Distal Phalanges

## Thigh

The thigh contains one bone:

Femur

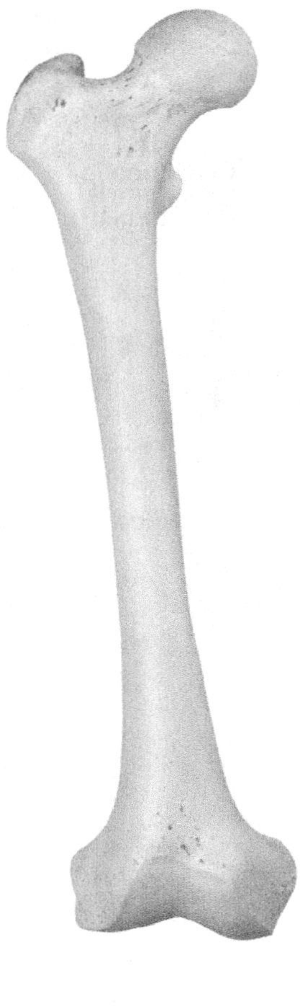

## Leg

The leg contains two bones:

Tibia
Fibula

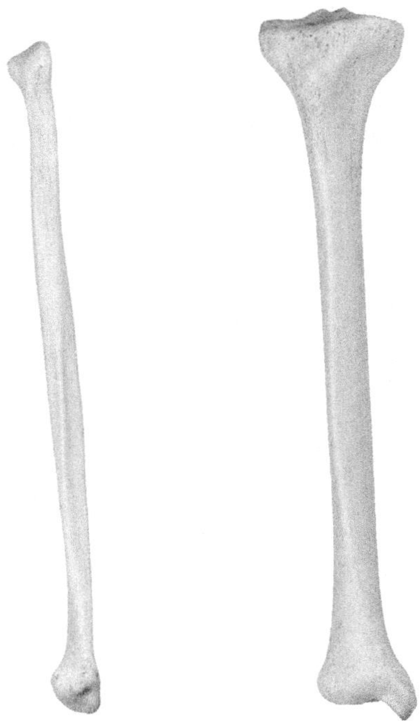


## Ankle

The ankle is located distally to the leg, and it consists of the bones of the **tarsals**:

Calcaneus
Talus
Navicular
Cuboid
Cuneiform I
Cuneiform II
Cuneiform III

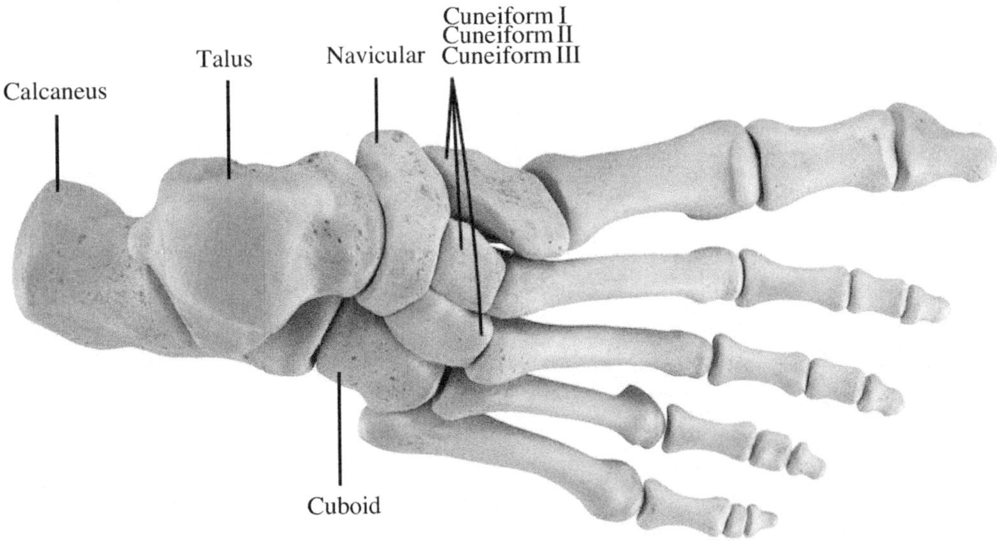

## Foot

The foot contains **19 bones** in each foot:

Metatarsals(5 bones)
Phalanges(14 bones)

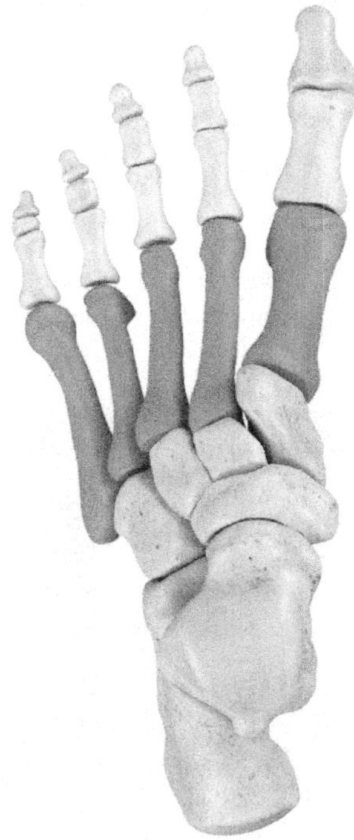

Metatarsals

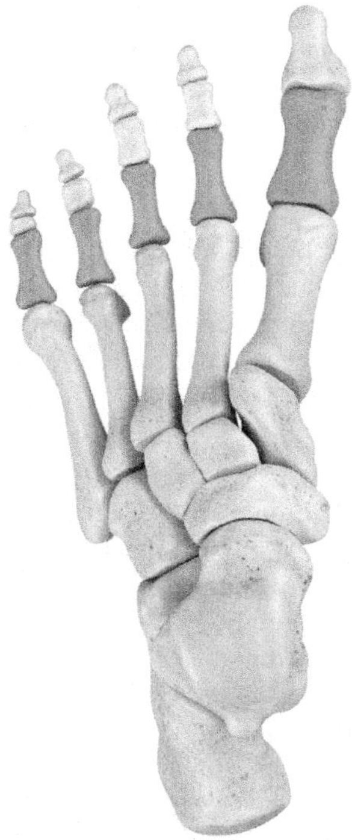

Proximal Phalanges

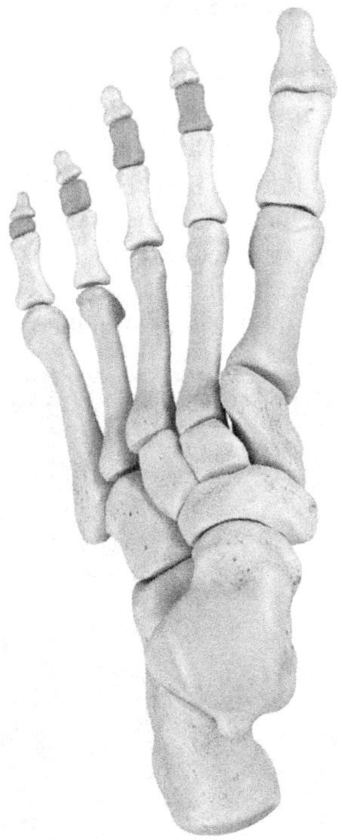

Middle Phalanges

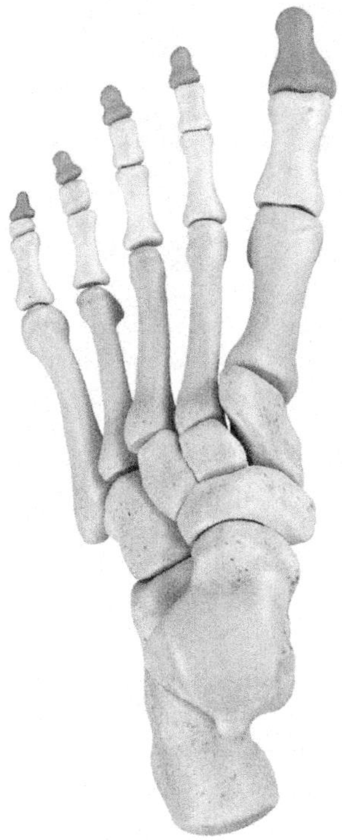

Distal Phalanges

## Medical Tests and Equipment

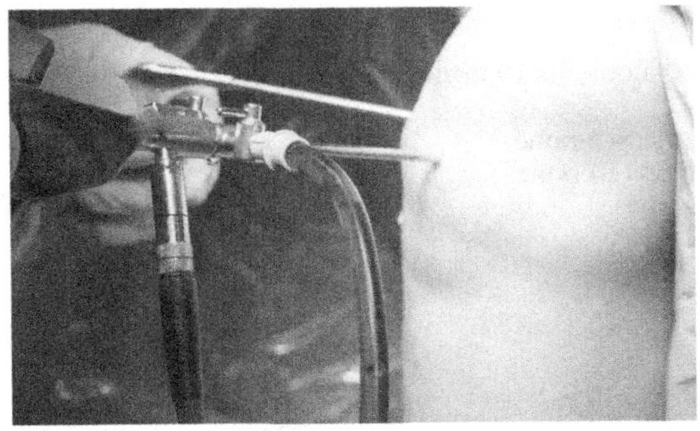

**Arthroscopy**: Arthroscopy is used to view the inner structures of a joint. It is performed by making a small incision, and inserting a tube with a camera attached directly into the joint. This allows a view of any structural damage that may occur, such as torn ligaments. If surgery is being performed, it may be performed arthroscopically, where all the instruments being used are inserted into the joint through small holes, without making a large incision.

**Bone Graft**: A bone graft, similar to a skin graft, is the removal of a small amount of bone tissue from one part of the body, placing the removed tissue on another bone that may be lacking in sufficient tissue. This can be done if part of a bone is removed during surgery, or in cases such as joint replacements to help the new structures anchor in to the bone more securely. The new bone sets, and the area where the graft is located becomes stronger.

**Computerized Axial Tomography(CT/CAT Scan)**: Computerized Axial Tomography, also known as CT or CAT Scan, is an imaging technique in which a snapshot is taken of a part of the body on a given body plane. This allows viewing of structures in the body from differing points of view. CT is extremely similar to MRI, but uses X-ray to produce images instead of magnetic fields.

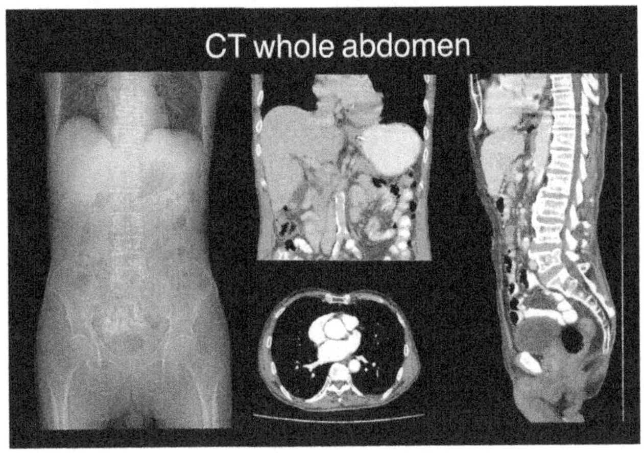


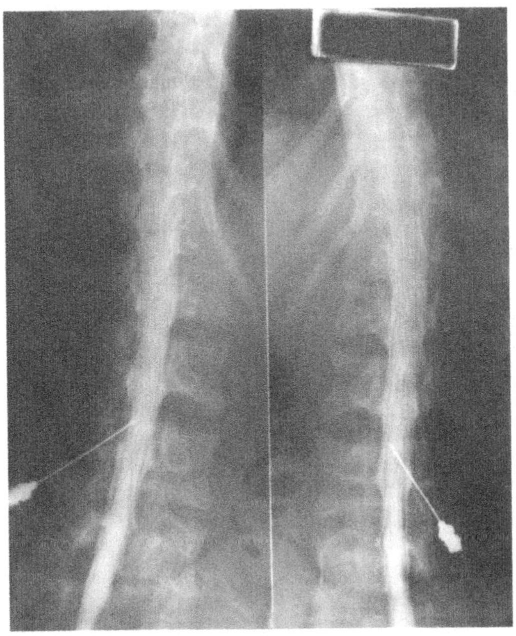

**Myelogram**: A myelogram is an imaging procedure used to view problems that may be occurring in the spinal canal. Special dyes are injected into the spinal column, and the patient is given X-rays, which allow the structures inside the spinal canal to be properly viewed. Myelograms are used to examine conditions such as herniated discs, infections such as meningitis, and tumors in the brain or spinal cord.

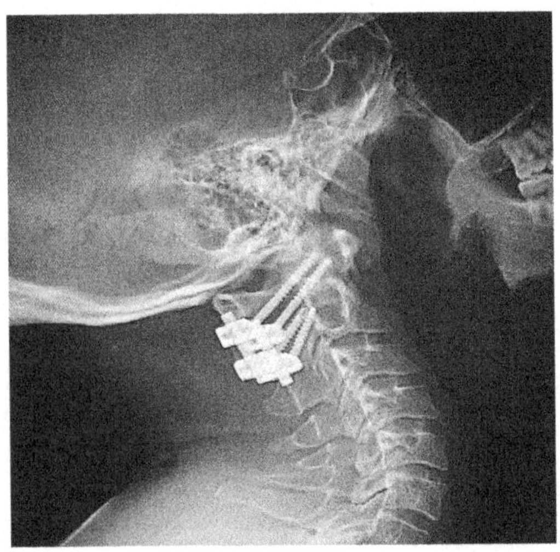

**X-Ray**: An X-ray is an imaging technique using radiation to view structures that light typically does not pass through. Structures most commonly viewed using X-rays are bones and metals. X-rays allow visual examination of structures that may be broken, damaged, or infected.

# Skeletal System Pathologies

## Ankylosing Spondylitis

*(ankyl/o: crooked; spondyl-: spine; -itis: inflammation)*

Ankylosing Spondylitis is an **autoimmune disorder**, similar to rheumatoid arthritis(page 239), in which the body's immune system attacks and destroys the **annulus fibrosus** of the **intervertebral discs**. Over time, the curvature in the vertebrae is lost. Because the intervertebral discs are destroyed, the space between vertebral bodies lessens, eventually allowing the vertebral bones to sit directly atop one another. Movement between these bones is severely reduced, and eventually the bones can fuse together, which eliminates any movement between the bones at all.

A person with ankylosing spondylitis may appear to be hunched forward, and may present with kyphosis(page 233) as a result. Another name for ankylosing spondylitis is "Bamboo Spine" because after fusion, the vertebrae resembles a bamboo stalk.

### *Causes*

Ankylosing spondylitis is caused by the body's immune system attacking the intervertebral discs for unknown reasons.

### *Symptoms*

Pain is an extremely common symptom of ankylosing spondylitis, especially in the neck, base of the skull, and lumbar region. Lack of mobility is a secondary symptom, usually the result of pain.

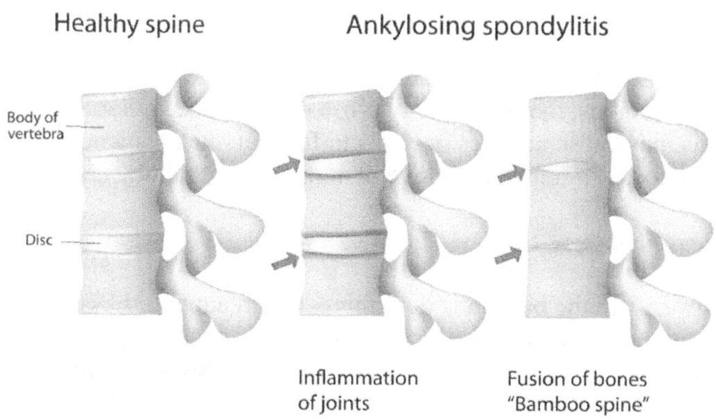


### *Treatments*

Non-steroidal anti-inflammatory medications may be prescribed to help reduce pain and inflammation in affected areas. Physical therapy, massage therapy, stretching, and range-of-motion exercises are all helpful in maintaining mobility in the vertebral joints and preventing bones from fusing together.

If the condition is severe, surgery may be performed to remove fused bone, or to insert metal rods to correct posture.

### *Contraindications*

Massage is indicated for ankylosing spondylitis. Stretching and range-of-motion exercises should be performed within the client's pain tolerance. If the client has difficulty lying supine due to kyphosis, side-lying position may be needed.

## Baker's Cyst

A Baker's Cyst is a **small sac** filled with **synovial fluid** that forms on the **back of the knee**. Another name for this is "Popliteal Cyst". A Baker's Cyst is usually the result of an **injury** in the knee joint.

### *Causes*

Tearing of the meniscus or ligaments in the knee can cause an overproduction of synovial fluid in the joint. If too much synovial fluid is produced, a sac can form around it on the back of the knee.

### *Symptoms*

Pain and stiffness in the knee are common symptoms experienced. The popliteal region can feel swollen and bulge out due to the cyst being present.

***Treatments***

Typically, a Baker's Cyst goes away on its own without treatment. However, if the cyst causes pain or discomfort, treatments are available. Medications may be prescribed to reduce inflammation, the fluid may physically be drained by a doctor, or ice may be applied to reduce inflammation. If the cause of the cyst is known, such as torn cartilage, an arthroscopic surgery may be performed to repair or clean up the tissue, which may aid in the cyst draining.

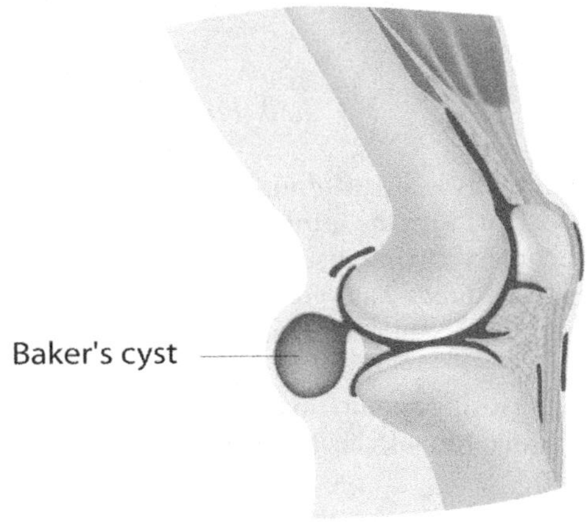


***Contraindications***

A Baker's Cyst is considered a local contraindication. Massage may be performed, but massaging the cyst itself should be avoided.

## Bunion

A Bunion is a **subluxation** of the **big toe**, the result of the toe pushing back against the first metatarsal. Excessive force against this bone causes the big toe to subluxate medially, creating a **large bump**.

***Causes***

Tight fitting shoes may contribute to the development of bunions. Rheumatoid arthritis(page 239) may also contribute. Foot injuries may also play a role.

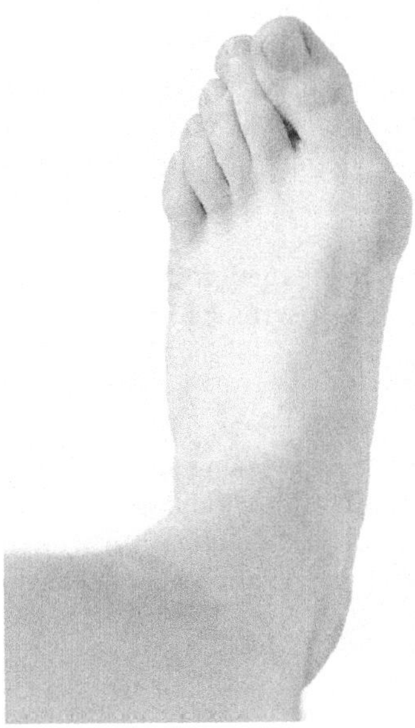

***Symptoms***

Pain and swelling may present in the area of the bunion. With bunions, the big toe may cross under the second toe. This may cause calluses or corns to form on the area where these toes rub together. Movement in the big toe may reduce.

***Treatments***

How severe the bunion is determines the treatment. Less severe bunions may require only changing shoes or applying a splint to help reset the toe. More severe forms of a bunion may require surgery to correct the placement of the toe.

***Contraindications***

Massage is generally not contraindicated for a bunion. However, if the client is experiencing pain as a result of the bunion, massage in the area should be avoided.

## Bursitis

*(burs-: bursa; -itis: inflammation)*

Bursitis is a condition that results in **inflammation** of a **bursa**, a small sac filled with synovial fluid.

***Causes***

Bursae are located all over the body, typically between a tendon and bone to prevent friction and irritation. When there is repeated stress placed on the bursa, it can become inflamed. Bursitis may affect many different joints, including the knee, shoulder, elbow, hip, and ankle.

Bursitis is most often caused by repetitive motions in the affected joint, which may irritate the bursa. Trauma may also result in bursitis, such as fractures or tendonitis.

***Symptoms***

Typically, a joint affected with bursitis will be inflamed and painful to move. The inflammation may be moderate or severe.

***Treatments***

Bursitis is easily treatable, primarily with rest and ice. Depending on the severity, the bursa may also need to be surgically drained or removed, or injected with corticosteroids to reduce the inflammation.

***Contraindications***

Bursitis is considered a local contraindication for massage. Cold packs may be used to help decrease inflammation in the area.

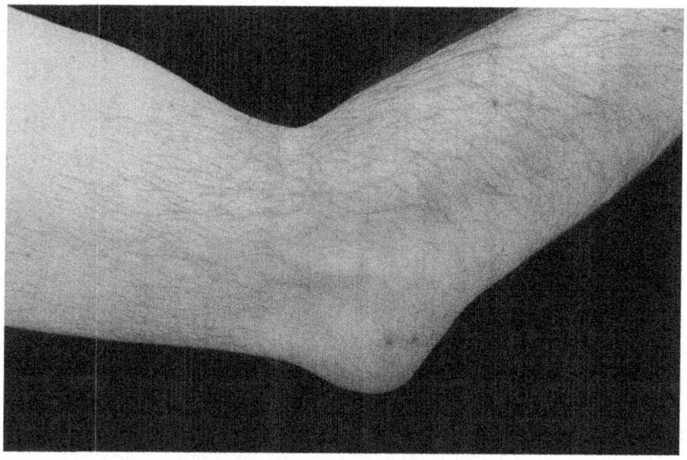

Inflammation of olecranon bursa

## Chondromalacia Patellae

*(chondr/o: cartilage; malacia: softening of tissue)*

Chondromalacia Patellae, also known as "**Runner's Knee**", is a **degenerative disorder** affecting the **cartilage** on the posterior side of the **patella**, which can increase friction and irritation in the knee. Younger adults are most likely to develop chondromalacia patellae due to being more physically active than older adults.

***Causes***

Over-use of the knee may contribute to the development of chondromalacia patellae, resulting in constant friction between the patella and femur. Excessive stress in the joint may lead to irritation. Weak thigh muscles can also contribute.

***Symptoms***

Pain in the knee is a common symptom of chondromalacia patellae. The pain may feel like grinding in the joint.

***Treatments***

Resting the knee joint can help reduce irritation, and allow any damage in the knee or on the cartilage of the patella to heal. Strengthening the thigh muscles can also help to prevent chondromalacia patellae in the future. In more severe cases, surgery may be performed to help realign the patella if it is not aligned properly on the femur.

***Contraindications***

Chondromalacia patellae is considered a local contraindication due to pain and inflammation in the area.

## Dislocation

A dislocation is when a bone at an articulation becomes **displaced** from its normal location. A dislocation, in the acute stage, results in immobilization of the joint and temporary deformation. It may also be painful and result in inflammation around the joint.

***Causes***

Dislocations are most commonly the result of trauma to the joint, which pushes a bone out of place. The most common areas for dislocations are the fingers and shoulder, but dislocations may occur in many other joints as well, such as the knee or hip.

Dislocations may result in tearing of tendons, ligaments, muscles, or in the case of the shoulder or hip, the labrum(circular cartilage surrounding the joint). The dislocated joint, while most commonly returns to normal strength and function after being relocated, may become prone to dislocations in the future. This may cause arthritis to develop.

***Symptoms***

Dislocations are extremely painful, and often present with deformity of the joint and an inability to move the joint. Inflammation may be present in some cases.

***Treatments***

Treatment of a dislocation in the acute stage primarily involves trying to get the bone back to its normal position, known as reduction. After the joint has returned to its normal position, it is typically immobilized for a number of weeks to reduce recurrence of dislocation and to help the tissues around the joint to heal. If the dislocation is severe and unable to be returned to position, surgery may be required.

***Contraindications***

In the acute stage, a dislocation is considered a local contraindication. If the joint has healed, massage may be performed on the area with caution. Stretching and range-of-motion should be avoided because the joint is much weaker after a dislocation.

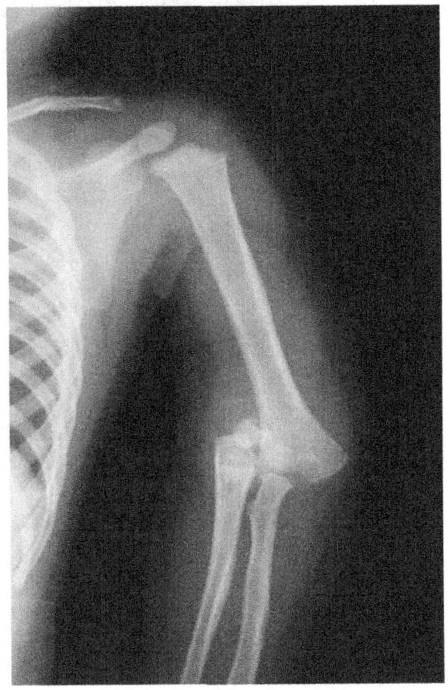

Dislocation of the elbow joint

## Fracture

A fracture is a **break** in a bone. There are several different types of fractures, including transverse, greenstick, oblique, and spiral.

***Causes***

Fractures are the result of trauma to a bone. Despite many different types of fractures, every fracture is categorized as one of the following: Simple or Compound. A **simple** fracture is a fracture that **does not break through** the skin, and does not damage any surrounding tissue. A **compound** fracture, which is much more severe, **breaks through** the skin and damages surrounding tissues. Compound fractures are much more prone to infection due to exposure to the outside environment.

***Symptoms***

Fractures result in deformity of the affected bone, pain, immobilization of the area, and inflammation. In the case of compound fractures, external bleeding may also occur.

Despite most fractures being the result of blunt trauma, certain diseases that weaken the bones may also cause fractures, such as osteoporosis.

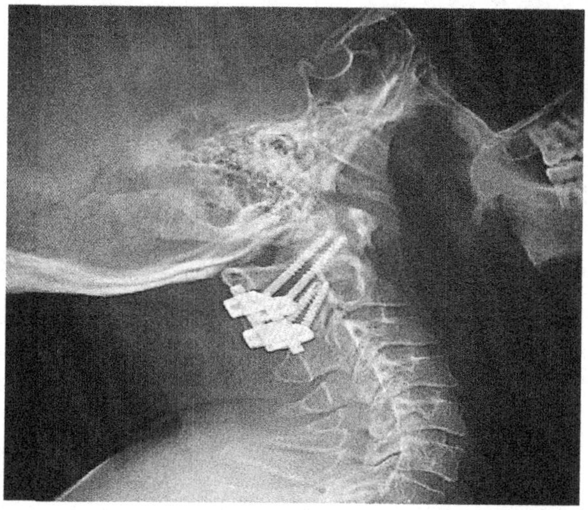

Fusion of C1-C2 to repair fracture

***Treatments***

Fractures should be treated immediately. A cast or splint may be applied, depending on which bone is fractured. Other fractures, such as vertebrae fractures, may need more extensive treatment, including metal plates or bone grafts.

***Contraindications***

In the acute stage, a fracture should be considered a local contraindication. After the fracture has healed, massage may be performed on the area. If metal plates, rods, screws, or pins have been placed in the bone, caution should be taken in the area, but massage may still be performed.

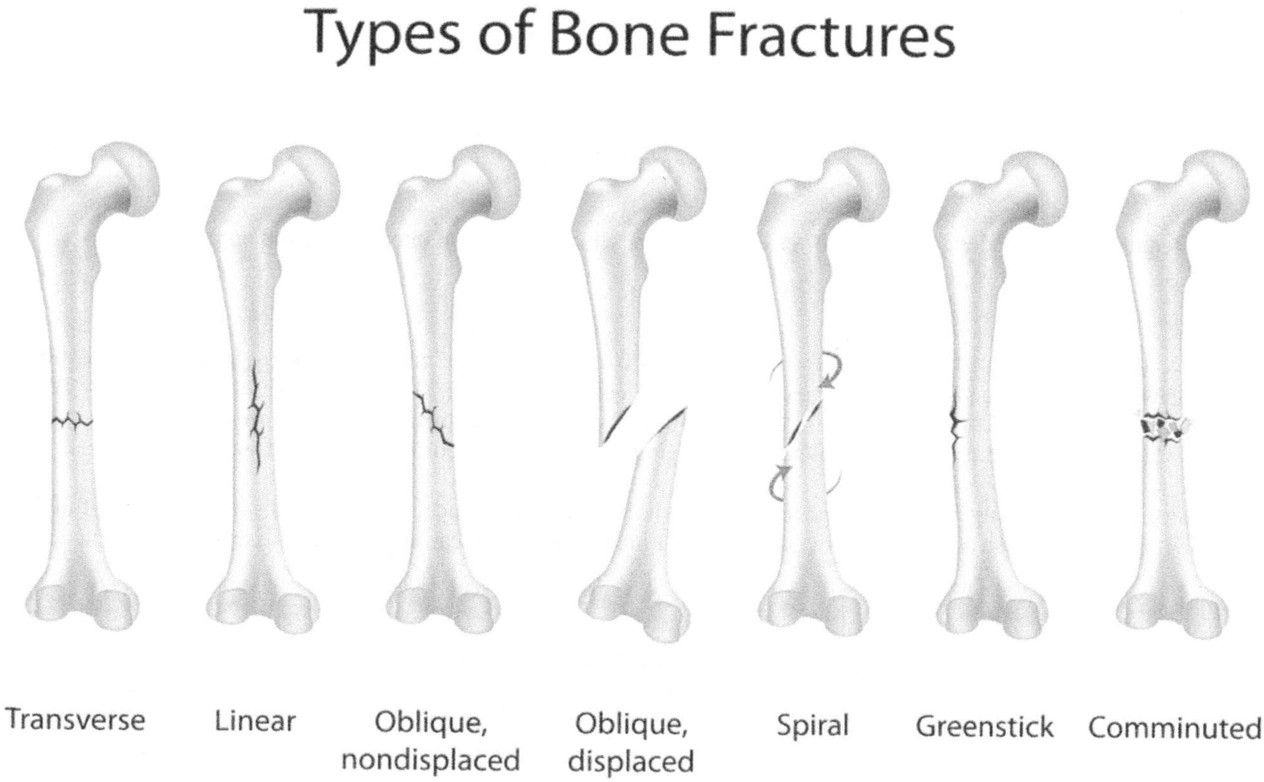


## Gout

Gout is a form of arthritis, mostly seen around the base of the **big toe**, but may also affect other joints in the body, such as the hands and fingers.

***Causes***

Gout is the result of an over-abundance of **uric acid** crystals in the body. Gravity pulls the uric acid crystals down the body, where they collect in the most distal points in the limbs, the big toes, hands and fingers. Gout is typically the result of the kidneys not excreting enough uric acid, or the body producing too much uric acid.

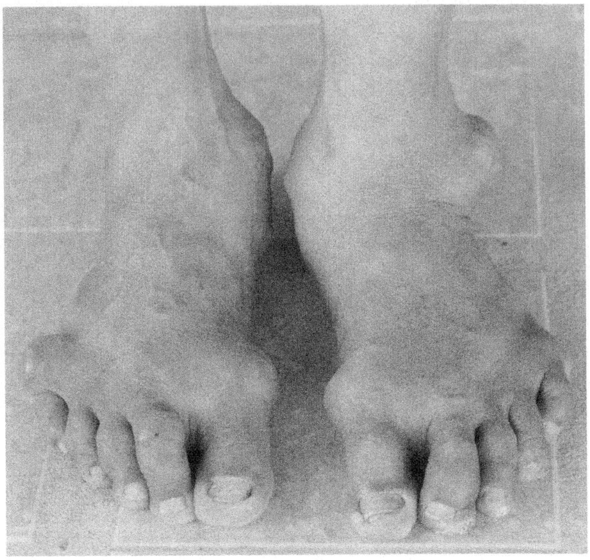

***Symptoms***

Gout may be extremely painful in the acute stage as the crystals collect in the joints. Inflammation may set in, which can increase the pressure and pain in the joint. Loss of range-of-motion may also occur. Untreated, gout may result in kidney stones.

***Treatments***

Treatments for gout include non-steroidal anti-inflammatory drugs and/or corticosteroids to reduce pain and inflammation. Gout may also require the use of certain medications that prevent the creation of uric acid in the body.

***Contraindications***

Gout is considered a local contraindication.

## Herniated Disc

A herniated disc is a condition affecting the vertebral column, which may cause intense pain and numbness.

***Causes***

An intervertebral disc, located between two vertebrae, is made of two parts: the nucleus pulposus, and the annulus fibrosus. The nucleus pulposus is a gelatinous substance located in the center of the disc. The annulus fibrosus is the part of the disc made of thick cartilage. If a tear occurs in the **annulus fibrosus**, the **nucleus pulposus** may **protrude** through the torn section, which may place pressure on spinal nerves emerging from the spinal cord. This is a herniated disc.

A herniated disc is primarily caused by degeneration of a disc, which takes place gradually. This makes injury of the disc much easier in actions such as lifting and twisting. Other times, trauma may cause a herniated disc, such as in car accidents.

***Symptoms***

Herniated discs may result in pain and/or numbness due to the disc placing pressure on the spinal nerves. Because numbness may occur, weakness in the muscles innervated by the nerves may also set in due to impaired function.

***Treatments***

Treatment for a herniated disc varies depending on the severity. Pain medication may help control pain. Muscle relaxers may help take pressure off the area of the herniation. Physical therapy may also contribute to lessening the effects of the herniated disc. Very rarely, surgery may be required.

***Contraindications***

Herniated discs are considered local contraindications. The area around the hernia may be massaged, but the disc itself should be avoided.

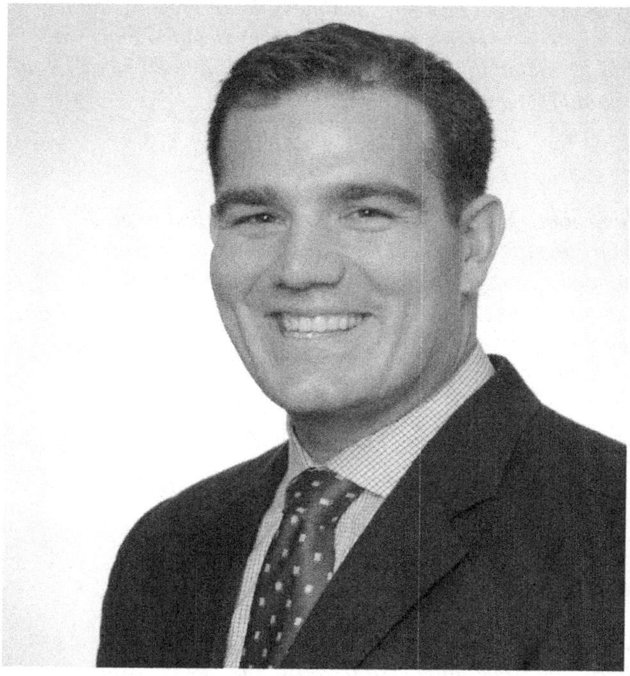

**Ross Tucker, Former Professional Football Lineman, Herniated Disc**
Host of the Ross Tucker Football Podcast
Twitter: @RossTuckerNFL

You had a herniated disc, correct?

*Two of 'em! I had surgery in Buffalo, L4-L5, and L5-S1, discectomy, laminotomy, and foraminotomy. My career ended with a herniated C5-C6 in my neck, which bruised my spinal cord with the Redskins in 2007. So in the span of four years, I had two that were REALLY herniated, and one that they said didn't look real good, so they cleaned it up with my L4-L5 surgery.*

So you had a lot going on, is what you're telling me.

*Yeah, most guys have some issues. Some guys have bad shoulders, some have bad ankles, some have bad knees, some get concussed a lot. Mine was the spine. We're all machines that break down, and my spine was the part of the machine that broke down.*

How long into your career did it take before you suffered one of those spinal injuries?

*I remember first tweaking my back in high school. I don't remember anything happening with my back in college. I think the summer before I had the herniated disc, I was working out doing drills, and I had vicious back spasms. It was actually the night of my engagement party, and I was in all kinds of pain. Later that year, it ended up gettin' me. Midway through the year it started to really bother me, and by the end of the year they were giving me an MRI, and we knew I had an issue.*

When you tweaked your back in high school, did you ever get that checked out?

*No, I just went to a chiropractor, because my mom went to a chiropractor. It was really on an as-needed basis.*

Did the injury take place at any of the spots you hurt your back in later on?

*I think so, yeah. I think it was the low back, the same area. Just kind of the precursor, the first time I had a bulge or something.*

Where were you when your back started giving you problems in your professional career?

*Buffalo Bills.*

After it happened, you went to the trainer, I assume?

*Well, I didn't say anything when I hurt it over the summer, because I was back home in Pennsylvania. I thought I just pulled a muscle and it was back spasms, so I didn't think anything of it. During the season, I don't think I said anything initially about my back, but it kept getting worse and worse. I didn't like it, I wasn't feeling good, so they X-rayed it, X-rayed it again, and finally X-rayed it a third time when I told them, "Look, I can't even tie my shoes!" I was heavily medicated to play those games at the end of that year.*

How long into the season was it before you went to the trainer to get it looked at?

*I don't remember it bothering me until halfway through the season. I don't remember saying anything for a couple weeks.*

What did the X-rays show, if anything?

*The X-ray showed nothing. After the MRI, I remember the radiologist asking if I had any numbness down my leg, and I actually wasn't! I didn't have any tingling, pain, or numbness down my leg, just pain in my back. They decided they were just going to monitor it. So after the season, every month they would fly me up there for another MRI. I noticed when I was driving, my leg would get so tired. My ankle and tibialis anterior would just get so tired.*

It sounds like you got a little bit of drop foot because of it.

*It felt like that, almost! Even when I would drive around the neighborhood, I would put cruise control on just to go 20 MPH because it was that tiring. They finally gave me an EMG(electromyelograph), and they realized I was only getting 35% of the nerve signal down my leg. That's when they said, "You need surgery." Before that, they thought it might get better, it might heal, but after the EMG they said I need surgery as soon as possible. During the surgery, they took care of L4-L5, and while they were in there, they cleaned up L5-S1. I remember them saying that my nerve was kinked, and that's what was causing the pain. I felt better after the surgery. It definitely helped.*

So they determined beforehand it was L4-L5, L5-S1?

*They determined beforehand it was L4-L5. When they did the surgery, they saw L5-S1 was trending in a bad direction as well. So the doctor just freed up more room for that nerve also.*

What kind of surgery did they perform on each one of those segments?

*Both of them were a discectomy, where you shave the disc. They also did a laminotomy, which is where they hollow out or shave the lamina of the vertebra, and a foraminotomy, which is almost the same thing. All of those things were done and designed to create more space for my nerves, so they wouldn't get kinked, and my disc wouldn't be herniated.*

After you had the surgery, how long did you continue playing, and did you experience any symptoms?

*I felt better, but I would say it took me a full year before I felt as close to normal. I never really felt as if I got back to 100%, but it took a year for me to get back as far as I could. That next season, I always felt stiff, and I didn't feel like myself. By the next year, I felt like I could move pretty well, and I was back to being decently explosive.*

How long was it until you suffered the neck injury?

*I had the surgery in April 2005, played 2006, but I got cut and was out of the league the whole year. I came back in 2007, and hurt my neck in the third preseason game against the Ravens, and that was it.*

What happened during that play where you hurt it?

*It was a wedge, on a kickoff return. I hit a linebacker hard, I got a really bad stinger. I thought that's all it was. It turned out to be more than that.*

So after that, you went to the trainer, you got another X-ray and MRI done, and what did it show?

*It showed I had a herniated disc in my neck at C5-C6, and they did manual tests with my toes and fingers. They'd flick them, and after they flicked them, they'd shake for a while. That was proof that my spinal cord was bruised. I remember asking the doctor what he thought. There were a couple surgical options, but I asked, "What do you think, man? What if I was your son?" He said, "Well, I'd tell you you're 28, you went to Princeton, and it's time to get a real job." That was actually good for me, because nobody would have signed me again after that anyway. I kind of needed that closure, so I was almost glad to get that closure. And that was it. I had to rehab that for a while, a good six months, maybe up to a year.*

So you didn't have any surgery for this injury?

*Nope!*

What kind of exercises were you doing during physical therapy?

*More stretching than anything else. I think the stretching was designed to calm the nerve down and make it a little looser there.*

So they were doing a lot of traction too?

*Yes, a lot of stretching, and a lot of traction to try to increase space to get the disc off the nerves.*

Have you had any MRIs done recently to take a look at your neck?

*I have not, and I have not needed to. If I got an MRI on anything, it would be on my back. My neck is pretty good! My neck, knock on wood, doesn't really ever bother me, but my back is very much a part of my life. I have to be very conscious of what I do, where I sit, certain body positions.*

When you receive massages, do you have the therapist stretch you out, do traction or joint mobilization on the vertebrae, or just work on the surrounding muscles a bit?

*More work on the surrounding muscles, with a heavy emphasis on the low back and glutes, and any areas I think create issues. I go to a chiropractor more for traction or joint manipulation. Chiropractor is more as-needed, massage is about once a month.*

Do you have any massage performed on your neck?

*Yeah, for sure. That's usually another point of emphasis, my neck and traps. I like to get those muscles relaxed and loose.*

Is there anything you'd tell a massage therapist not to work on in regards to your back or neck issues?

*No. The only thing I tell them not to work on is my big toes, because I had turf toe, and if they work on my big toes, that really hurts.*

## Kyphosis

*(kyph-: hill; -osis: condition)*

Kyphosis is a condition affecting the **thoracic** vertebrae, resulting in **hyper-curvature**. Another name for kyphosis is "Dowager's Hump".

***Causes***

A kyphotic curvature in the vertebrae is a curvature that moves posteriorly. If the curvature is exaggerated, it is known as kyphosis. Kyphosis has many different causes. Kyphosis may be caused by extremely tight muscles(such as **pectoralis minor** and **serratus anterior**) pulling the scapulae anteriorly, which rounds the back. It may also be the result of bone degeneration(osteoporosis), disc degeneration(ankylosing spondylitis), or even birth defects.

***Symptoms***

Kyphosis may cause pain in the back, and difficulty in movement and breathing as a result. It may also result in the lumbar vertebrae losing its curvature, a condition known as **flat back**.

***Treatments***

Kyphosis may vary from mild to severe, depending on the cause. Treatments include exercises that strengthen the muscles of the back, stretching of tight muscles that may contribute to kyphosis, braces to keep the vertebrae properly aligned, and possibly even surgery if it's warranted.

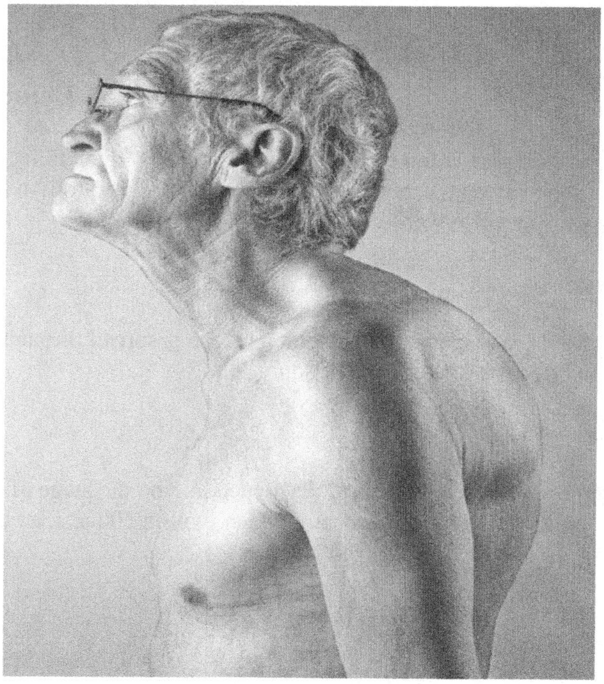

***Contraindications***

Kyphosis is not contraindicated for massage. A person with kyphosis may be uncomfortable lying supine, and may need to be placed into side-lying position for comfort. Massage of the pectoralis minor and serratus anterior muscles may help the scapulae return to their normal locations, which can help straighten the vertebrae.

## Lordosis

*(lord-: curve; -osis: condition)*

Lordosis is a condition affecting the **lumbar** vertebrae, resulting in **hyper-curvature**. Another name for lordosis is "Swayback".

***Causes***

A lordotic curvature in the vertebrae is a curvature that moves anteriorly. If the curvature is exaggerated, it is known as lordosis. Lordosis has many different causes. Lordosis may be caused by tight muscles(such as **psoas major**, **iliacus**, **quadratus lumborum**, and **rectus femoris**), weak muscles(such as **rectus abdominis** and the **hamstrings**), obesity, or bone diseases(such as osteoporosis). Pregnancy is also a common cause of lordosis, but the condition typically subsides post-pregnancy.

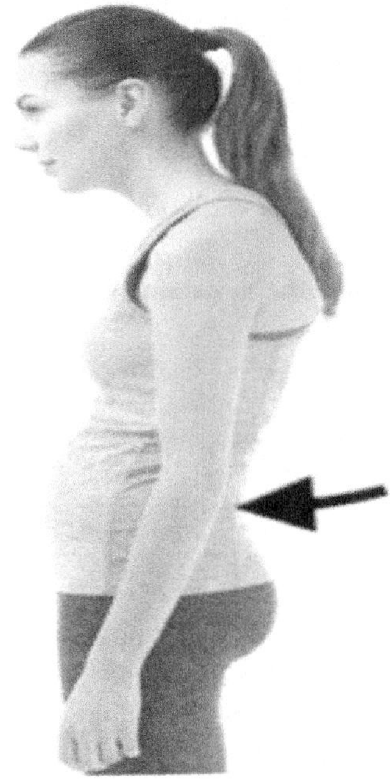

***Symptoms***

Lordosis may place excessive pressure on the vertebrae, and alter a person's stance and gait. Lordosis may result in pain in the back, and cause difficulty moving.

***Treatments***

Treatment primarily includes strengthening weak muscles, stretching tight muscles, and lifestyle changes such as adjusting posture, diet, and exercise.

***Contraindications***

Lordosis is not contraindicated for massage. Stretching exercises on the psoas major, iliacus, and quadratus lumborum muscles may help return the lumbar spine back to its normal curvature.

## Lyme Disease

Lyme Disease is a **bacterial infection** spread by **deer ticks**, and contracting the infection is much more common in grassy or wooded areas where deer ticks are found. The condition may affect a person for months, and lead to symptoms that may last for years afterwards.

***Causes***

The bacteria responsible for Lyme Disease is spread through a bite from deer ticks. The bacteria is usually only transmitted if the bite lasts longer than 36 hours.

***Symptoms***

Symptoms of Lyme Disease vary depending on the stage of infection. In the early stages, a bump may appear where the person has been bitten. Sometime later, within 30 days, a rash may appear that forms a **bullseye pattern**. It may spread outward from that area over a few days. A person may experience flu-like symptoms when the rash appears. In advanced stages, conditions may begin occurring such as pain and inflammation in joints, meningitis, and paralysis in different parts of the body such as the face.

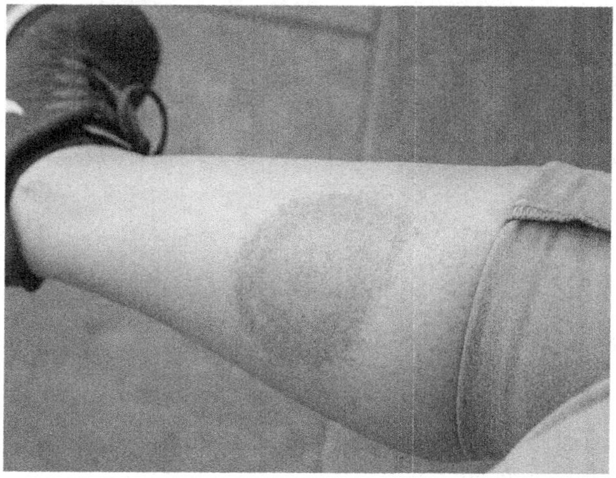

***Treatments***

Lyme Disease is a bacterial infection, and therefore is treated with antibiotics. Advanced stages of Lyme Disease, where there may be some sort of paralysis, require the use of intravenous antibiotics. Otherwise, oral antibiotics may be taken. The course of treatment usually lasts up to three weeks to completely destroy all bacteria.

***Contraindications***

Massage largely depends on the symptoms a client is experiencing. Lesser symptoms, such as aches and joint inflammation, may allow for massage while avoiding general local contraindications. If a client is experiencing flu-like symptoms, the massage should be postponed until the client is feeling better.

## Osgood-Schlatter Disease

Osgood-Schlatter Disease is a repetitive strain injury, caused by over-use of the **patellar** tendon.

***Causes***

Osgood-Schlatter Disease primarily affects adolescents, particularly those involved in sports. Over-use of the **quadriceps** during activities such as running and jumping can cause tightness in the patellar tendon. When the patellar tendon tightens, it pulls proximally on the tibial tuberosity. Because the bone is still growing, the force of the patellar tendon on the tibial tuberosity can cause an **over-growth of bone**, resulting in a bony lump. Males are more likely to develop this condition than females, but instances in females are increasing as participation in sports by females increases.

***Symptoms***

Osgood-Schlatter Disease may cause pain, but it varies from person to person. The pain may be mild, or it may be more intense, making movement of the knee difficult.

Despite complications from Osgood-Schlatter Disease being rare, inflammation of the area may persist over time. The bony lump produced by increased bone production may also remain.

***Treatments***

Treatment is mild, usually nothing more than pain relievers, rest, and ice. Exercises that stretch the quadriceps are recommended.

***Contraindications***

In the acute stage, massage of the tibial tuberosity is a local contraindication. If the client is beyond the age of 21, and bone is no longer being produced at the tibial tuberosity, massage on the area may be performed.

In the acute stage, massage and stretching techniques should be performed on the quadriceps to loosen the muscles and take pressure off the patellar tendon, which can reduce the excessive development of bone at the tibial tuberosity.

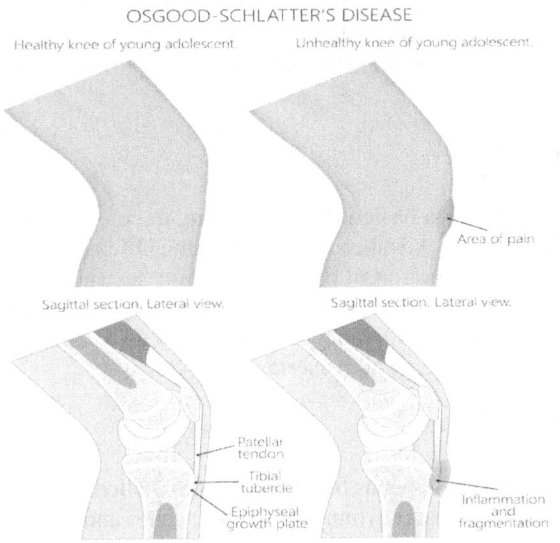


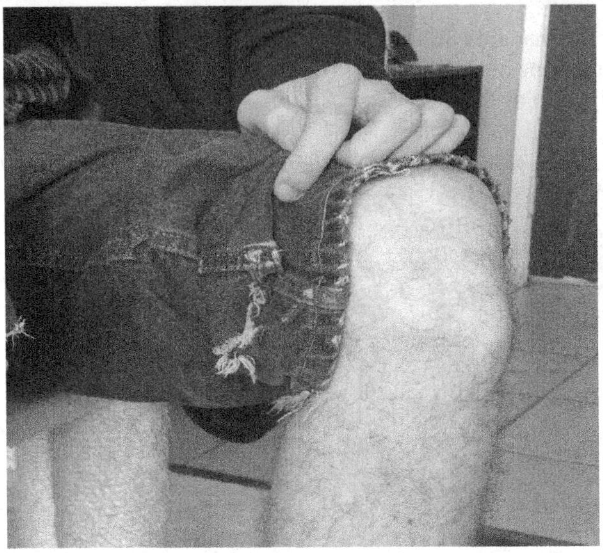

## Osteoarthritis

*(osteo-: bone; arthr-: joint; -itis: inflammation)*

Osteoarthritis is the most common form of arthritis, which is **inflammation** of a **joint**.

***Causes***

Osteoarthritis, also known as "**wear-and-tear arthritis**", is caused by damage to the **hyaline cartilage** separating one bone from another. The cartilage between bones reduces friction between the bones, and absorbs shock in the joint. Over time, the articular cartilage may begin to break down and wear away. This causes irritation in the joint and increases friction between the bones, which causes inflammation. As this persists, damage to the bone may take place. The most common location of osteoarthritis is the knee, but in massage therapists, it may also affect the carpometacarpal joint of the thumb(saddle joint).

***Symptoms***

Osteoarthritis may cause pain, difficulty moving the affected joint, and bone spurs in the joint due to increased friction between the bones. When the condition advances to the point of the joint being mostly unusable, joint replacement surgery may be recommended.

***Treatments***

Treatment includes non-steroidal anti-inflammatory drugs, lifestyle and dietary changes if caused by obesity, and alternative methods such as yoga.

***Contraindications***

In the acute stage, massage is considered a local contraindication for any form of arthritis because it can bring more blood into the area and increase inflammation. In the post-acute stage, massage should be performed on the area usually affected to bring fresh blood and nutrients into the area, and to increase production of synovial fluid in the joint. This can help reduce irritation in the joint and lessen the effects of arthritis.

DESTRUCTION OF CARTILAGE

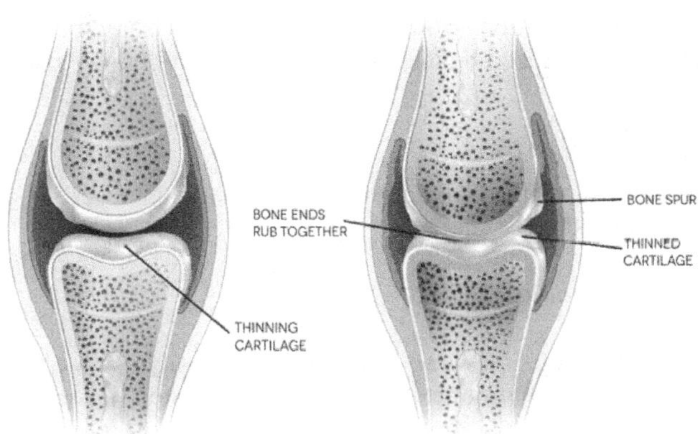

## Osteomyelitis

*(oste/o: bone; myel-: canal; -itis: inflammation)*

Osteomyelitis is a **bacterial infection** of the bone, occurring inside the **bone canal**. The bacteria can enter the bone through the blood supply, or through direct exposure of bone tissue in cases such as fractures. If not treated promptly, necrosis of bone tissue may result, or a person may experience septicemia.

***Causes***

When the body has a bacterial infection of some sort, such as pneumonia, the bacteria may enter the blood stream and end up in the bone canal. This provides a place for bacteria to reproduce, resulting in infection of the bone.

If a person suffers a compound fracture, the bone is exposed to air, dirt, and debris. Bacteria can enter the bone through the wound, and if the bone is not properly cleaned, a bacterial infection may result.

***Symptoms***

A person with osteomyelitis may experience no symptoms if the infection is not severe. More advanced cases present with fever, pain in the infected bone, and inflammation in the area of infection.

***Treatments***

If the infection is severe, surgery may be performed to drain the infection from the bone. If necrosis of bone tissue has taken place, the dead tissue is removed and the area is cleaned to ensure the infection is gone. Antibiotics will be prescribed to combat the infection.

***Contraindications***

Osteomyelitis is an absolute contraindication, as massage may help spread the bacterium throughout the body.

## Osteoporosis

*(osteo-: bone; por-: porous; -osis: condition)*

Osteoporosis is a condition that causes **weakness** and **degeneration** in the **bones**.

***Causes***

Osteoporosis mainly affects post-menopausal women. After menopause, a woman's body produces less **estrogen**. Estrogen, during growth stages of a person's life, helps the bones grow and mature. When estrogen levels drop post-menopause, osteoclast levels increase, and more bone is destroyed than is created. When this occurs, the bones become brittle, weak, and prone to fracture.

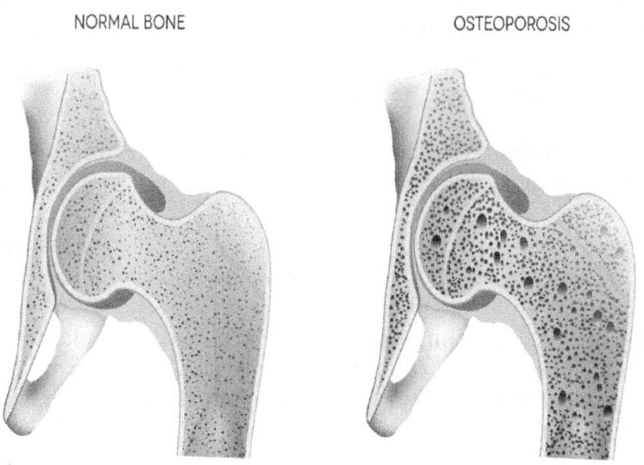


Osteoporosis, in addition to making bones brittle, may also contribute to the development of kyphosis and back pain. One of the most common places for fracture to occur is in the neck of the femur. The femur, which is normally the strongest bone in the body, should be able to support roughly 2,000 pounds of pressure per square inch. When the femur becomes weakened, it makes it incredibly easy to break. If a fracture takes place around the hip joint, joint replacement surgery is often required.

***Symptoms***

In the early stages of osteoporosis, there are usually no symptoms. As bone loss increases over time, a person may experience back pain, hunched posture(kyphosis), and bones that fracture easier than usual. These symptoms often become worse as the disease progresses and more bone tissue is lost.

***Treatments***

Treatments for osteoporosis include estrogen replacement therapy, and weight-bearing exercise earlier in life before any symptoms of osteoporosis surface. Weight-bearing exercise, such as squats and dead-lifts, helps to strengthen the bones, which substantially reduces the risk of developing osteoporosis in older age.

***Contraindications***

Massage is indicated for osteoporosis. However, precautions should be taken, such as performing a lighter massage, and not performing techniques such as tapotement to avoid damaging bone.

## Paget's Disease

Paget's Disease is a condition in which bone is **not properly replaced** after normal bone cells have died. This can result in bones becoming **brittle**, and may increase the chances of fracture occurring. The most common sites where bones are affected are the skull, vertebral column, pelvis, and lower limbs.

***Causes***

There is no known cause of Paget's Disease. It may be a genetic disorder.

***Symptoms***

Paget's disease is largely asymptomatic, until bones become too fragile. Once the bone has become weak, pain may be experienced, including headaches, compression of spinal nerves emerging from the spinal cord, and the development of arthritis due to the bones of the lower limbs becoming misshapen.

***Treatments***

Because Paget's disease is very similar to osteoporosis, treatment is extremely similar. Medications may help reduce bone brittleness. Surgery may be an option to help repair bones that have become deformed or fractured.

***Contraindications***

Paget's disease is not contraindicated for massage. Massage may be implemented as part of a person's physical therapy plan to help treat symptoms.

## Plantarfasciitis

*(plantar-: sole of the feet; fasci-: fascia; -itis: inflammation)*

Plantarfasciitis is **inflammation** of the fascia on the **plantar surface** of the foot. It is usually the result of **over-stretching** of the plantarfascia, connecting the calcaneus to the toes, which results in tearing. The tearing is usually small, but constant injury to the plantarfascia may cause pain. It is a common injury in athletes, people who are flat-footed, and people who are obese.

***Causes***

Plantarfasciitis is the result of the plantarfascia being stretched further than it normally does, causing small tears.

***Symptoms***

Stabbing pain in the foot is a common symptom, occurring near the calcaneus. The pain usually subsides when the foot is not in use.

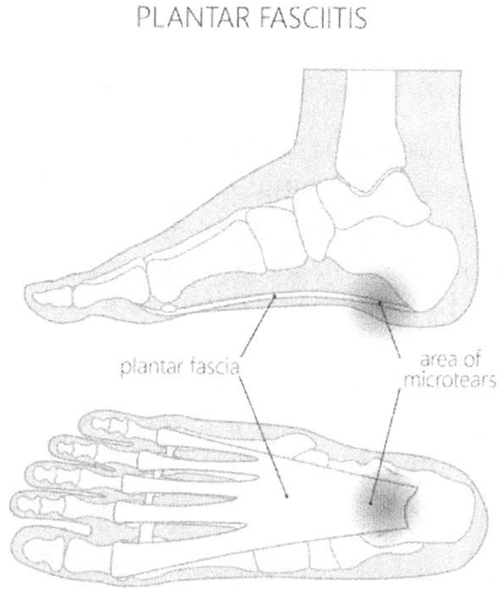


***Treatments***

PRICE(protect, rest, ice, compression, elevation) is extremely useful in aiding the healing of plantarfasciitis. Splints may be used to return the foot back to its normal position, taking pressure off the plantarfascia. Pain relievers may be taken to aid with any discomfort and pain a person may be experiencing.

***Contraindications***

Plantarfasciitis is considered a local contraindication in the acute stage.

## Rheumatoid Arthritis

Rheumatoid Arthritis is an **autoimmune** disorder, resulting in **inflammation**, **pain**, and **deformity** of the **joints** around the **hands and wrists**.

***Causes***

Around synovial joints, there is a membrane called the synovial membrane, which supplies joints with synovial fluid. In rheumatoid arthritis, the body's immune system attacks the **synovial membranes**, destroying them. This is especially common in the metacarpophalangeal joints. After the synovial membranes have been destroyed, extremely thick, fibrous material replaces them, which not only makes movement painful and difficult, but can also cause deformity, turning the fingers into an adducted position.

***Symptoms***

Rheumatoid arthritis can produce pain and discomfort in the affected joints, as well as cause pain and stiffness after long periods of inactivity in the joints. Fever and fatigue may also be symptoms of general rheumatoid arthritis. Less commonly, some people may experience symptoms in structures completely unrelated to the affected joints, such as the eyes, heart, lungs, and kidneys.

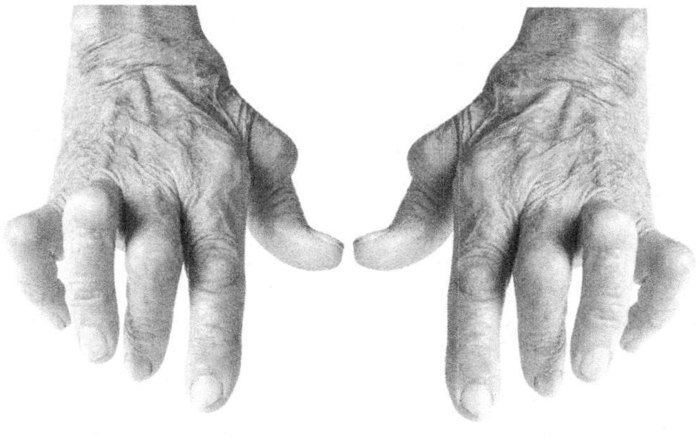

***Treatments***

There is no cure for rheumatoid arthritis, but treatments include non-steroidal anti-inflammatory drugs, corticosteroids, and physical therapy.

***Contraindications***

In the acute stage, rheumatoid arthritis is considered a local contraindication, as the pain may be too intense for the client to receive massage on the affected area. In general, however, a client with rheumatoid arthritis may receive massage to help ease pain associated with inflammation if the body can tolerate a light-to-medium pressured massage.

## Scoliosis

*(scoli-: crooked; -osis: condition)*

Scoliosis is a condition causing the vertebral column, usually in the thoracic region, to be pulled into a **lateral** position.

***Causes***

The causes of scoliosis are unknown, but there may be a hereditary link. Scoliosis typically develops around the beginning stages of puberty. Scoliosis is mostly mild in severity, but can become much more prominent, which can put incredible strain on the ribs, vertebrae, and hips. With scoliosis, one hip may be higher than the other, which causes a discrepancy in gait. Tight muscles may also contribute to the development of scoliosis, as seen in cases such as a hypertonic rhomboid major and minor unilaterally, which pulls the vertebrae to one side.

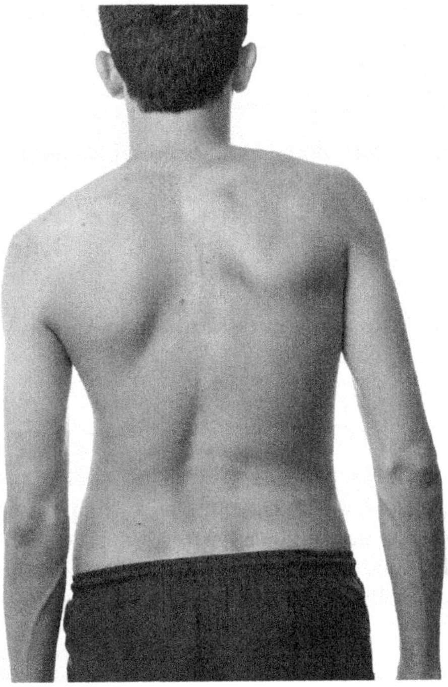

***Symptoms***

If scoliosis is severe, damage to the heart or lungs may occur, due to the deformity of the rib cage. Back pain may also persist.

***Treatments***

Treatment, while commonly unnecessary, may include the use of braces to correct posture, the use of chiropractic therapy, massage therapy, or in severe cases, surgery with metal rod implantation.

***Contraindications***

Scoliosis is indicated for massage. In instances where scoliosis is caused by hypertonic muscles, such as the rhomboids unilaterally, massage may help loosen the muscles and allow the bones to realign themselves. If surgery has been performed and metal rods have been placed in the back, massage should be performed lighter on the area, and the use of cold packs should be avoided.

## Shin Splint

Shin Splints, also known as **Medial Tibial Stress Syndrome**, is pain felt along the medial side of the anterior tibia. It is common in people who **run**, **dance**, or are **athletes**.

***Causes***

During physical activity, such as running, the muscles on the anterior leg may become strained, and the periosteum may experience tearing. This can cause pain along the medial tibia. There are many reasons why a person may experience shin splints, from improper running technique, to wearing the wrong shoes.

***Symptoms***

Sharp pain on the medial tibia is the main symptom of shin splints. The pain may also be a dull ache in some people if it's less severe.

***Treatments***

PRICE(protect, rest, ice, compression, elevation) is the preferred treatment for shin splints. Correcting foot technique and improper footwear is key in preventing shin splints in the future.

***Contraindications***

Massage is indicated for shin splints, depending on the pain tolerance of the client. If the pain is too much, do not massage the area.

## Spondylosis

*(spondyl/o: spine; -osis: condition)*

Spondylosis is a general term describing any degeneration of the spine. For specific examples, see: Osteoarthritis, page 236; Ankylosing Spondylitis, page 225.

## Sprain

A sprain is an injury to a **ligament**.

***Causes***

Sprains are much less likely to be caused by repetitive motions, unlike strains. Sprains typically occur quickly, causing tears in a ligament. Like strains, sprains may be broken down in severity by using grades: grade 1, grade 2, and grade 3.

A grade 1 sprain is caused by stretching of a ligament, but does not cause major tearing. Common grade 1 sprains may be caused by activities such as running. After 24/48 hours, the ligament should return to normal, and any pain and/or inflammation should subside.

A grade 2 sprain, such as a high ankle sprain, causes tearing of a ligament and presents with bruising and inflammation. Grade 2 sprains may require surgery to repair, or they may heal on their own, depending on the severity of the tear.

A grade 3 sprain is a complete rupture of a ligament, and much like a grade 3 strain, does require surgery to repair. The most common form of grade 3 sprain is a torn anterior cruciate ligament(ACL, the ligament holding the femur and tibia together), most commonly caused by sports or automobile accidents.

***Symptoms***

Symptoms of sprains are very similar to symptoms of strains, including inflammation, pain, and potential bruising depending on the grade of sprain. If the sprain is severe, a pop in the joint may be heard or felt at the time of injury.

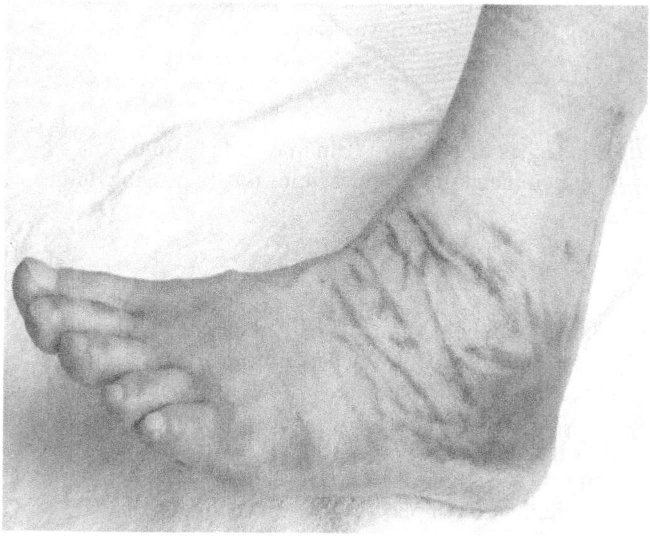

***Treatments***

Sprains take much longer to heal than strains, due to ligaments being avascular, compared to muscles and tendons, which have a rich blood supply. Treatment for sprains vary depending on the severity of the sprain. The less severe, the more likely it is that rest, ice, and elevation will suffice. Surgery is only required when there is no chance of the ligament repairing itself.

***Contraindications***

In the acute stage, sprains are local contraindications. If inflammation has subsided from a first degree sprain, gentle massage in the area may be performed to bring fresh blood and nutrients into the area and speed healing. Contrast therapy may be performed in addition to gentle massage to reduce any inflammation that may occur due to the massage.

## Temporomandibular Joint Dysfunction

Temporomandibular Joint Dysfunction(TMJD) is a condition affecting the mandible, causing simple tasks such as **chewing** to become **painful** and **difficult**.

***Causes***

The temporomandibular joint is the joint that connects the mandible to the temporal bone. Between the bones, there is a small disc of cartilage, used to prevent friction between the bones and to make movement smooth. If there is arthritis in the joint, or the disc is damaged, it can result in Temporomandibular Joint Dysfunction. This can cause pain, difficulty in moving the jaw, and produce a clicking sensation when the jaw opens. Often times, the muscles that connect to the mandible(temporalis, lateral pterygoid) may tighten and pull the mandible out of place.

***Symptoms***

Temporomandibular Joint Dysfunction can produce pain in the face, a clicking or popping sound when closing the mouth, and difficulty in opening the mouth. The jaw may become locked while open.

***Treatments***

Treatments vary depending on the primary cause, ranging from prescription muscle relaxants and pain relievers, to physical and massage therapy.

***Contraindications***

Massage is indicated for Temporomandibular Joint Dysfunction. Massage of the temporalis may help the jaw realign and reduce the pain and clicking.

## Whiplash

Whiplash is an injury to the neck, resulting from a quick, forceful movement of the head forward and back. This results in the tendons and ligaments in the neck to become stretched further than normal, damaging the tissue and making the neck much less stable than normal.

***Causes***

The most common cause of whiplash is a car accident. Injuries during sport or physical abuse may also cause whiplash. Shaking a baby may result in whiplash, and is one of the reasons shaking a baby should never happen.

***Symptoms***

The neck can become stiff and painful, especially upon movement. Headaches may occur. Pain may radiate to the shoulders, and range-of-motion may be restricted. Numbness may be experienced in the upper limbs due to possible injury to nerves emerging from the brachial plexus.

***Treatments***

Rest and ice are effective treatments for whiplash. The use of pain relievers can help eliminate pain associated with the condition. Inflammation in the area may be present, and contrast therapy on the neck may be performed to assist with reduction of inflammation. Physical therapy may also be performed to help strengthen the tendons and ligaments affected.

***Contraindications***

In the acute stage, massage is considered a local contraindication for a client with whiplash. Once the symptoms have subsided, gentle massage in the area may be performed. Stretching of the neck should be avoided to prevent injuring the tissue.

# Skeletal Pathologies

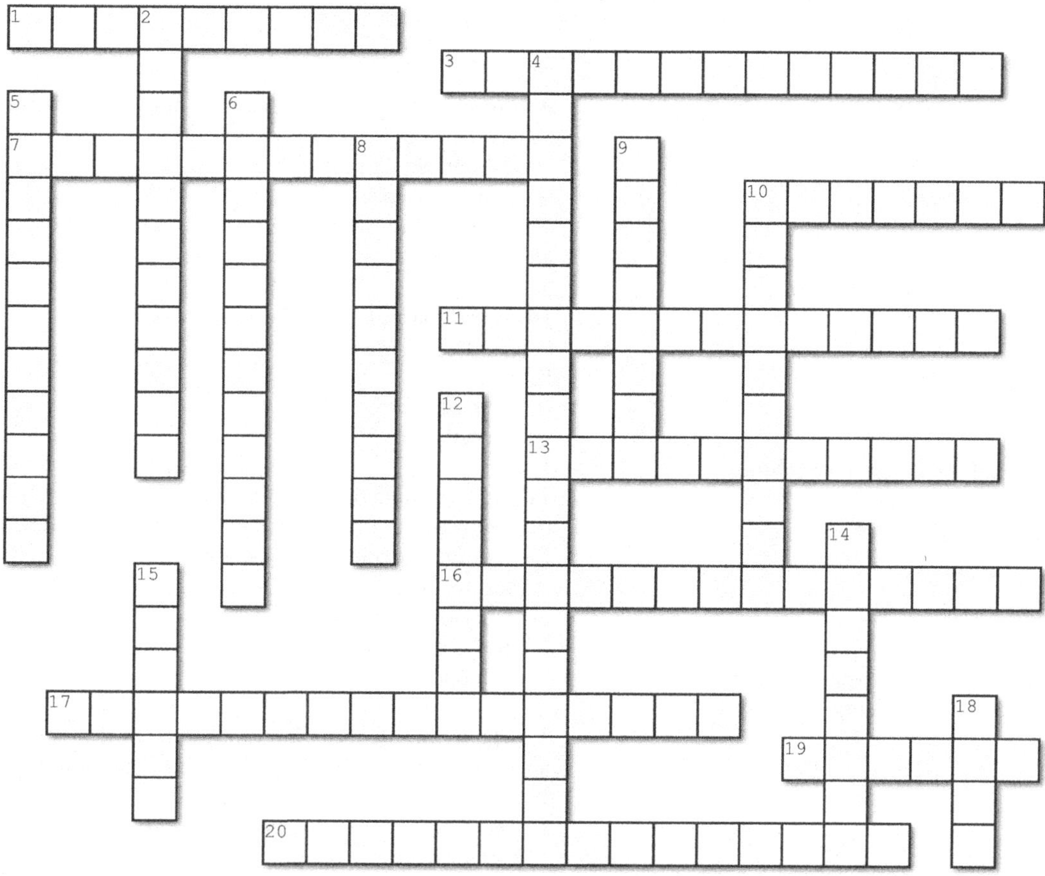

**Across**

**1.** Lateral curvature of the vertebrae, usually found in the thoracic region
**3.** Protrusion of the nucleus pulposus through the annulus fibrosis
**7.** Weakness of bones due to bone tissue not being replaced after normal bone cells have died
**10.** Inflammation of a bursa, typically caused by damage to a bursa
**11.** Bacterial infection inside the bone canal
**13.** A bone becoming displaced from its normal location
**16.** Inflammation of a joint caused by degeneration of cartilage, which increases friction between the bones
**17.** Inflammation of the fascia on the plantar surface of the foot
**19.** Subluxation of the big toe
**20.** Over-use of the quadriceps, resulting in the patellar tendon pulling on the tibial tuberosity and producing more bone

**Down**

**2.** Bacterial infection spread by deer ticks that may damage joints
**4.** Autoimmune disorder that attacks the synovial membranes surrounding joints, replacing them with fibrous tissue
**5.** General term for degeneration of the spine
**6.** Weakness and degeneration of bone tissue caused by a decrease in estrogen levels in the body
**8.** Tearing of the periosteum along the medial shaft of the tibia
**9.** Hyper-curvature of the thoracic vertebrae
**10.** Formation of a fluid-filled sac in the popliteal region
**12.** Hyper-curvature of the lumbar vertebrae
**14.** A break in a bone
**15.** An injury to a ligament
**18.** Inflammation caused by an excessive amount of uric acid collecting in the distal areas of the body

Answer Key on Page 288

# Skeletal Quiz

1. Most common form of arthritis
A. Rheumatoid arthritis
B. Gouty arthritis
C. Osteoarthritis
D. Periostitis

2. Epiphyses are covered in the following
A. Elastic cartilage
B. Periosteum
C. Hyaline cartilage
D. Mesentery

3. Lateral curvature of the thoracic vertebrae
A. Swayback
B. Dowager's hump
C. Scoliosis
D. Bamboo spine

4. If a person were to fall forward, landing on their outstretched arms, the shoulder joint could most likely become dislocated in which direction
A. Medially
B. Anteriorly
C. Distally
D. Posteriorly

5. The second cervical vertebrae is also called the
A. Occiput
B. Atlas
C. Axis
D. Dens

6. Hyper-curvature in the thoracic region
A. Swayback
B. Dowager's hump
C. Scoliosis
D. Bamboo spine

7. Shearing of the anterior cruciate ligament most commonly results from force placed on the femur, causing it to move too far in which direction
A. Posteriorly
B. Medially
C. Anteriorly
D. Laterally

8. The nucleus pulposus is located in
A. Stratum germinativum
B. Vertebral bodies
C. Squamous epithelium
D. Intervertebral discs

9. Chronic inflammation located at the tibial tuberosity, caused by overuse of the quadriceps
A. Osgood-Schlatter disease
B. Graves' disease
C. Raynaud's disease
D. Knock-knee

10. Which part of a long bone is the diaphysis
A. Shaft
B. End
C. Articular surface
D. Growth plate

11. Autoimmune disorder in which the intervertebral discs degenerate over time, which can eventually lead to vertebrae fusing together and motion at these joints to be lost
A. Scoliosis
B. Ankylosing spondylitis
C. Rheumatoid arthritis
D. Osteoporosis

12. Bacterial infection that presents with flu-like symptoms, and a bullseye rash at the location of contraction
A. Lyme disease
B. Osgood Schlatter disease
C. Osteomyelitis
D. Paget's disease

13. Subluxation of the big toe, forcing the toe laterally
A. Bursitis
B. Osteoporosis
C. Potts fracture
D. Bunion

14. Autoimmune disorder that attacks synovial membranes throughout the body, replacing them with thick, fibrous material
A. Osteomyelitis
B. Rheumatoid arthritis
C. Paget's disease
D. Ankylosing spondylitis

15. Fluid filled sac formation located in the popliteal region
A. Osgood-Schlatter disease
B. Paget's disease
C. Baker's cyst
D. Rheumatoid arthritis

Answer Key on Page 289

# Urinary System and Pathologies

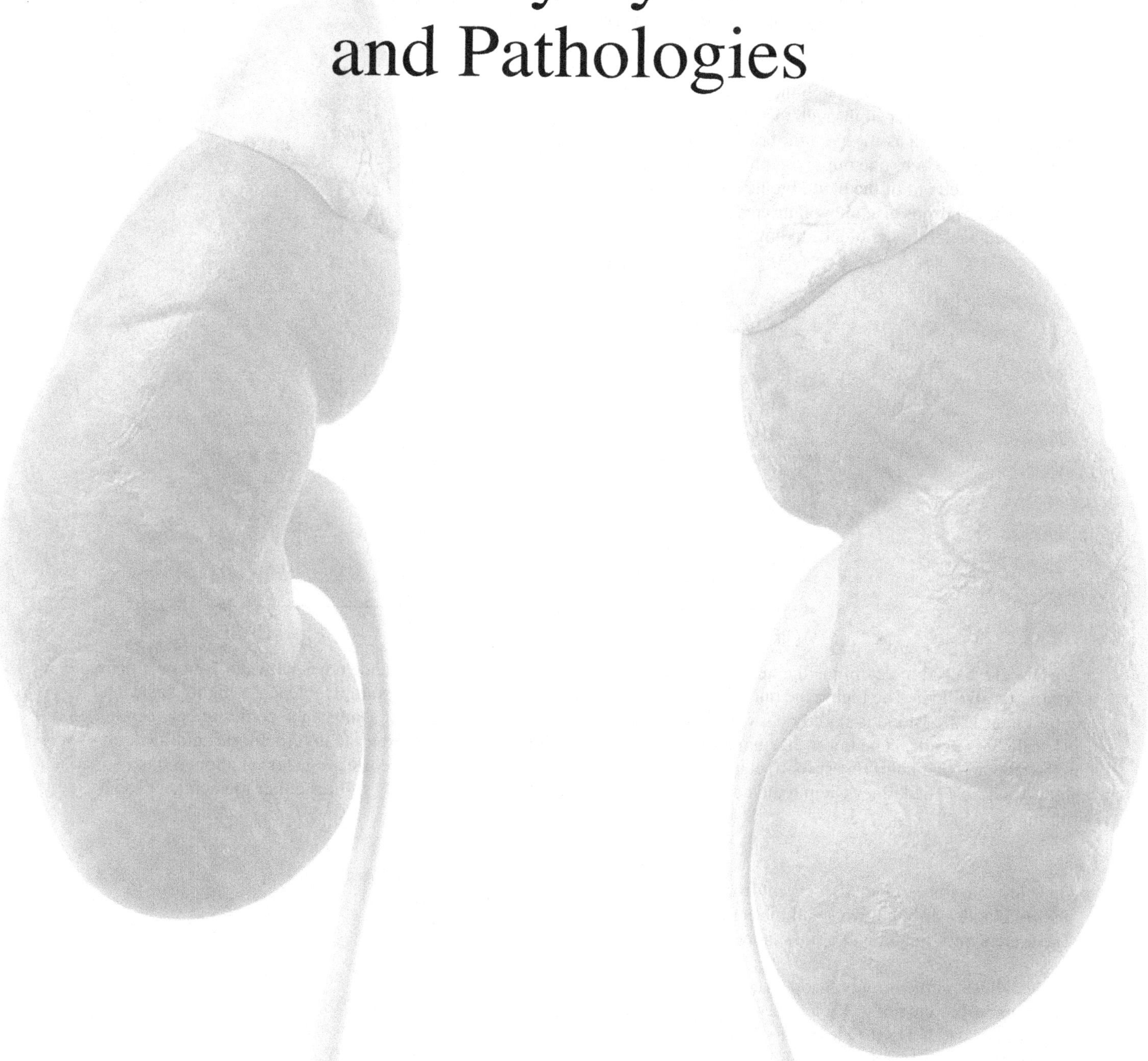

# Urinary System

The Urinary System is primarily responsible for **elimination** of **waste** from the body. It also assists in regulating the **pH level** of the body, and may also assist in reabsorption of substances back into the body. The four main structures of the Urinary System are (in descending order) the **kidneys, ureters, urinary bladder,** and **urethra**.

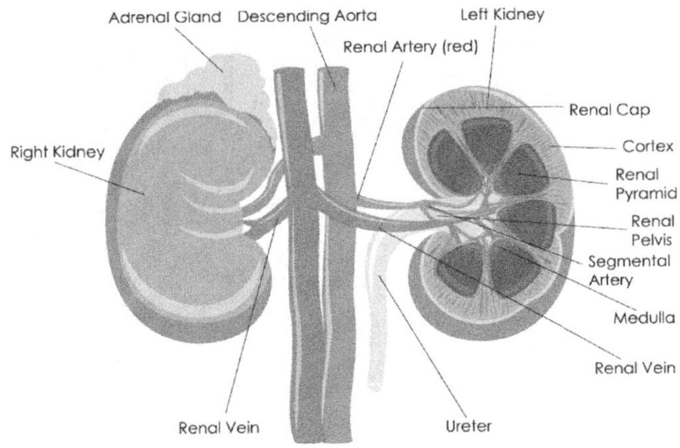


Blood enters the kidneys through the renal arteries. Inside the kidneys, blood is **filtered** through the **nephrons**, which extracts waste products such as **urea** out of the blood. Inside each kidney, there are over one million nephrons. The waste products filtered out of the blood by the nephrons become **urine**. The nephrons also allow nutrients and water to be reabsorbed back into the blood stream.

## The pH Scale

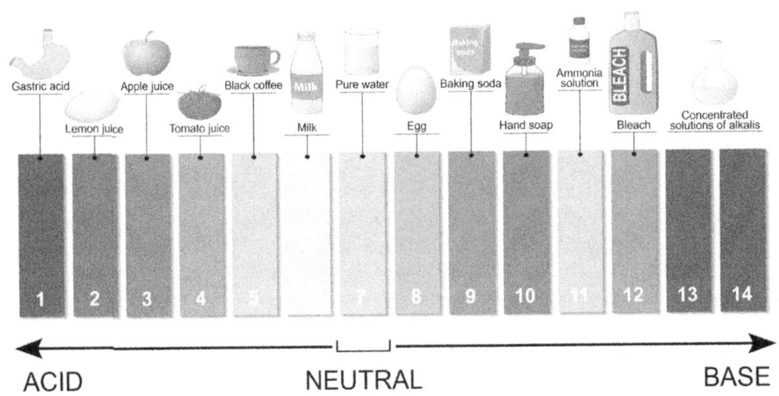


A **pH scale** is used to determine the **acidity** or **alkalinity** of a substance. If a substance reads between **7-14** on a pH scale, it is base, or **alkaline**. The higher the number, the more alkaline a substance is. An example, bleach is highly basic, and comes in at 12.6. Blood is slightly basic, and comes in at 7.4. On the other hand, if a substance comes in between **0-7** on a pH scale, it is **acidic**. The lower the number, the more acidic a substance is. An example, hydrochloric acid(the kind of acid in the stomach that helps digest food) comes in at 2.0, so it is highly acidic. Black coffee registers at about 5.0, so it is slightly acidic. The kidneys help regulate substances in the body that make the body's fluids either too acidic or too basic by filtration.

Once urine has been created, it is sent from the kidneys to the urinary bladder through two small tubes known as ureters. The ureters only function as a **passageway** for urine.

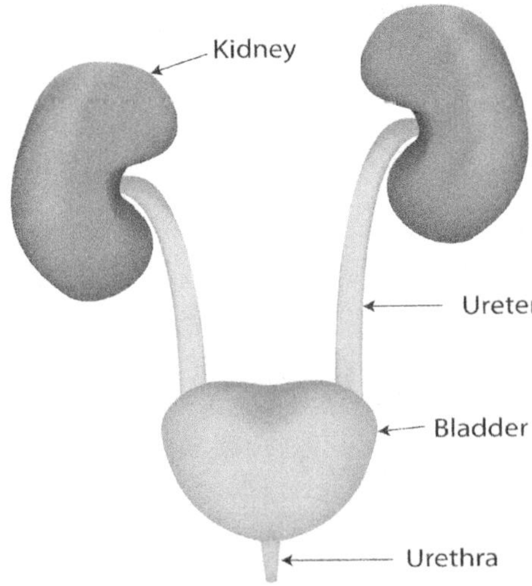


Urine collects in the urinary bladder, until it is ready to be eliminated from the body. The urinary bladder expands as more urine is added to it. The urinary bladder can typically hold between 300-500 ml of fluid. Once urine is released from the urinary bladder, it passes through the urethra.

The urethra, much like the ureters, is a small tube that has one function: **transporting urine** from the urinary bladder **out of the body**.

**Medical Tests and Equipment**

**Catheter:** A catheter is a small tube inserted into a part of the body to help fluid drain. The most common form is a urinary catheter. These are inserted into the urethra and into the urinary bladder. From there, fluid is able to drain freely from the bladder.

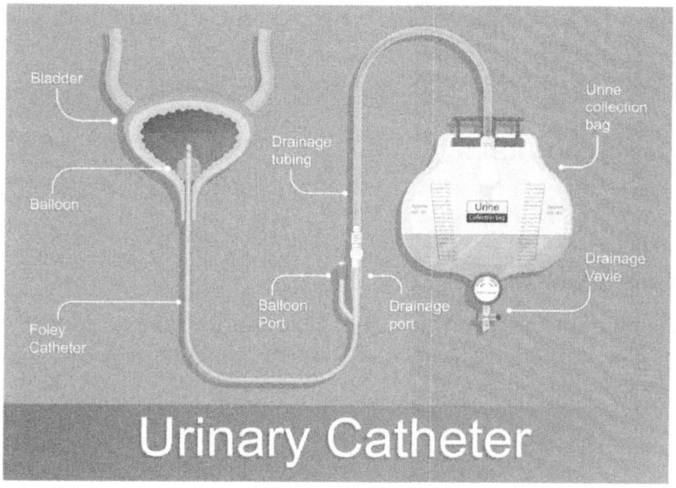


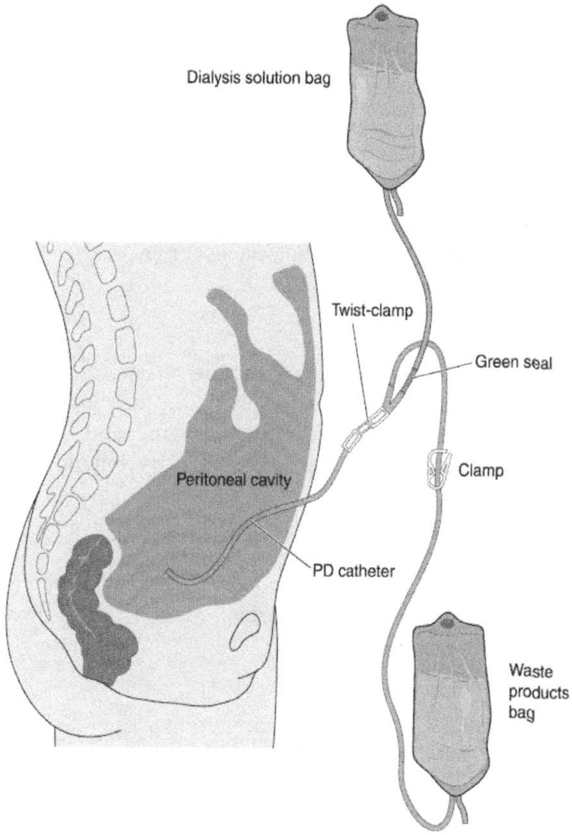


**Dialysis**: Dialysis is used when the kidneys are no longer able to properly function and filter waste products from the blood. Dialysis is meant to mimic the kidneys, pulling waste from the blood and filtering blood back into the body. There are two types of dialysis: hemodialysis and peritoneal dialysis. Hemodialysis is performed by drawing blood from the body, which is cycled through a machine. The dialysis machine contains a permeable membrane that filters the blood, known as a dialyzer. When the waste from the blood has been filtered, the blood is returned to the body. Peritoneal dialysis is performed by administering a catheter into the peritoneum. Dialysate, a fluid, is placed in the body, and it's this fluid that draws waste from the blood. The peritoneum acts as the filter. The waste is removed from the body, and blood never leaves the body like it does with hemodialysis.

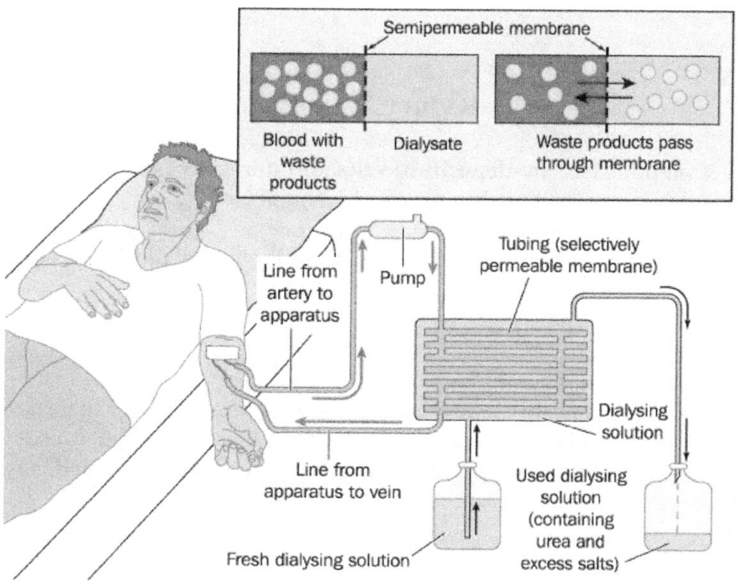

**Lithotripsy**: Lithotripsy is the use of sound waves administered via ultrasound to break up or destroy deposits building up in the body, such as kidney stones and gallstones. Lithotripsy is typically only performed if one of these deposits is too large to pass from the body on its own. The sound waves produced break up the deposit, and allow it to be passed normally. These sound waves are produced by a machine known as a lithotripter.

**Urinometer**: A urinometer is a device placed inside of a tube of urine that measures the specific gravity of urine. This can give information about the content of the urine, the filtering ability of the kidneys, etc. The weight of urine can help determine if there is too much protein in the urine.

## Urinary System Pathologies

### Cystitis

*(cyst-: bladder; -itis: inflammation)*

Cystitis is a **bacterial infection** resulting in **inflammation** of the **bladder**. Often, it can involve the entire Urinary System, and is then known as a Urinary Tract Infection(UTI). Cystitis is most common in women, as the female urethra is shorter than the male urethra, giving bacteria a shorter passage to the bladder.

#### *Causes*

Cystitis is caused most commonly by E. Coli entering the urethra, then reproducing. The increased amount of bacterium in the urethra causes the infection to spread upwards into the bladder. Cystitis can cause numerous symptoms, including blood in the urine, burning sensations while urinating, and a frequent urge to urinate. If untreated, the infection may spread to the kidneys. When this happens, it is known as pyelonephritis.

#### *Symptoms*

Symptoms of cystitis include a frequent urge to urinate, a painful burning sensation upon urination, urinating small amounts at a time, fever, and blood in the urine.

#### *Treatments*

Because cystitis is a bacterial infection, it is treated with antibiotics.

#### *Contraindications*

In the acute stage of infection, massage is contraindication for cystitis. Once the infection has cleared, massage may be performed.

### Kidney Stones

Kidney Stones, also known as nephrolithiasis, are **deposits** of **salts and minerals** created inside the kidney, which are hard and rough. They vary in size, and may cause many differing health complications.

Kidney stones are more common in people who are obese or have a family history of kidney stone development. Diet may play a role as well.

#### *Causes*

Kidney stones may be caused by numerous factors. Most commonly, they are caused by increased amounts of calcium oxalate, which is found in many types of food. Excessive amounts of calcium oxalate can cause stones to develop. Uric acid may also produce stone s if a person does not drink enough fluids. A high protein diet may contribute to the development of uric acid stones.

Less commonly, struvite stones may form, which are the result of bacterial infections of the urinary tract.

***Symptoms***

Kidney stones are largely asymptomatic until they leave the kidney and enter the ureter. When this occurs, pain may be felt around the abdomen, groin, back, and sides. Painful urination may take place as the stone blocks the ureter. The urine may have a pink or brown appearance due to blood in the urine. An inadequate amount of urine may be produced due to blockages.

***Treatments***

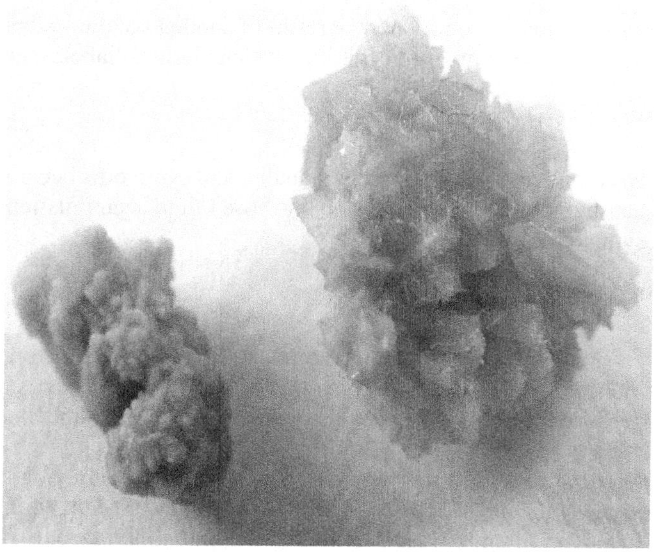

Many treatment options are available. In less severe cases, increasing water intake can help flush the kidneys of the increased calcium and help move the stones out of the body. To aid in moving the stone out of the body, a doctor may prescribe medications that help to relax the smooth muscle in the ureter, known as alpha blockers.

In more severe cases, stones may be destroyed while still inside the body using a treatment known as **extracorporeal shock wave lithotripsy**. The stones are broken down using sound waves, and then are able to be passed out of the body easier. If the stones are too big to be destroyed using sound waves, they may be removed surgically.

***Contraindications***

Kidney stones are not considered a contraindication for massage therapy.

## Pyelonephritis

*(pyel/o: renal pelvis; nephr/o: kidney; -itis: inflammation)*

Pyelonephritis is a **bacterial infection** of the **kidney**, usually beginning in the urethra or bladder. The infection spreads upwards through the ureters and into the kidneys. Pyelonephritis is considered a serious condition, and if suspected, should be seen by a doctor immediately for treatment.

***Causes***

Bacteria enters the urethra. Usually, urinating cleans out the urethra. Rarely, it does not, and bacteria can reproduce in the urethra. The bacteria then can spread upwards into the bladder, then move further up into the ureters and kidneys. Women are more likely than men to develop urinary tract infections due to a shorter urethra.

***Symptoms***

Symptoms of an acute infection in the kidneys include pain in the back, groin, or abdomen, nausea, vomiting, fever, blood in the urine, burning during urination, and an urge to constantly urinate. Cloudy urine may also be a sign of an infection, especially if there is a foul odor.

***Treatments***

Antibiotics are used to combat pyelonephritis. Typically they are administered orally, but in more severe cases that require hospitalization, they may be administered via IV. Pain relievers may be used to aid with associated pain.

***Contraindications***

Pyelonephritis is considered an absolute contraindication. A client who suspects a kidney infection should seek medical treatment.

## Renal Failure

Renal Failure is **kidney failure**, where the kidneys stop functioning properly. This can lead to the body being **unable to eliminate waste**, electrolytes, and excessive fluid. This can lead to dangerous, even fatal levels of these substances in the body.

***Causes***

Renal failure is commonly the result of another condition damaging the kidney enough to impair function. Examples are hypertension, glomerulonephritis, pyelonephritis, diabetes, and polycystic kidney disease.

***Symptoms***

Usually, renal failure occurs gradually, and symptoms become more known as the kidney begins to lose function. Fatigue, nausea, vomiting, hypertension, increased fluid accumulation in the lower limbs, and loss of appetite are common symptoms.

***Treatments***

As the kidneys begin failing, treatment usually revolves around treating the symptoms to try and slow the disease. Once the kidneys have experienced too much damage and the body is unable to eliminate waste and fluid effectively, dialysis may be performed to remove these substances, either through the blood or through the peritoneum.

Kidney transplants may be performed. Instead of removing the damaged kidneys, a doctor will leave the damaged kidneys in the body and attach another kidney. Despite not functioning optimally, the damaged kidneys can still assist the new kidney in filtering waste and fluid, even though it may only be a small amount.

***Contraindications***

Because massage may increase the load on kidneys by helping rid the body of waste, massage is considered an absolute contraindication in clients with renal failure. There is debate amongst kidney specialists on this matter, though, and some believe massage therapy does not do harm in people with renal failure.

## Urethritis

*(urethr/o: urethra; -itis: inflammation)*

Urethritis is **inflammation** of the **urethra**, usually caused by a **bacterial** infection. It is extremely treatable.

***Causes***

Urethritis is caused by a bacterial infection. Bacteria enters the urethra and reproduces, resulting in an infection. The infection may spread up the urinary tract, and may lead to cystitis or pyelonephritis if left untreated.

Less commonly, urethritis may be caused by herpes simplex.

***Symptoms***

Pain upon urination is the primary symptom of urethritis. A less common symptom is inability to effectively urinate, known as dysuria. Discharge from the vagina may present, and the urine may contain blood.

***Treatments***

Because urethritis is most commonly caused by bacterial infection, antibiotics are prescribed to destroy the bacteria and prevent the infection from moving further into the urinary tract.

***Contraindications***

Massage is indicated for clients with urethritis.

# Urinary Pathologies

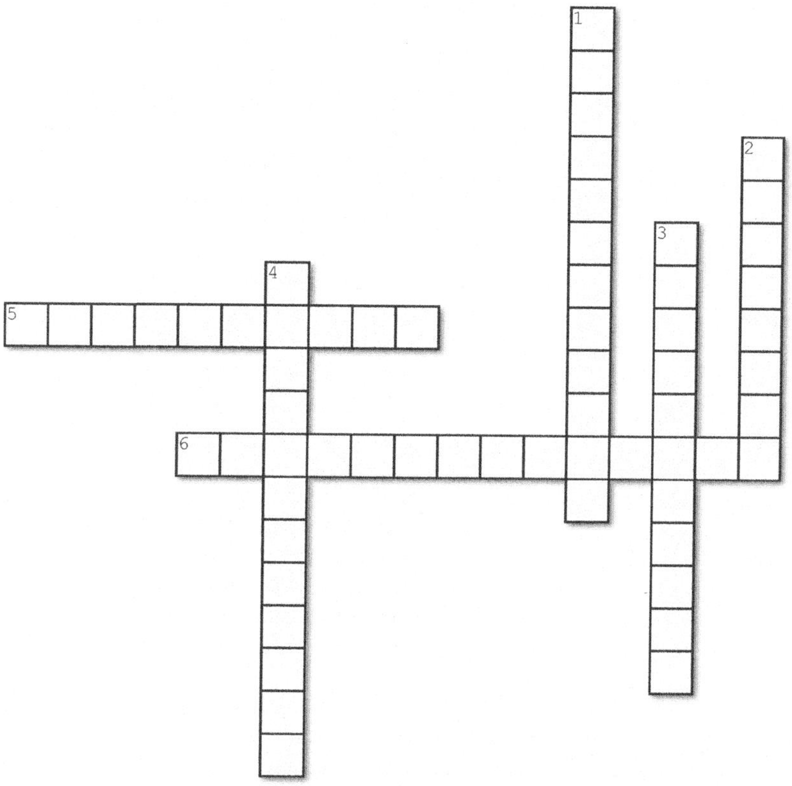


## Across

**5.** Bacterial infection resulting in inflammation of the urethra
**6.** Bacterial infection of the kidney

## Down

**1.** Proper functioning of the kidneys ceases
**2.** Bacterial infection resulting in inflammation of the bladder
**3.** Procedure used to break up stones and deposits in the kidneys to allow for easier passing
**4.** Deposits of salts and minerals in the kidney

Answer Key on Page 288

# Urinary Quiz

1. Balancing electrolyte and acid levels in the body is regulated by
A. Stomach
B. Bladder
C. Large intestine
D. Kidneys

2. Storage of urine is found in the
A. Kidneys
B. Gallbladder
C. Bladder
D. Urethra

3. If a substance is a 6 on a pH scale, that means the substance is
A. Neither acidic nor alkaline
B. Highly acidic
C. Slightly alkaline
D. Slightly acidic

4. When the kidneys experience failure, they are unable to properly filter waste. What treatment is utilized to allow waste to be filtered from the blood in place of the kidneys
A. Dialysis
B. Chemotherapy
C. Lithotripsy
D. Catheterization

5. Pyelonephritis
A. Blockage of ureters by kidney stones
B. Bacterial infection in the kidneys
C. Failure of the kidneys to filter waste
D. Inflammation of the urinary bladder

6. Procedure used to break kidney stones into smaller pieces, allowing for easier passing
A. Urinometer
B. Lithotripsy
C. Dialysis
D. Angioplasty

7. Inflammation of the urethra, caused by bacterial infection
A. Glomerulonephritis
B. Pyelonephritis
C. Cystitis
D. Urethritis

8. Medication used to treat cystitis and pyelonephritis
A. Antibiotics
B. Diuretics
C. Antifungals
D. SSRI's

9. Cystitis is caused by
A. Kidney stones blocking the entrance to the bladder
B. Bacterial infection in the bladder
C. Renal failure
D. Excessive waste being produced by the kidneys

10. Urine flows from the kidneys through the ureters on its way to the
A. Urethra
B. Bladder
C. Bloodstream
D. Liver

11. Medication used to increase the amount of urine being produced
A. Statins
B. Antihistamines
C. Diuretics
D. Beta blockers

12. Nephroliathiasis is another term for
A. Pyelonephritis
B. Renal failure
C. Cystitis
D. Kidney stones

13. All of the following are infectious conditions except
A. Kidney stones
B. Pyelonephritis
C. Urethritis
D. Cystitis

14. Form of dialysis in which the blood is filtered through a dialysis machine and placed back in the body
A. Peritoneal dialysis
B. Hemodialysis
C. Nephrodialysis
D. Urethral dialysis

15. Urea and ammonia are filtered from the blood by the
A. Large intestine
B. Bladder
C. Kidneys
D. Spleen

Answer Key on Page 289

# Cancer

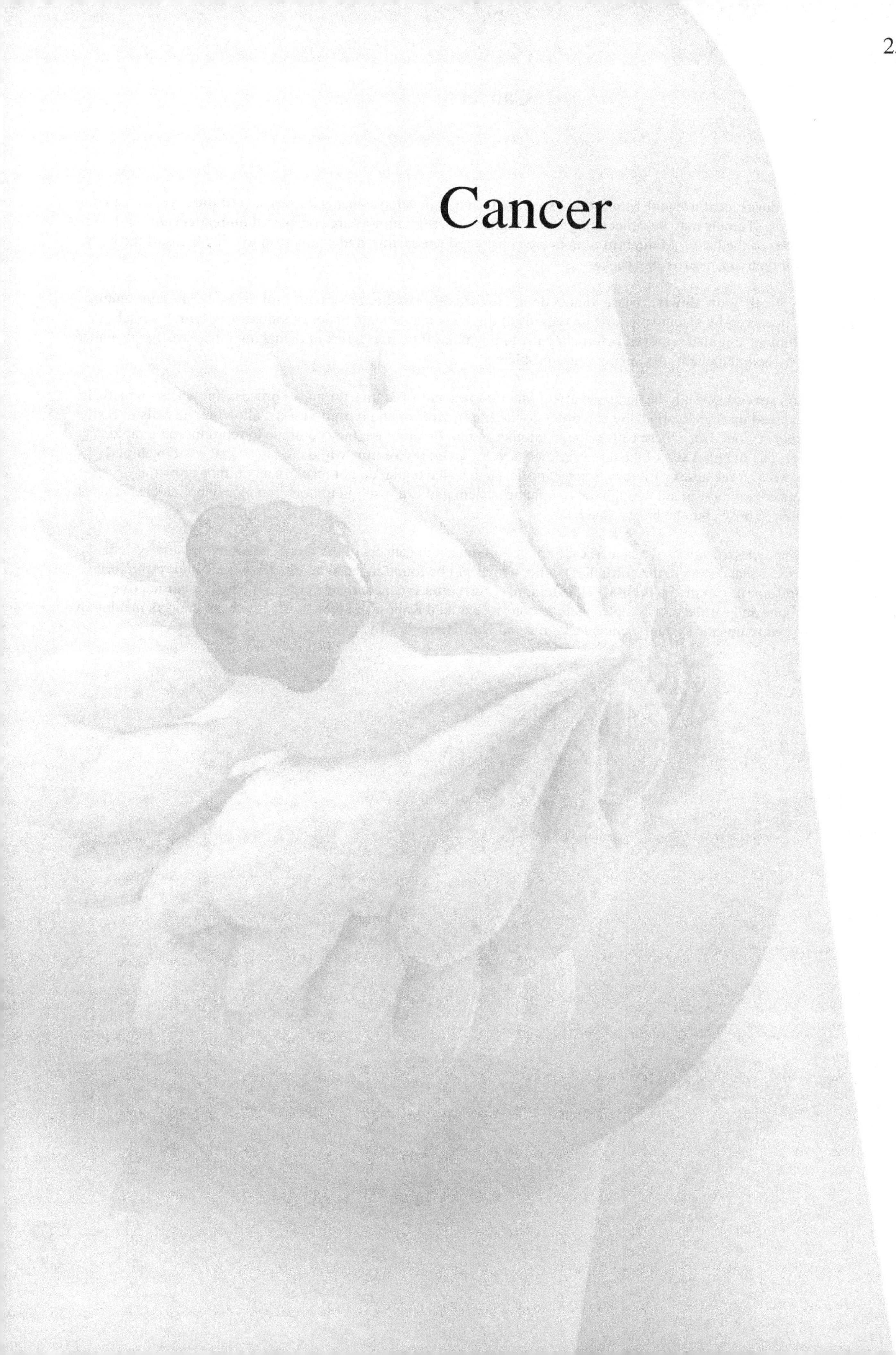

# Cancers

When the body produces an **abnormal amount** of a **specific tissue**, it develops what is known as a **tumor**. Tumors are also known as neoplasms. Tumors may be either benign or malignant. **Benign** tumors are considered **noncancerous**, and do not spread to other areas of the body. **Malignant** tumors are considered **cancerous**, and will spread to other areas of the body. The most common type of cancer is skin cancer.

**Benign** tumors typically grow **slowly**. These tumors do not invade other tissues or structures in the body. Benign tumors may cause harm, however, by placing pressure on regions of the body that contain major blood vessels, lymph vessels, or nerves. Benign tumors are often removed before they get to this point if there is a risk of damaging other structures. Other benign tumors may be left alone if they do not cause problems.

**Malignant** tumors **spread** through the body and affect other tissues and structures through a process known as **metastasis**. Cancerous cells spread through the body by entering into the **blood stream** and **lymph vessels**, allowing the cells to easily transport to another region. Once these cells settle in another region or structure, they continue to reproduce at a rapid, uncontrolled rate. The **original site** of the tumor is known as the **primary tumor**, while the tumor that has **developed elsewhere** is known as a **secondary tumor**. Some cancers, such as leukemia, do not result in any tumor growing. Malignant cancers commonly spread through the lymphatic system and can result in tumors in major lymph nodes. This is especially common in areas like the breasts and neck.

There are three main classifications for cancer: carcinoma, sarcoma, and cancers of the blood stream/lymphatic system. **Carcinoma** is cancer that occurs in the **epithelial tissue**, which can be found in the skin, digestive tract, and respiratory tract. A common form of carcinoma is basal cell carcinoma. **Sarcoma** is cancer that occurs in the body's **connective tissues**, such as bone and cartilage. Examples include bone cancer and Kaposi's Sarcoma. Examples of cancers that involve the bloodstream and lymphatic system include leukemia and Non-Hodgkin's Lymphoma.

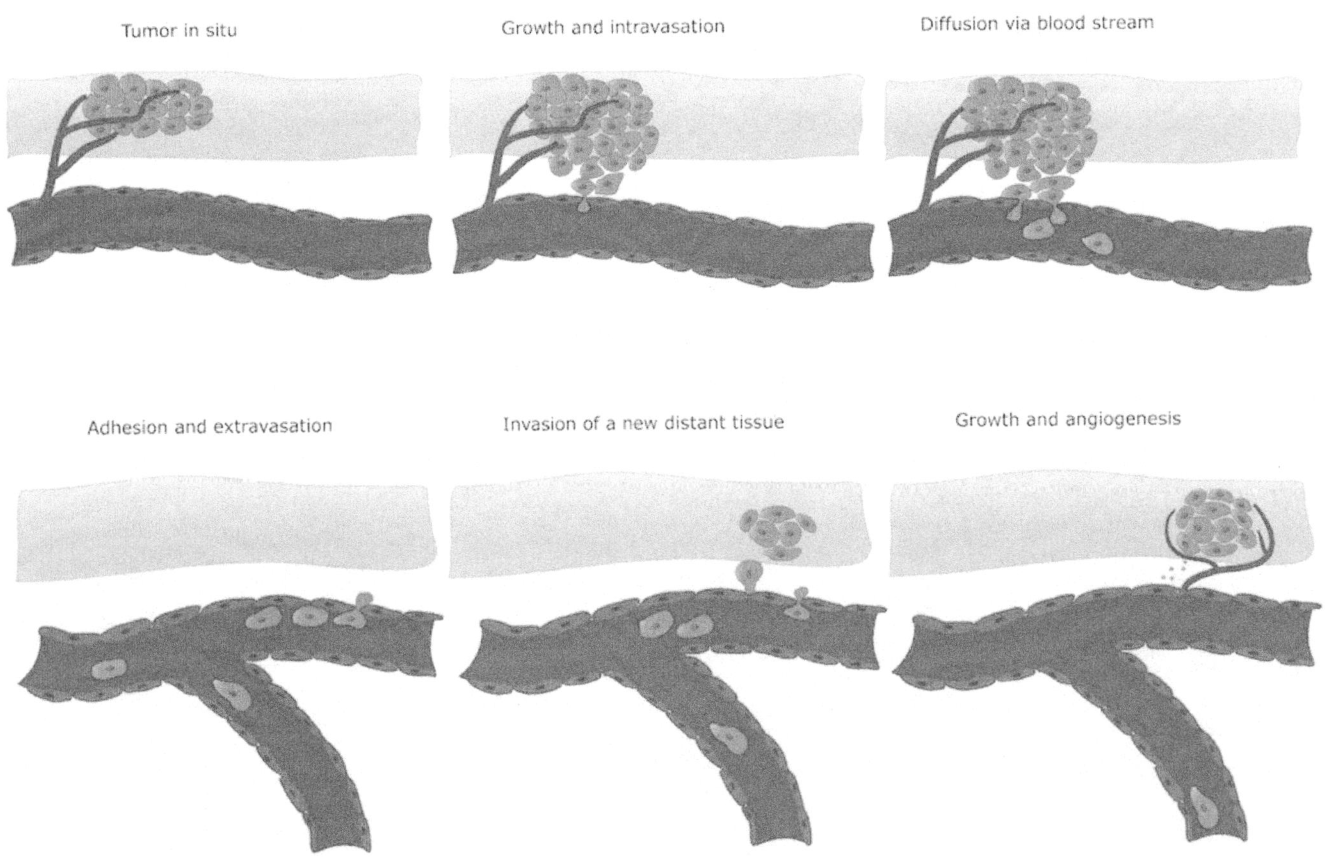

**Medical Tests and Equipment**

**Chemotherapy**: Chemotherapy is the use of certain chemicals to destroy cancerous cells and tumors in the body. Chemotherapy may be administered at different times and different ways, depending on the cause of the cancer. It may be used to destroy some cancer cells and shrink a tumor to aid with pain relief, or to make surgery on the tumor more successful. After a tumor is removed, chemotherapy may be used to destroy any remaining cancerous cells in the body and prevent it from recurring or spreading elsewhere. Chemotherapy is usually given intravenously, but may also be given orally or topically.

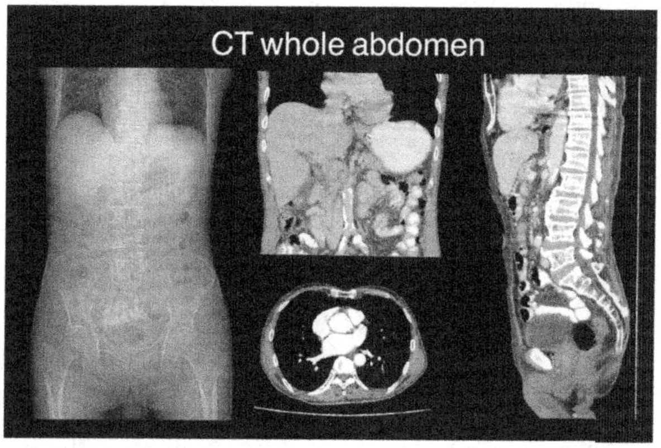


**Computerized Axial Tomography(CT/CAT Scan)**: Computerized Axial Tomography, also known as CT or CAT Scan, is an imaging technique in which a snapshot is taken of a part of the body on a given body plane. This allows viewing of structures in the body from differing points of view. CT is extremely similar to MRI, but uses X-ray to produce images instead of magnetic fields.

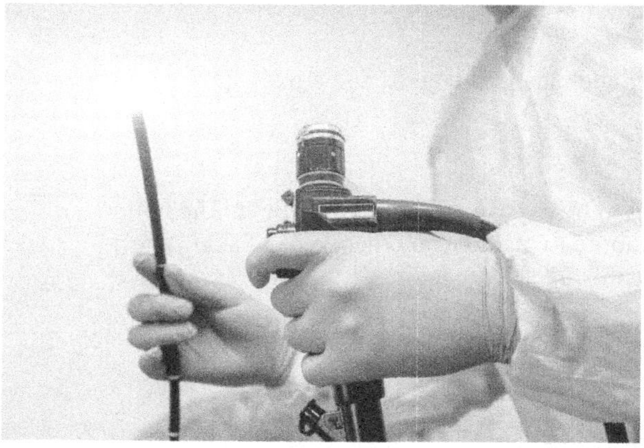

**Endoscopy:** An endoscopy is a procedure in which a tube is inserted into a part of the digestive tract with a camera and light attached, allowing a doctor to see inside the organs. Commonly, this is performed to view the esophagus, stomach, and small intestine. An endoscope used to view the large intestine is known as a colonoscopy.

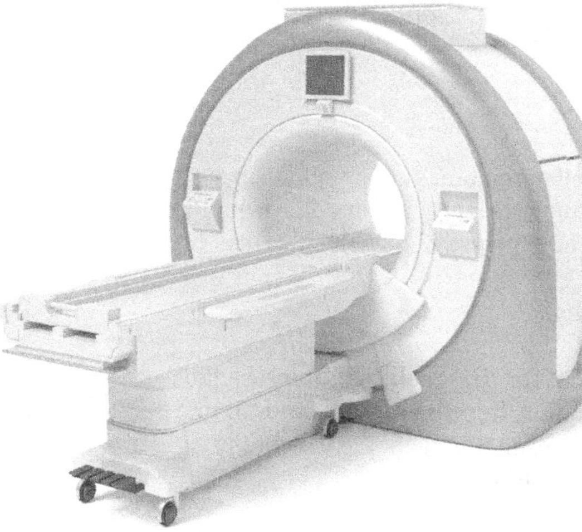

**Magnetic Resonance Imaging(MRI)**: Magnetic Resonance Imaging is the use of high powered magnetic fields to help produce images of structures and organs inside the body. These images are typically much more detailed than X-rays, especially when viewing organs. MRI is used to help diagnose conditions such as tumors, issues with the digestive system, and issues with the heart and blood vessels. The MRI machine is a large tube in which a person lies for an extended period of time, which allows a thorough image to be produced.

**Mammogram**: A mammogram is a procedure used to detect breast cancer in patients who are not showing any symptoms. It uses an X-ray to view the internal breast tissue. A mammogram is typically performed by placing the breast between two glass plates that compress the tissue. Compressing the tissue allows the X-ray to view all of the breast without missing anything.

**Mohs Surgery**: Mohs surgery is a type of surgery performed on skin cancer. During this treatment, thin layers of a tumor in the skin are removed one at a time, until eventually nothing but healthy tissue remains. This type of procedure is done to reduce the amount of damage done to surrounding tissues while ensuring the tumor has been effectively removed. The area may be stitched closed, receive a skin graft, have skin pulled over from an adjacent area to cover the site, or may be left to heal on its own.

**Radiation Therapy**: Radiation therapy is a type of treatment used to destroy cancerous tissue. It is performed by exposing the affected portion of the body to a highly concentrated beam of radiation. The machine responsible for administering the radiation is pointed directly at the spot to be treated, and uses X-rays to destroy cancerous cells. It may also destroy healthy tissue, however. Radiation therapy may also be used to make tumors smaller and prevent a tumor from growing or spreading before surgery may be performed.

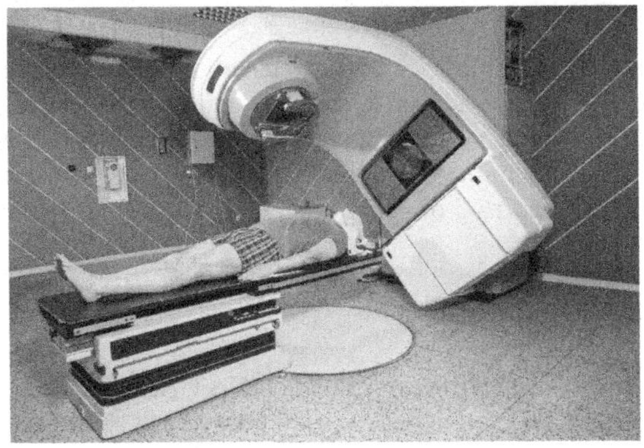

# Cancers

## Basal Cell Carcinoma

*(carcin-: cancer; -oma: tumor)*

Basal Cell Carcinoma is a type of **skin** cancer typically seen around the face, head, neck, and arms.

***Causes***

Basal cell carcinoma is the most common form of skin cancer, caused by exposure to ultraviolet light. The tumor grows **extremely slowly**, which makes basal cell carcinoma much more treatable than other types of skin cancer. Because it is much more treatable, it is considered the **least serious** form of skin cancer.

Basal cell carcinoma is considered a malignant form of cancer, due to its ability to spread to the tissues immediately surrounding it. It will very rarely spread to other organs, however.

***Symptoms***

Basal cell carcinoma tumors may appear to have blood vessels in them, and vary in color from black to brown to pink. These growths may bleed easily.

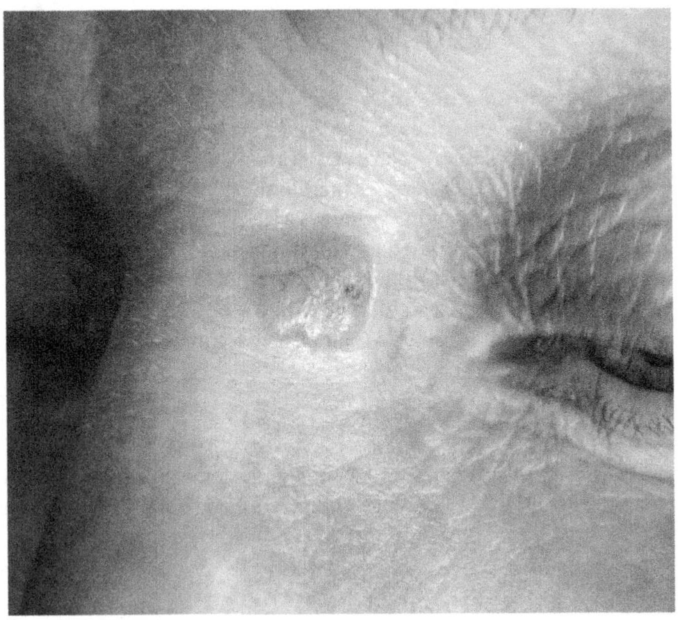

***Treatments***

Treatment for basal cell carcinoma includes surgical excision of the tumor, freezing the tumor, or in more serious cases, medications that prevent the cancerous cells from spreading to other tissues.

***Contraindications***

Massage is indicated for a client with basal cell carcinoma. However, the tumor is a local contraindication, and massage around the area should be avoided to prevent spreading of cancerous tissue through increased blood and lymph flow.

**Colin, Basal Cell Carcinoma**

When were you first diagnosed, and what symptoms were you experiencing at the time that led you to getting checked out?

*I was diagnosed in the last quarter of 2011 with basal cell carcinoma on the left portion of my nose. In 2007, during the last few months of college, I had developed a bump on my nose(what ended up being cancer) that I had originally thought was a pimple, and then a mole or wart. I finally wanted to get it cut off for aesthetic reasons. When the specialist cut it off of my nose, he told me not to worry about it, and that it was nothing. A week later, I got a call at work, and he told me what it was, and not to worry too much about it.*

How big was it?

*The growth was a fairly prominent bump on my nose, perhaps a few millimeters across.*

Did you notice it getting larger over time?

*It never really grew, but I did try to pop it or remove it myself a few times, and so it bled from time to time. LOL. Turns out, you can't pop cancer.*

What color was it? Did it change color over time?

*It was skin-toned, though it sometimes turned a lighter red color when it was agitated for whatever reason.*

Did you notice any vascularity in it?

*I don't recall seeing any veins or anything, no.*

Was it or the area around it tender or painful?

*It wasn't tender unless I messed with it a lot, which I sometimes did in an effort to get it to go away.*

How was it removed?

*It was removed by blade. Once they realized it wasn't surface level, and actually cancer, they then dug in and scooped out whatever else was there. They actually left my scar open for a full week without stitching me up, so that they could make sure they got it all, and wouldn't mess up my scar. Still, my scar is noticeable(not that I really mind).*

What do you think was the cause of the growth?

*The cause of the growth is likely sun exposure. I grew up on Long Island, and we were always outside, at the pool, at the beach, riding bikes, playing ball, whatever. I was telling someone recently that I honest to God don't remember my parents telling me to put sunscreen on a single time when I wasn't at the beach. And, as I'm Italian, we have that olive skin that can really withstand sun. So, the doctors think that's the culprit, which is ironic, 'cause as an adult I'm a total shut-in.*

After it was determined that it was basal cell, did your doctor give you any treatment recommendations or future preventative measures you could take to avoid more tumors in the future?

*I was recommended to stay out of the sun or use skincare stuff that will help block UVs.*

Was there any medication you received afterwards?

*I was given some ointment and antibiotics after the surgery, but it was a long time ago, so I don't remember what they were.*

Do you schedule regular visits to a dermatologist, and if so, how often?

*In early 2012, I was given the all-clear, and I've only been back to the dermatologist twice(in the last two years, ironically) for check-ups. Everything seems fine.*

## Bladder Cancer

Bladder cancer is cancer affecting the **urinary bladder**. Tumors grow in the **lining** of the bladder. Bladder cancer occurs in men more often than women, and a person is more likely to develop bladder cancer if they smoke.

Urothelial carcinoma is the most common form of bladder cancer, in which the cells on the inner lining of the bladder produce uncontrolled. However, these cells may grow in any portion of the urinary tract.

### *Causes*

Common causes include smoking, chronic bladder infections or diseases, and exposure to chemicals that can accumulate in the bladder. Less commonly, a parasitic infection may result in bladder cancer.

### *Symptoms*

Symptoms are similar to other more common bladder conditions, including blood in the urine, pain upon urination, and pain in the pelvis or back. Frequent urination may also be a sign of bladder cancer.

### *Treatments*

Treatment depends on the severity of the cancer. If the cancer is caught early, treatment may only require chemotherapy and/or radiation therapy to destroy the tumor. If the tumor is large enough, surgery to remove the tumor and cancerous tissue may be performed. If too much of the bladder is removed, a new bladder may be reconstructed. If the bladder is completely removed, men will typically have the prostate and seminal vesicles removed as well. Women will have the uterus, ovaries, and fallopian tubes removed. This is done to prevent spreading of cancerous tissue to any of these other structures.

STAGES OF BLADDER CANCER

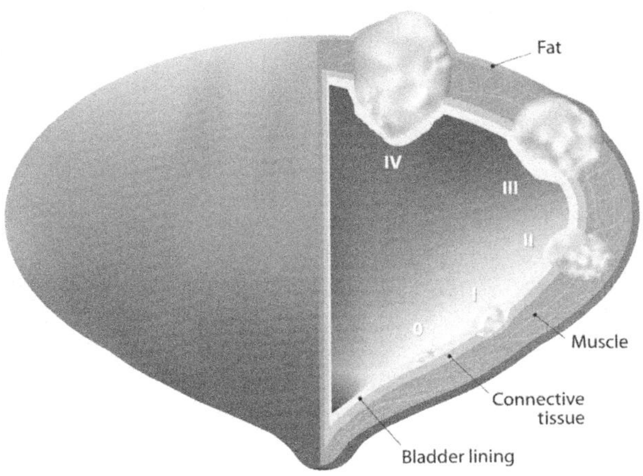


### *Contraindications*

A massage therapist should obtain a doctor's note approving massage. Afterwards, massage may be performed, avoiding any tumors, lymph nodes, or other areas affected.

## Bone Cancer

Bone cancer is cancer of the **bone**, most commonly taking place in **long bones** and the **pelvis**. Bone cancer does not include cancers such as leukemia which begin elsewhere in the body and then spread into the bone tissue.

There are three types of bone cancer: Chondrosarcoma, Ewing Sarcoma, and Osteosarcoma. In chondrosarcoma, the cancerous tissue is produced in cartilage*(chondr/o: cartilage)*. The other two both begin in bone, while Ewing Sarcoma may begin in the periosteum.

### *Causes*

There are no known causes of bone cancer.

### *Symptoms*

Tumor growth in the bone results in pain in the bone. The bone may become weakened and more prone to fracture. Inflammation in the area of the tumor may present.

*Treatments*

Treatment for bone cancer depends on the stage of the cancer and size of the tumor. Smaller tumors are removed along with any affected bone tissue. The bone tissue is replaced by bone from another part of the body. In larger tumors, amputation of the limb may result if too much bone tissue needs to be removed.

Chemotherapy and radiation therapy to kill any remaining cancerous tissue will be prescribed.

*Contraindications*

A massage therapist should obtain a doctor's note approving massage. Afterwards, massage may be performed, avoiding any tumors, lymph nodes, or other areas affected.

## Brain Cancer

Brain cancer is the growth of a **malignant tumor** in the **brain**. These tumors may originate in the brain or tissues around it(primary brain tumor), or spread to the brain from other parts of the body(secondary brain tumor).

*Causes*

Primary brain tumors are usually the result of some sort of genetic mutation which causes brain tissue in certain regions of the brain to grow abnormally. Secondary brain tumors occur when a cancer elsewhere in the body metastasize to the brain, and a tumor grows as a result. Many types of malignant cancers can cause secondary brain tumors, including breast cancer, lung cancer, and malignant melanoma.

*Symptoms*

Symptoms vary depending on location and size of the tumor. Common symptoms include headache, nausea, vomiting, problems with speech, problems with balance, blurred vision, double vision, seizure, confusion, and changes in personality or behavior.

*Treatments*

Some tumors are able to be removed surgically, while some are not. This all depends on the location of the tumor. If the tumor is able to be removed, a surgeon will remove as much of the tumor as possible, and the patient will then be treated with chemotherapy and radiation therapy to try and destroy the remaining cancerous tissue.

After surgery, rehabilitation may be sought to regain any lost functions such as speech or motor skills.

*Contraindications*

A massage therapist should obtain a doctor's note approving massage. Afterwards, massage may be performed, avoiding any tumors, lymph nodes, or other areas affected.

## Breast Cancer

Breast cancer is cancer of **breast tissue**, including **lymph nodes and vessels** in the **breast** and **axillary region**. Breast cancer is the second most common form of cancer diagnosed in women, behind skin cancer. Breast cancer is much more common in women, but it can also occur in men.

Breast cancer can spread throughout the breast and to other regions of the body, and is considered a malignant form of cancer.

*Causes*

Breast cancer occurs when breast tissue begins growing abnormally, forming a tumor that feels like a lump under the skin.

Breast cancer may be a genetic disorder, or may be the cause of unspecified environmental factors. Women who are older in age tend to develop breast cancer more often than younger women.

***Symptoms***

Symptoms include a lump in the breast that does not feel the same as tissue surrounding it, a nipple that has recently become inverted, change in size or appearance of the breast, dimpling of the skin of the breast, the skin of the breast and/or areola becoming scaly or flaky, and the skin of the breast becoming red. If any of these symptoms occur, a person should be seen by a medical professional.

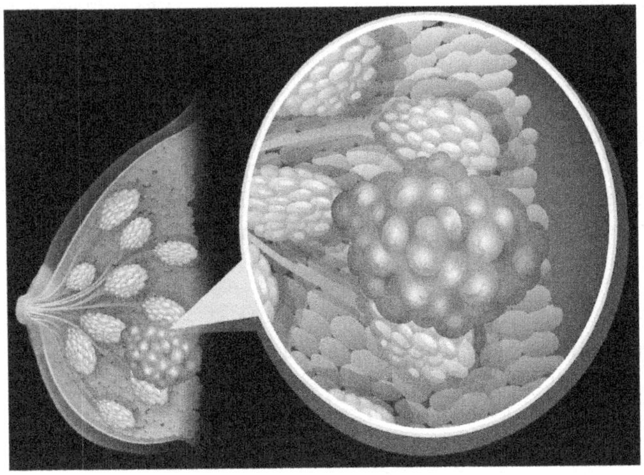

***Treatments***

Treatment is based on the severity of the tumor growth. Surgery to remove the tumor will likely be performed after locating it via mammogram and ultrasound. If a large amount of breast tissue is involved, the breast may be completely removed, known as a mastectomy. Lymph nodes may also be removed to prevent any cancerous tissue from spreading to other parts of the body. Chemotherapy and radiation therapy are performed to kill the remaining cancerous cells.

***Contraindications***

A massage therapist should obtain a doctor's note approving massage. Afterwards, massage may be performed, avoiding any tumors, lymph nodes, or other areas affected.

## Cervical Cancer

Cervical cancer is cancer of the **cervix**, the neck-like passageway between the vagina and the uterus.

***Causes***

Cervical cancer is most commonly caused by the **human papilloma virus(HPV)**. In a small percentage of women, the body does not develop an immunity to the virus. The virus attacks the cells of the cervix, which in turn, transforms them into cancerous cells.

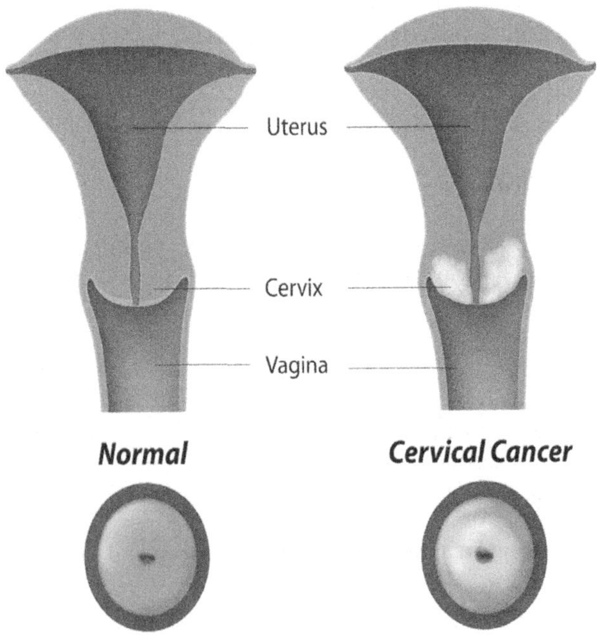


***Symptoms***

Cervical cancer is typically asymptomatic in early stages. As the cancer progresses, bleeding from the vagina may occur. Pain during intercourse may present, with a watery discharge that may contain blood.

***Treatments***

Treatment depends on the severity of the cancer. In early stages, the cancer is usually removed with the uterus and cervix, but the rest of the reproductive system is left intact. In more advanced cases, the uterus, cervix, vagina, and lymph nodes in the groin are removed. Chemotherapy and radiation therapy are used to destroy any remaining cancerous cells and prevent spreading of the cancer.

***Contraindications***

A massage therapist should obtain a doctor's note approving massage. Afterwards, massage may be performed, avoiding any tumors, lymph nodes, or other areas affected.

## Colon Cancer

Colon cancer is the formation of tumors in the **large intestine**. Colon cancer typically occurs in people over the age of 50, and in people with gastrointestinal disorders such as Crohn's Disease(page 77). It begins as benign tumors in the large intestine known as adenomatous polyps. These tumors may eventually grow and spread, becoming malignant. The most common locations for colon cancer to spread are the liver, brain, and lungs.

***Causes***

There is no known cause of colon cancer. It may occur more in people who eat a diet high in fat and low in fiber more commonly than others.

***Symptoms***

Symptoms are largely asymptomatic in early stages, and only appear as the cancer progresses. A person with colon cancer may experience bloody stools, diarrhea or constipation lasting longer than a month, pain in the abdomen, cramping in the abdomen, and feeling as if the bowels haven't completely emptied after defecation.

***Treatments***

Treatment depends on the stage of the cancer. Early stages may require only removal of the polyps without removing a portion of the large intestine. As the cancer grows and spreads, it may affect the lining of the large intestine. If this is the case, surgery to move that specific part of the large intestine may be performed. Depending on the amount of large intestine removed, a person may need to have a hole placed in the abdomen to allow a place for feces to empty from the body. This is known as a colostomy.

In addition to removal of the cancer and possible removal of portions of the large intestine, chemotherapy and radiation therapy are used to destroy any remaining cancerous cells in the body.

***Contraindications***

A massage therapist should obtain a doctor's note approving massage. Afterwards, massage may be performed, avoiding any tumors, lymph nodes, or other areas affected.

## Hodgkin's Lymphoma

*(lymph-: lymph; -oma: tumor)*

Hodgkin's Lymphoma is a malignant cancer affecting the lymphatic system, specifically the **lymph nodes** in the **upper limb**, **chest**, and **neck**. Hodgkin's Lymphoma usually follows lymph channels in a predictable manner, moving from one lymph node to the next.

***Causes***

Hodgkin's Lymphoma is caused by an excessive amount of B cells being produced. These cells, known as **Reed-Sternberg cells**, are larger than normal and contain multiple nuclei, as opposed to non-cancerous B cells, which are smaller and only contain one nucleus.

***Symptoms***

Symptoms of Hodgkin's Lymphoma include swelling of lymph nodes in the neck, upper limb, and axilla that may be painless, weight loss, fever, and fatigue. A person may also experience sensitivity to alcohol.

***Treatments***

Surgery isn't usually performed for a patient with Hodgkin's Lymphoma. Instead, chemotherapy and radiation therapy are used to destroy the cancerous lymphocytes. Bone marrow transplants may also be performed to stimulate the production of non-cancerous cells.

***Contraindications***

A massage therapist should obtain a doctor's note approving massage. Afterwards, massage may be performed, avoiding any tumors, lymph nodes, or other areas affected.

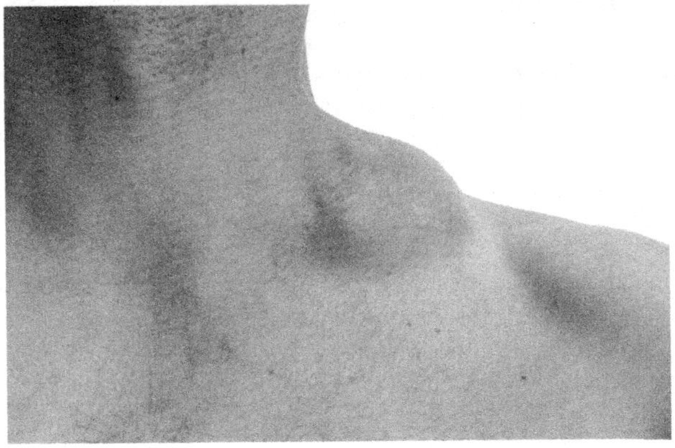

## Kaposi's Sarcoma

Kaposi's Sarcoma is a cancer of the **linings** of **blood** and **lymph vessels**, most commonly seen with the development of tumors in the **face**, **legs**, and **feet**. These tumors can appear purple, red, or brown, and are known as lesions. The cancerous cells may metastasize and affect other tissues or organs such as the lungs or liver.

***Causes***

Kaposi's Sarcoma is caused by the **human herpesvirus 8(HHV-8)**. HHV-8 usually does not result in any symptoms, unless a person has a weakened immune system. A person infected with **HIV** has the highest risk of developing Kaposi's Sarcoma due to the immune system being weakened by the virus. This allows HHV-8 to multiply and develop into cancer.

***Symptoms***

Symptoms of Kaposi's Sarcoma include the development of lesions in the skin and on mucous membranes such as the mouth, nausea, vomiting, problems eating or swallowing, coughing, shortness of breath, and swelling in the limbs, face, or groin.

***Treatments***

Antiretroviral therapy may be used to treat the lesions that develop. It may also prevent further lesions from developing. Lesions may be surgically removed, and chemotherapy and radiation therapy may be performed to kill the cancerous cells. If the cancer has spread to other organs, those organs may be treated by surgically removing the tumors.

***Contraindications***

A massage therapist should obtain a doctor's note approving massage. Afterwards, massage may be performed, avoiding any tumors, lymph nodes, skin lesions, or other areas affected.

## Leukemia

*(leuk/o: white; -emia: blood condition)*

Leukemia is a cancer of the **bone** and **lymph** involving **excessive production** of **non-functioning leukocytes**. These leukocytes do not function the way normal leukocytes should, leaving the body with a compromised immune system. These cancerous cells may spread to other parts of the body such as the liver and brain.

***Causes***

There is no known cause for the development of leukemia.

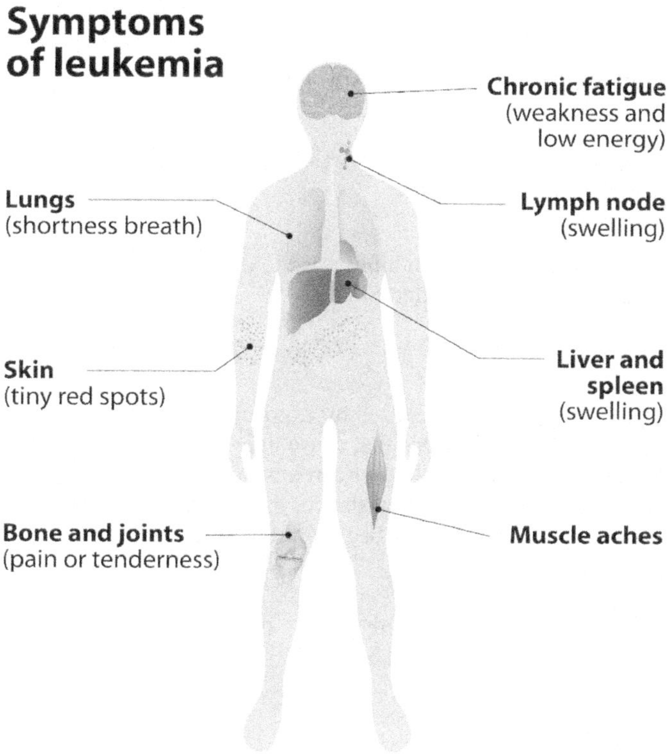


*Symptoms*

Common symptoms of leukemia include pain in the bone, swollen lymph nodes, fatigue, fever, chills, increased likelihood of developing infections, the appearance of small red spots in the skin, and bruising or bleeding easily. A doctor should be seen if any of these symptoms persist.

*Treatments*

Treatment for leukemia largely depends on the advancement of the condition. If the cancer has metastasized to other parts of the body, treatment would be performed on those areas in conjunction with treating the leukemia. Chemotherapy and radiation therapy are used to target and destroy cancerous cells throughout the body. After chemotherapy and/or radiation therapy, stem cell transplant may be performed to supply the bone with stem cells that grow healthy marrow, which produces functioning leukocytes. Bone marrow itself may also be transplanted into the patient to accomplish the same goal.

*Contraindications*

A massage therapist should obtain a doctor's note approving massage. Afterwards, massage may be performed, avoiding any tumors, lymph nodes, or other areas affected.

## Liver Cancer

Liver cancer is the development of **tumors** in the **liver**. The most common form of liver cancer is **hepatocellular carcinoma**, in which the cancer begins in the cells of the liver.

Cancer originating elsewhere that spreads to the liver occurs much more commonly than cancer originating in the liver itself.

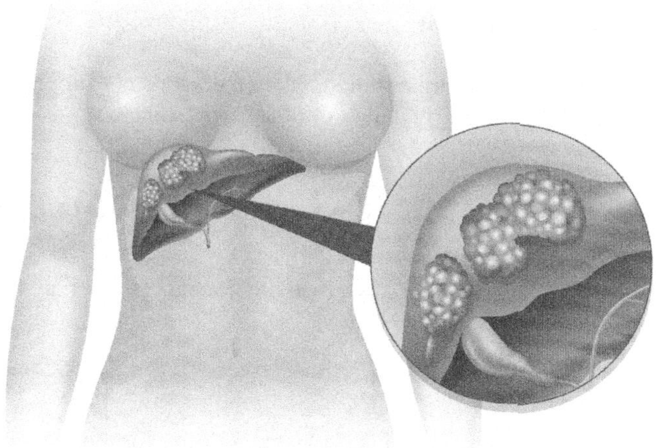

*Causes*

Most of the time, the exact cause of liver cancer is unknown. Certain diseases, such as hepatitis B or C, cirrhosis, and diabetes, may damage the liver and lead to the development of cancer. Drinking alcohol in excess may also damage the liver and contribute.

*Symptoms*

Liver cancer is typically asymptomatic until later stages. Symptoms may include nausea, vomiting, weight loss, pain and swelling in the abdomen, and jaundice.

*Treatments*

Treatment for liver cancer largely depends on the stage of the cancer. Surgery may be performed to remove the tumor if it does not damage the liver too severely. In more advanced cases, a liver transplant may be sought. Other treatments include radiation therapy to target and kill cancer cells, chemotherapy drugs injected into the tumor, freezing the cancer cells, using electric currents to destroy the cancer cells, and injecting the tumor with pure alcohol to kill cancer cells.

***Contraindications***

A massage therapist should obtain a doctor's note approving massage. Afterwards, massage may be performed, avoiding any tumors, lymph nodes, or other areas affected.

## Lung Cancer

Lung cancer is the development of **tumors** in the **lung**. People who **smoke** are at a much higher risk to develop lung cancer than anyone else. Lung cancer is the leading cause of cancerous death in the United States.

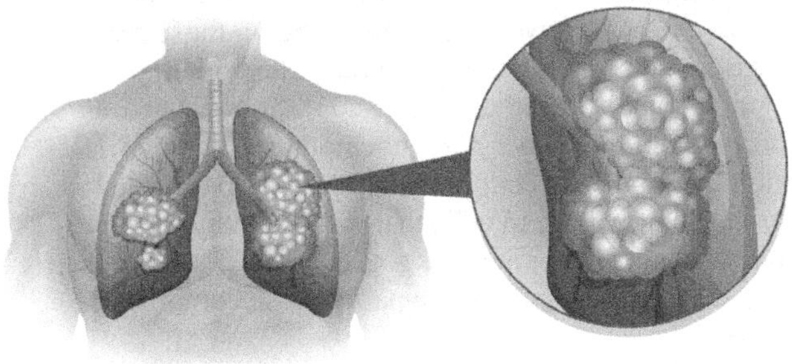

***Causes***

Lung cancer is primarily caused by exposure to carcinogens being inhaled. Carcinogens that cause lung cancer may be found in cigarette smoke. Other carcinogens may include radon and asbestos. These substances damage the tissue of the lungs, which in turn may begin reproducing unnaturally, causing cancer.

Lung cancer may spread to other areas and organs of the body, including the liver and brain.

***Symptoms***

Lung cancer is usually asymptomatic in early stages. As the condition progresses, however, symptoms may begin to appear and worsen over time. Symptoms include coughing that may produce blood, shortness of breath, and chest pain. Hoarseness may occur due to excessive coughing.

***Treatments***

Treatment largely depends on the stage of the cancer. The earlier stages of cancer may only require surgical removal of a small portion of the lung to take out the tumor. Advanced stages involving larger tumors may require an entire lobe of a lung to be removed, or in extreme cases, having the entire lung removed.

After the tumor is removed, radiation and chemotherapy may be performed to destroy any remaining cancerous cells.

***Contraindications***

A massage therapist should obtain a doctor's note approving massage. Afterwards, massage may be performed, avoiding any tumors, lymph nodes, or other areas affected.

## Malignant Melanoma

*(melan-: black; -oma: tumor)*

Malignant Melanoma is a type of **skin** cancer that may affect any part of the skin, and can also affect other tissues such as the eyes and internal organs.

***Causes***

Malignant melanoma is the **least common** form of skin cancer, but it is the **most serious**. It is caused by exposure to ultraviolet light. The cells in the body that produce skin pigment, **melanocytes**, become stimulated by exposure to ultraviolet light, and reproduce, causing darker skin. In malignant melanoma, the melanocytes reproduce uncontrolled. This uncontrolled reproduction results in a tumor, and these cancerous cells can easily spread throughout the body and damage other organs and tissues.

Dermatologists use the ABCDE method to diagnose malignant melanoma:

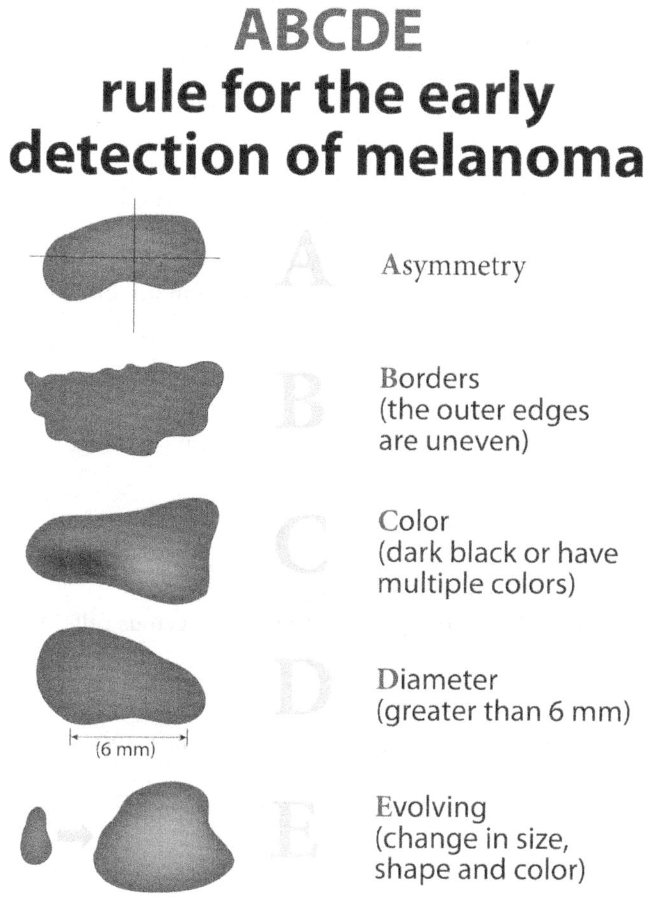


A: Asymmetrical; moles are typically symmetrical, but melanoma tumors have an unusual shape, and the sides don't match.

B: Borders; the borders of the growth change over time and are uneven. This is a sign of significantly increased melanin production.

C: Color; moles are typically some shade of brown. If there are multiple shades or colors, or if the tumor is black, this may be a sign of increased melanin production.

D: Diameter; if a growth is 6mm or greater in diameter(the distance through it), this may be a sign of melanoma.

E: Evolving; moles typically look the same over time. If a mole or growth begins to evolve or change in any way, this may be a sign of melanoma.

Malignant melanoma most commonly begins to appear on a part of the body that doesn't have any prior lesions, like moles. If a new growth appears where there was nothing prior, this may be a sign of melanoma. Less commonly, moles may become cancerous.

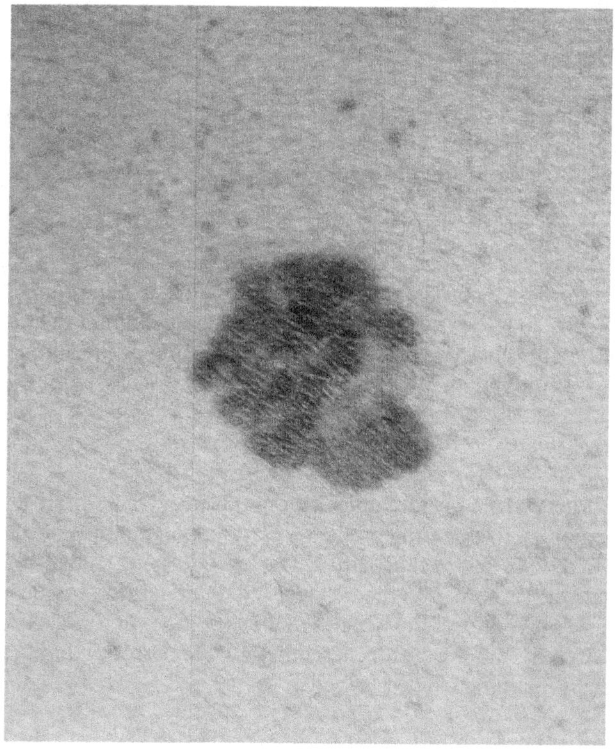

***Symptoms***

Symptoms of melanoma are all included in the ABCDE's.

***Treatments***

Malignant melanoma, if caught early enough, is easily treatable. Later stages, where it has grown beyond the skin, need more advanced treatments, including surgery to remove any tumors or cancerous lymph nodes, chemotherapy, and radiation therapy.

***Contraindications***

A client with malignant melanoma should obtain permission from a doctor before proceeding with any type of massage, because the cancerous cells are easily spread throughout the body through the blood and lymph. The site of tumor growth should be avoided.

## Non-Hodgkin's Lymphoma

*(lymph-: lymph; -oma: tumor)*

Non-Hodgkin's Lymphoma is a type of cancer of the **Lymphatic System**, caused by the development of tumors by **lymphocytes**.

***Causes***

In the body, lymphocytes, like every cell, go through their normal life cycle, and die when they are supposed to. In Non-Hodgkin's Lymphoma, the **lymphocytes don't die**, but **continue reproducing**. This causes an **excessive amount** of **lymphocytes** to build up in the lymph nodes.

***Symptoms***

People with Non-Hodgkin's Lymphoma may experience swollen lymph nodes around the neck, groin, and axilla, fatigue, weight loss, and fever.

***Treatments***

Oftentimes, Non-Hodgkin's Lymphoma isn't serious, and treatment is only required when it becomes advanced. Advanced Non-Hodgkin's Lymphoma is treated with chemotherapy and radiation therapy to destroy the cancerous cells.

***Contraindications***

A massage therapist should obtain a doctor's note approving massage. Afterwards, massage may be performed, avoiding any tumors, lymph nodes, or other areas affected.

## Oral Cancer

Oral cancer is a cancer of the **mouth**, and may affect several different structures related to the mouth. These structures include the gums, lips, tongue, hard palate, soft palate, and inner lining of the cheek. Oral cancer may spread to other regions of the body, most commonly the cervical lymph nodes, the liver, the brain, and the lungs.

***Causes***

Oral cancer occurs when the cells inside the mouth are damaged in some way, changing the DNA, causing them to grow abnormally. Common reasons for this to occur is **smoking**, using **chewing tobacco**, **excessive alcohol consumption**, and over-exposure of **ultraviolet light** on the lips from the sun.

***Symptoms***

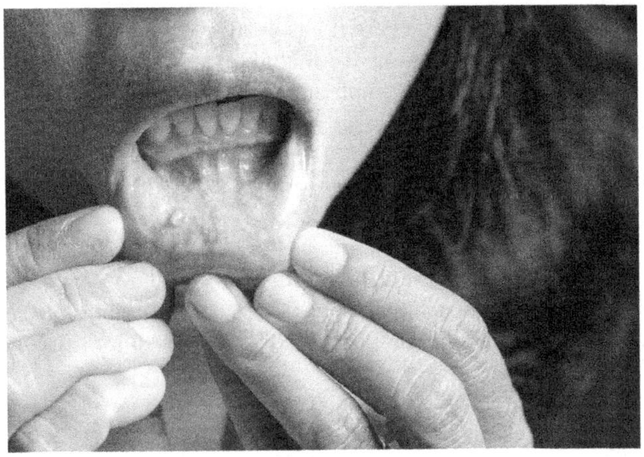

Common symptoms may include a sore inside the mouth that bleeds and does not heal, pain in the tongue, pain in the jaw, problems chewing or swallowing, thickening of the skin inside the mouth, and a sore throat.

***Treatments***

Surgery is the best treatment for oral cancer. The tumor is removed. Depending on the size, reconstruction of parts of the mouth, such as the hard palate, may be performed. If the cancer has spread to the cervical lymph nodes, the tumor may be removed from the neck as well. After the tumor has been removed, radiation and chemotherapy are performed to kill any remaining cancerous cells.

***Contraindications***

A massage therapist should obtain a doctor's note approving massage. Afterwards, massage may be performed, avoiding any tumors, lymph nodes, or other areas affected.

## Ovarian Cancer

Ovarian cancer is cancer that originates in the **ovaries**. As the cancer grows, it may spread into the regions around the ovary, the abdomen and pelvis. At this stage, it is much more difficult to treat.

***Causes***

The exact cause of ovarian cancer is unknown. Age may play a role, as the majority of cases affect women between the ages of 50 and 60.

***Symptoms***

Early stages of ovarian cancer are largely asymptomatic. Symptoms usually appear as the cancer grows and spreads to other parts of the body, including weight loss, swelling in the abdomen, constipation, and frequently needing to urinate.

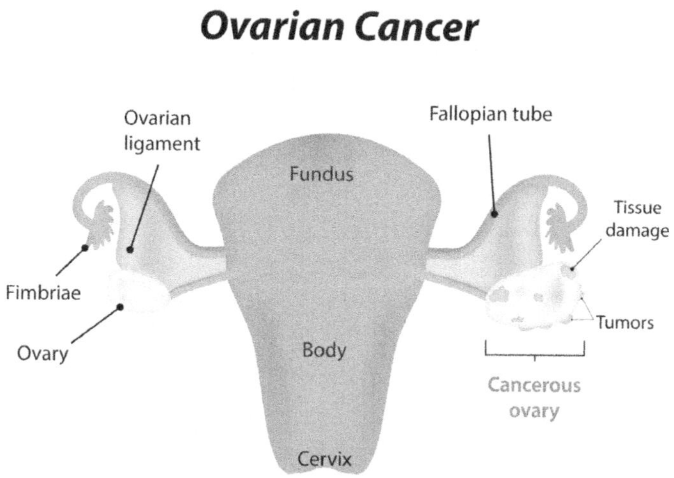


***Treatments***

Surgery is the most common form of treatment for ovarian cancer. Depending on the advancement of the cancer, surgery may be performed to remove one ovary, both ovaries, both ovaries and the uterus, and surgery to remove tumors from other parts of the body. After surgery, chemotherapy is typically performed to destroy any remaining cancerous cells.

***Contraindications***

A massage therapist should obtain a doctor's note approving massage. Afterwards, massage may be performed, avoiding any tumors, lymph nodes, or other areas affected.

## Pancreatic Cancer

Pancreatic cancer is cancer that grows in the **pancreas**, which can metastasize rapidly into other tissues and organs, such as the liver.

***Causes***

The exact cause of pancreatic cancer is unknown. People who are more likely to develop pancreatic cancer include those who **smoke**, are **obese**, have **diabetes**, and have **chronic pancreatitis**.

***Symptoms***

Early stages of pancreatic cancer may be asymptomatic. As the cancer progresses, a person may experience pain in the abdomen, loss of appetite, loss of weight, fatigue, jaundice, and diabetes.

***Treatments***

Treatment largely depends on the stage of the cancer. Typical treatment focuses on removing the tumor from the pancreas. If the tumor is too large, or has affected too much of the pancreas, the entire pancreas may be removed. The spleen may also be removed, as it may contain cancerous cells. After the tumor has been removed, chemotherapy and radiation therapy may be performed to destroy any remaining cancerous cells.

***Contraindications***

A massage therapist should obtain a doctor's note approving massage. Afterwards, massage may be performed, avoiding any tumors, lymph nodes, or other areas affected.

## Prostate Cancer

Prostate cancer is cancer of the **prostate**, which is responsible for producing seminal fluid. This form of cancer may be **benign**, but it does carry the risk of metastasizing to other areas of the body, such as the bones and lymph nodes.

***Causes***

There is no known cause of prostate cancer. People who are obese have a higher risk of developing prostate cancer. As a person ages, the chances they get prostate cancer increases.

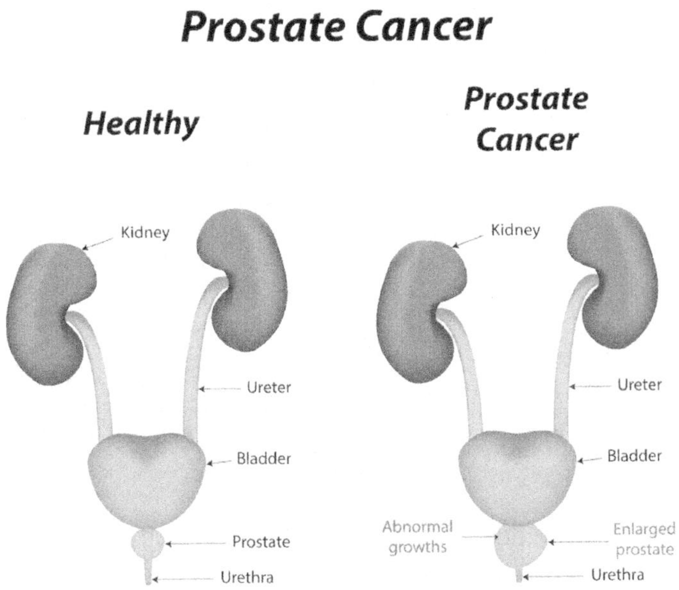


***Symptoms***

Early stages of prostate cancer are usually asymptomatic. As the condition progresses, symptoms may begin appearing, such as blood in the semen, difficulty urinating, a weak urine stream, erectile dysfunction, and pain in the pelvis. If the cancer has spread, the person may also experience pain in the bone.

***Treatments***

If the cancer is in the early stages and is not causing problems, or doesn't appear to be spreading, treatment may not be necessary. In this case, the cancer is carefully monitored, and if changes occur, treatment then may be sought. Treatment involves surgically removing the prostate and lymph nodes in the immediate area. Chemotherapy and radiation therapy may be used to kill any remaining cancerous cells in the body.

***Contraindications***

A massage therapist should obtain a doctor's note approving massage. Afterwards, massage may be performed, avoiding any tumors, lymph nodes, or other areas affected.

## Squamous Cell Carcinoma

Squamous Cell Carcinoma is a form of **skin** cancer that in many cases is not serious, but has the ability to spread to other parts of the body. Squamous cell carcinoma is **more serious** and **less common** than **basal cell carcinoma**, but **not as serious** and **more common** than **malignant melanoma**.

***Causes***

Squamous cell carcinoma, much like basal cell carcinoma and malignant melanoma, is most often caused by exposure to ultraviolet light. Tumors most commonly develop on areas of the body commonly exposed to sunlight, such as the head, neck, arms, and hands. Tumors may be flat, scaly, and firm, and appear around the mouth, in the mouth, and on the lips.

***Symptoms***

Squamous cell carcinoma tumors are typically shaped like a dome, and tend to bleed easily. They appear red and scaly, with a rough texture. If the tumor is large, pain may be present around the area.

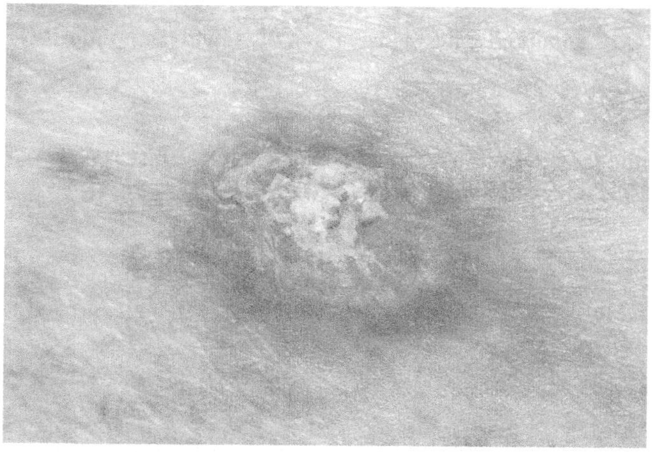

*Treatments*

Much like basal cell carcinoma, treatment for squamous cell carcinoma is relatively easy, with several different methods, from surgical excision and freezing of the tumor, to radiation therapy for more advanced tumors.

*Contraindications*

A client with squamous cell carcinoma may receive massage, but the site of the tumor should be avoided due to possible spreading of cancerous tissue.

## Stomach Cancer

Stomach cancer is a cancer of the **inner lining** of the **stomach**. Stomach cancer may metastasize to neighboring structures, such as the spleen, liver, and pancreas.

*Causes*

While there is no known direct cause of stomach cancer, it is strongly suspected that **gastroesophageal reflux disease(GERD)** may play a role by damaging the lining of the stomach and esophagus. Smoking, and a diet high in sodium may also contribute to the development of stomach cancer.

*Symptoms*

Symptoms of stomach cancer include a feeling of fullness in the stomach, bloating, fatigue, chronic heartburn, nausea, vomiting, and weight loss.

*Treatments*

Treatment is largely dependent on the stage of the cancer. Surgery is the main treatment of stomach cancer. In the early stages, surgery may be performed to only remove the tumor from the inner lining of the stomach. As the cancer advances, surgery may be performed to remove the tumor and a portions of the stomach the cancer has damaged. In later stages, if the cancer has grown large enough, the entire stomach may be removed. In addition to the tumor being removed, the lymph nodes around the stomach are also removed. Chemotherapy and radiation therapy are used to destroy any remaining cancerous cells.

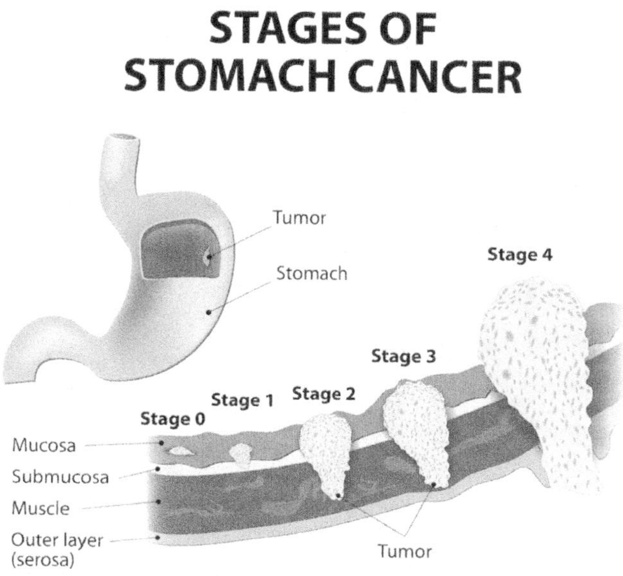


*Contraindications*

A massage therapist should obtain a doctor's note approving massage. Afterwards, massage may be performed, avoiding any tumors, lymph nodes, or other areas affected.

## Throat Cancer

Throat cancer is the growth of tumors in the **pharynx** or **larynx**. Less commonly, it can also affect the **tonsils** or **epiglottis**.

### *Causes*

Common causes for throat cancer include the use of **cigarettes** and **heavy drinking**. Gastroesophageal reflux disease may damage the tissues in the throat and make them more susceptible to developing tumors.

### *Symptoms*

Common symptoms of cancers of the throat include coughing, trouble swallowing or speaking, pain in the throat or ear, and loss of weight associated with not eating due to pain in the throat.

### *Treatments*

Treatment of throat cancer is dependent on the stage and location of the tumor. If the tumor is smaller and only on the top layer of tissue, surgery may be performed to only remove the tumor. If the tumor is larger and deeper in the tissue, entire segments of the throat may be removed, including the larynx. Chemotherapy and radiation therapy are used to kill any remaining cancerous cells.

### *Contraindications*

A massage therapist should obtain a doctor's note approving massage. Afterwards, massage may be performed, avoiding any tumors, lymph nodes, or other areas affected.

# Cancer

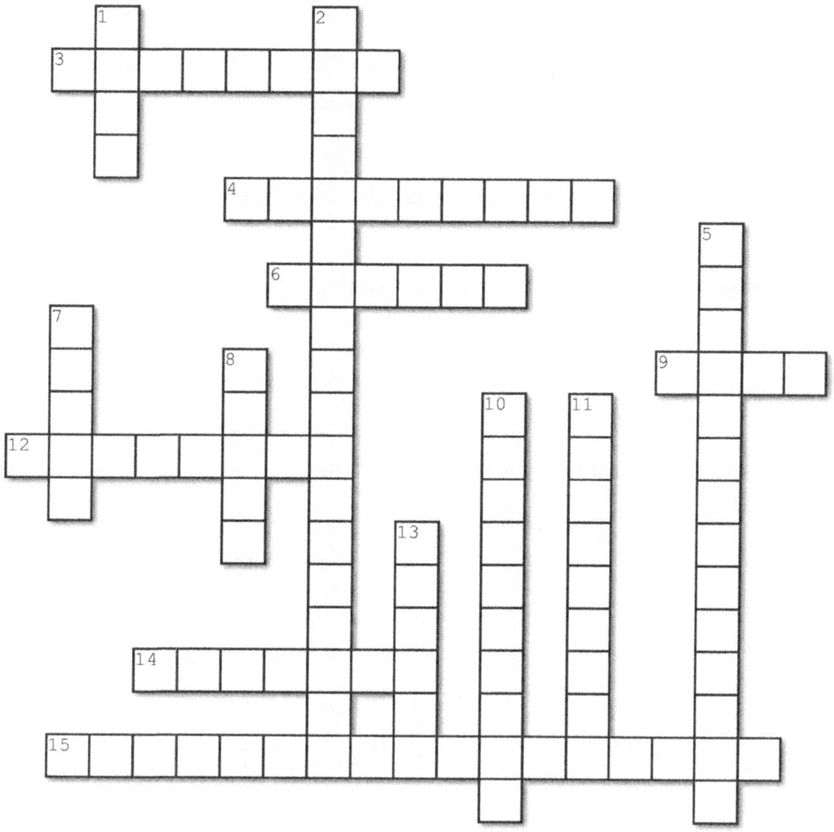

## Across

**3.** Type of cancer caused by the human papilloma virus
**4.** A tumor that spreads to other parts of the body
**6.** A tumor that does not spread
**9.** Osteosarcoma is a form of this type of cancer
**12.** Cancer of the blood in which the body produces excessive amounts of non-functioning white blood cells
**14.** Cancer that affects connective tissue
**15.** Least common, most serious, fastest growing form of skin cancer

## Down

**1.** This condition is commonly seen in people who have developed stomach cancer
**2.** Most common, least serious, slowest growing form of skin cancer
**5.** Type of cancer that can occur in people with compromised immune systems, such as AIDS patients
**7.** Hepatitis and cirrhosis may lead to the development of this type of cancer
**8.** An abnormal amount of a specific tissue
**10.** Using these may increase the chances of a person developing oral, throat, or lung cancer
**11.** Cancer that affects epithelial tissue
**13.** Second most common form of cancer diagnosed in women

Answer Key on Page 288

# Cancer Quiz

1. The leading cause of lung, oral, and esophageal cancer
A. Industrial dust
B. Cigarette smoking
C. Asbestos
D. Cystic fibrosis

2. Basal cell carcinoma is what type of tumor
A. Idiopathic
B. Malignant
C. Benign
D. Lymphatic

3. Over-production in melanocytes results in a tumor known as
A. Sarcoma
B. Carcinoma
C. Melanoma
D. Lymphoma

4. The most fatal form of tumor is generally
A. Cystic
B. Benign
C. Malignant
D. Gangrenous

5. Basal cell carcinoma
A. Most common, most serious, fastest growing form of skin cancer
B. Least common, most serious, fastest growing form of skin cancer
C. Most common, least serious, slowest growing form of skin cancer
D. Least common, least serious, slowest growing form of skin cancer

6. Sarcoma is a type of cancer that affects what kind of tissue
A. Muscular
B. Nervous
C. Epithelial
D. Connective

7. Chondrosarcoma is a form of cancer found in
A. Bones
B. Lymph
C. Digestive tract
D. Lungs

8. Cervical cancer is most commonly caused by
A. Smoking
B. Yeast infection
C. Kaposi's sarcoma
D. Human papilloma virus

9. Common form of treatment for cancer that involves exposing one specific part of the body to concentrated beams of x-rays
A. Chemotherapy
B. Moh's Surgery
C. MRI
D. Radiation therapy

10. Normal cells growing uncontrollably results in
A. Inflammation
B. Cyst
C. Cancer
D. Edema

11. Hodgkin's Lymphoma presents with tumors located
A. In the upper limb, chest, and neck
B. In the stomach
C. In the skin
D. In the brain

12. Kaposi's sarcoma most commonly only forms when a person has
A. A weakened immune system
B. A smoking addiction
C. An alcohol addiction
D. An excessive amount of leukocytes

13. Blood in the semen and difficulty urinating may be a sign of
A. Non-Hodgkin's Lymphoma
B. Pancreatic cancer
C. Prostate cancer
D. Squamous cell carcinoma

14. Leukemia is a form of cancer in which
A. The body produces an excessive amount of non-functioning white blood cells
B. The liver produces an excessive amount of bile
C. The skin produces tumors due to a weakened immune system consistent with HIV infection
D. The urinary bladder produces tumors in the inner linings of the bladder

15. A cancer spreading from one location in the body to another makes it
A. Asymptomatic
B. Benign
C. Malignant
D. Asymmetrical

Answer Key on Page 289

# Psychological and Other Pathologies

# Psychological Disorders

## Addiction

Addiction is the **repeated use** of a **substance** or **behavior** that makes the person feel as if they need to constantly repeat this behavior by providing a rewarding sensation. Examples include alcohol addiction, nicotine addiction, opioid addiction, and gambling addiction. A behavior becomes an addiction when a person is **unable to stop themselves** from doing the action.

A person with substance or behavioral addiction carries an increased risk of developing depression or anxiety.

***Causes***

Family history may contribute to the development of addiction. Anxiety and depression may lead a person into addictive behaviors.

***Symptoms***

Addiction may lead to many health issues, including poor hygiene, and damage to the body and its organs by substance abuse. If a person stops taking the addictive substance or performing the addictive behavior, they may experience withdrawal symptoms such as seizures, sweating, change in personality and anger, depression, and increased likelihood of violence.

A person who is addicted may distance themselves from others and give up certain things in their life that may cost money in order to keep themselves supplied with their substance of choice. Commonly, an addict will deny that they are addicted, and may experience problems with personal relationships because of the addiction.

***Treatments***

Addiction is a mental health disorder, and is highly treatable with psychotherapy. Going to self-help and recovery groups may help a person cope with overcoming the addiction.

***Contraindications***

A person suffering from an addiction may receive massage therapy. If the client is under the influence of a substance at the time of the massage, the massage should be postponed and rescheduled.

If you or a someone you know is struggling with addiction, don't hesitate to call the Substance Abuse and Mental Health Services Administration National Helpline at 1-800-662-4357.

## Anorexia Nervosa

Anorexia nervosa is a condition marked by **severe weight loss** resulting from an unhealthy **restricting of caloric intake**. In conjunction with eating an inadequate amount of food, a person with anorexia may also try losing weight by taking diuretics, laxatives, and vomiting after eating. This can cause a severe lack of nutrition, resulting in the body thinning far beyond a healthy level.

***Causes***

Anorexia is a psychological disorder in which a person's perception of their weight is distorted. Contributing factors towards the development of anorexia include environmental influences that put an over-emphasis on being thin, and psychological issues such as obsessive compulsive disorder that make it easier to not eat by sticking to set goals.

***Symptoms***

Symptoms are wide-ranging, from severe thinness and weight loss, to problems with tooth decay from excessive vomiting.

A lack of proper nutrition can lead to fatigue, weakness, thinning hair, and dehydration. A person with anorexia may develop anemia, osteoporosis, abnormalities in hormone production and regulation, issues with kidney function, and muscle atrophy.

Psychologically, a person may withdraw socially, and try to hide their anorexia by wearing clothing to hide their weight loss. A person may become irritable and skip meals. When confronted, a person may deny skipping meals or lie about how much food they have eaten.

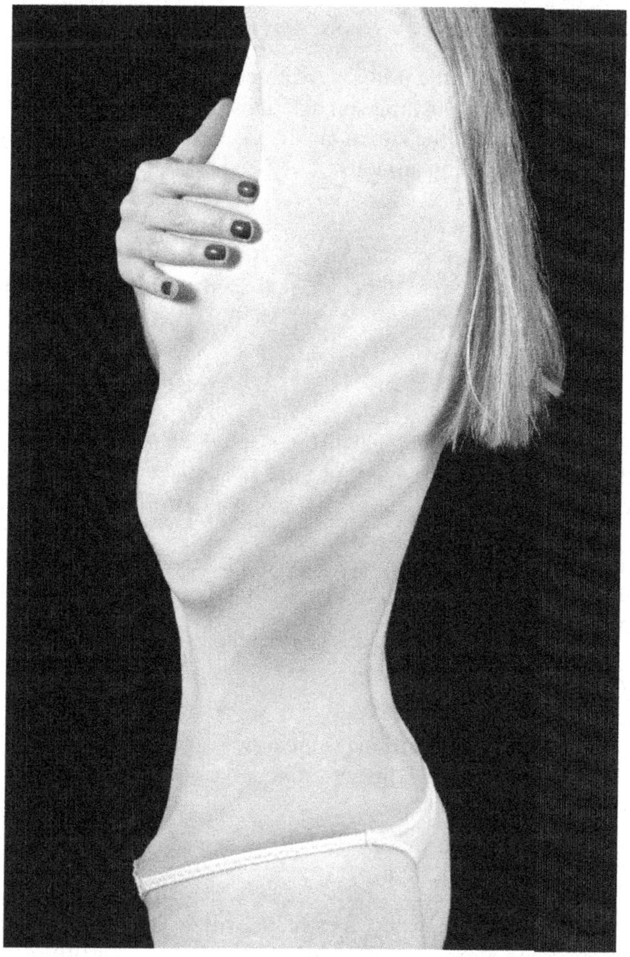

***Treatments***

Treatment for anorexia may include hospitalization in severe cases, where the body is not receiving adequate nutrition over a long period of time. While in the hospital, a person will be given fluids to balance dehydration and electrolyte levels, and be treated for issues possibly relating to the heart, liver, and kidneys. A feeding tube may be inserted to ensure a person is receiving enough nutrients.

Aside from a stay in the hospital, a person may be seen by a mental health professional to deal with underlying causes of anorexia. A person may work closely with a dietician to maintain a healthy diet.

***Contraindications***

Massage therapy is not contraindicated in clients with anorexia. A lighter massage should be performed to prevent damage to bones and other structures in the body.

## Anxiety Disorders

Anxiety disorders are a group of disorders in where a person experiences an **increased amount of anxiety**, often at a level where the person feels they are in a **life-or-death situation**. These anxious moments can adversely influence a person's daily life and relationships. Different types of anxiety disorders include panic disorder, social anxiety disorder, and general anxiety disorder.

A person with an anxiety disorder may also suffer from addiction, depression, chronic pain, or even attempt suicide.

***Causes***

Oftentimes, underlying medical issues may be the cause of anxiety disorders. Some examples include cardiovascular diseases, substance withdrawal, asthma, and hyperthyroidism. Medications may also induce anxiety.

***Symptoms***

Symptoms vary depending on the type of anxiety a person suffers from. General symptoms include nervousness, increased breathing and heart rate, shaking, trembling, digestive issues, and the inability to stop thinking about whatever it is that is putting a person into a state of anxiety.

Panic anxiety may leave a person with a feeling of fear or terror, and lead to chest pain, shortness of breath, and a rapid heart beat. Social anxiety may lead a person to avoid contact with others as a means to protect themselves from situations they might find themselves being embarrassed or self-conscious in.

*Treatments*

Psychotherapy is the primary treatment for anxiety disorders. Cognitive Behavioral Therapy is used to help treat social anxiety by exposing a person to situations they may experience in real life, giving them exposure and helping them learn how to cope with the situation when it arises. Medications may be prescribed, such as antidepressants, that can help a person from feeling anxious.

*Contraindications*

Anxiety disorders are not contraindicated for massage therapy.

## Bulimia

*(Greek "boulimia": ravenous hunger)*

Bulimia is a psychological disorder in which a person ingests abnormally large portions of food, followed by **purging** of the food ingested. Purging of food can be caused by self-induced vomiting, by consuming laxatives or diuretics, and/or excessive exercise. This is all done in an effort to avoid weight gain.

The use of self-induced vomiting and laxatives/diuretics is known as **Purging Bulimia**. These involve ridding the body of the ingested food in some way that doesn't allow it to be properly digested. The use of excessive exercise is known as **Non-Purging Bulimia**.

*Causes*

The exact cause of bulimia is unknown, although there are several contributing factors that may lead to the development of the condition. Stress, history of abuse, trauma, low self-esteem, and having a negative image of one's body can all be contributing factors.

*Symptoms*

Common symptoms may include dehydration, imbalances in electrolyte levels, fluctuating weight, lesions in the mouth due to excessive vomiting, chronic heart burn, and infertility.

People with bulimia may exhibit some of the following traits and behaviors: frequent bathroom usage after eating, eating privately, smelling of vomit, and lacking control when eating.

*Treatments*

Bulimia is most commonly caused by low self-esteem and negative body image. Therefore, the primary treatment is therapy to help the patient overcome these psychological issues.

*Contraindications*

Bulimia is not contraindicated for massage. Massage may help psychologically and improve self esteem and body image. A lighter massage may be indicated, as the client may have atrophied muscles and a weakened body due to lack of nutrients.

## Dementia

Dementia is a general term for symptoms that involve **loss of memory**, with diminished **social** and **critical thinking skills**. These skills may be impaired to the point where it affects a person's ability to function effectively on a daily basis. Dementia is caused by damage to neurons in the brain. There are numerous reasons for neurons to be damaged that can contribute to dementia.

*Causes*

Dementia may be permanent, or may be reversed, depending on the cause. Causes of dementia that involve permanent damage to the brain include progressive disorders such as Alzheimer's disease. Strokes may permanently damage the brain. Similar to strokes, injuries to the brain such as concussions may lead to brain damage.

Cases where dementia may be reversed include certain infections that cause high fever, autoimmune disorders such as multiple sclerosis, tumors in the brain, hypoxia, inadequate fluid intake, and hormonal problems such as having too much calcium in the body. As these conditions are treated, the dementia should go away.

***Symptoms***

Dementia is most commonly associated with memory loss. This can lead to problems communicating, focusing, using the body properly, and problem solving. A person may become depressed, develop anxiety or paranoia, and become easily irritated.

***Treatments***

Dementia itself can't be cured. Treating the underlying cause is the best way to treat dementia. This can include medications to help brain function, and physical therapy to help with any motor skills that may be affected.

***Contraindications***

Dementia is not contraindicated for massage therapy.

## Depression

Depression is a disorder affecting **mood**, causing a person to feel **sad**, usually over a prolonged period of time. A person may become disinterested in normal daily activities, and become more distant.

Depression usually develops during teenage years, but may occur at any time. If a person is experiencing depression, they should seek help from a mental health professional.

***Causes***

There are many different causes for depression, and no one person is the same as another. Causes include a change in the body's hormone levels, such as during and after pregnancy, changes in the function of neurotransmitters in the brain, and even may be genetically passed down.

***Symptoms***

Symptoms are wide-ranging, and people experience depression differently. Symptoms may include a feeling of sadness, fatigue, disinterest in eating, anxiety, insomnia, irritability, and consistently thinking about death and suicide. A person with depression may attempt suicide.

***Treatments***

If a person is diagnosed with depression, antidepressants known as selective serotonin reuptake inhibitors, or SSRIs, are usually prescribed to help manage hormone levels and increase serotonin levels in the blood. Talking with a mental health professional may help a person feel better. Exercise and a healthy diet may help with hormone imbalances and increase a person's self esteem, which can aid in lowering depression. Other relaxation techniques, such as massage therapy and yoga, may be sought.

***Contraindications***

Depression is not contraindicated for massage therapy. Massage may help relax a person with depression, increase self-esteem and body image, and help manage hormone levels in the body.

The National Suicide Prevention Lifeline is 1-800-273-8255

## Insomnia

*(in-: not; somnus: sleep)*

Insomnia is a disorder causing a **lack** of **sufficient sleep**. This may be the result of a person having difficulty falling asleep, staying asleep, or waking too early. This can lead to many health complications. There are many reasons a person's sleep may be affected. Stress is the most common cause of insomnia, making it difficult to "turn off" thoughts when it's time to sleep. Having an irregular sleep schedule may make it difficult for the body to adjust when it's time to sleep. Jet lag may also cause insomnia.

### *Causes*

Certain medications may interfere with normal sleep. Pain associated with medical conditions may also keep a person from sleeping.

### *Symptoms*

Common symptoms include trouble falling asleep, trouble staying asleep, waking too early, general fatigue, irritability, increased stress and anxiety, and depression. A person with insomnia may develop other health conditions as a result of not getting enough sleep, such as hypertension.

### *Treatments*

Determining the root cause of the insomnia and treating that is the primary treatment for insomnia. Reducing stress, getting a person on a set sleep schedule, increasing exercise, meditation, yoga, and massage therapy can all aid in eliminating insomnia. If these methods do not accomplish the goal, medications to help a person sleep may be prescribed. Over-the-counter sleep aids may help a person sleep, but should not be used long-term as a person may develop a dependency on them.

### *Contraindications*

Insomnia is not a contraindication for massage. Massage therapy may aid a person in reducing stress and helping them obtain a normal sleep cycle.

## Obsessive Compulsive Disorder

Obsessive Compulsive Disorder(OCD) is a chronic disorder in which a person experiences **uncontrollable thoughts**, **sensations**, and **behaviors**, which they feel the urge to repeat consistently. Examples of these behaviors include washing hands, cleaning, and speaking a name or phrase repeatedly.

### *Causes*

The exact cause of obsessive compulsive disorder is unknown. Depression may play a role, and there may be a genetic component, as it is more common in people who have close relatives with it.

### *Symptoms*

Obsessions are things a person repeatedly thinks about, such as cleanliness or things needing to be in an exact place or order. Compulsions are things done in relation to obsessions, such as washing hands repeatedly, counting, putting things in order, and performing certain tasks in a specific order. These obsessions and compulsions can have an adverse effect on people's daily lives.

### *Treatments*

Medication is commonly prescribed to help deal with obsessions and compulsions, such as antidepressants. Psychotherapy is also useful in helping a person control their compulsions and obsessions.

### *Contraindications*

Obsessive compulsive disorder is not contraindicated for massage.

# Other Pathologies

## Cataract

A cataract is a disorder affecting the eye, causing the **lens** to become **cloudy**. Clouding of the lens may make it difficult to see clearly, giving the vision a foggy, blurry appearance. This can make performing certain actions difficult, such as driving at night, and reading. People who smoke, are obese, or have diabetes are more likely to develop cataracts than others.

***Causes***

Cataracts are usually caused by either natural aging or injury to the eye or lens. Cataracts develop slowly, but eventually may affect vision enough to warrant treatment.

***Symptoms***

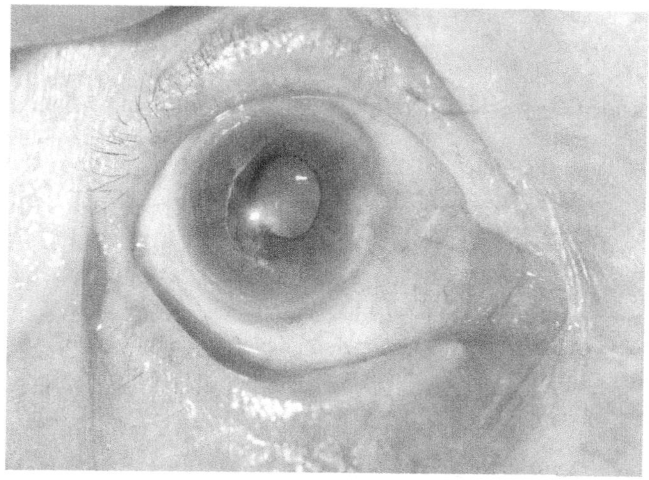

Common symptoms include cloudy vision, blurred vision, trouble seeing at night, requiring bright light to see properly, and experiencing double vision in one eye. These are caused by the cloudiness in the lens dispersing light entering the eye ineffectively.

***Treatments***

The only proper treatment for cataracts is surgery. During this surgery, the lens of the affected eye is removed, and a new lens is inserted in its place. This artificial lens becomes a permanent part of the eye, and after healing, allows the patient to see properly through the eye once again.

***Contraindications***

Cataracts are not contraindicated for massage.

## Conjunctivitis

*(conjunctiv/o: conjunctiva; -itis: inflammation)*

Conjunctivitis is **inflammation** and/or **infection** of the **conjunctiva**, the clear membrane that lines the inner eyelid and covers the sclera of the eye. Conjunctivitis is also known as **pinkeye**, due to the appearance of the conjunctiva when the blood vessels inside become irritated and inflamed.

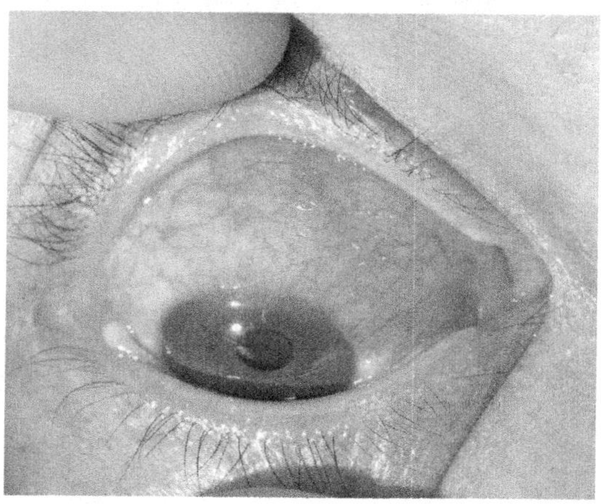

***Causes***

The most common cause of conjunctivitis is a bacterial or viral infection. In infants, conjunctivitis may occur if tear ducts become blocked. Allergens may also cause conjunctivitis.

***Symptoms***

The affected eye may appear red, producing a discharge. This discharge may crust over and make it difficult to open the eye in the morning after sleep. The eye may feel itchy. Vision is not affected by conjunctivitis, but an increased amount of tears may be produced.

***Treatments***

Treating conjunctivitis is dependent on the cause. If it is caused by bacteria, antibiotic eye drops are prescribed. Antiviral medications may be prescribed in certain cases, such as a herpes simplex outbreak.

If conjunctivitis is caused by an irritant such as contact lenses, a person will stop using contacts until the conjunctivitis clears up.

***Contraindications***

Conjunctivitis is generally not a contraindication, unless it is caused by bacteria or a virus. If this is the case, massage is considered an absolute contraindication, and should be rescheduled until after the condition has resolved.

## Glaucoma

*(Greek glaukos: bluish-green; -oma: tumor)*

Glaucoma is a **degenerative** eye disorder in which the **optic nerve** is progressively damaged by **increased pressure** in the eye, eventually resulting in blindness. It is more common in people over the age of 60.

***Causes***

Inside the eye, there is fluid known as aqueous humor that is normally produced and drained from the eye. In people with glaucoma, this fluid does not properly drain, but keeps being produced, which adds pressure inside the eye. This pressure damages the optic nerve. When the optic nerve is damaged extensively, vision is lost.

***Symptoms***

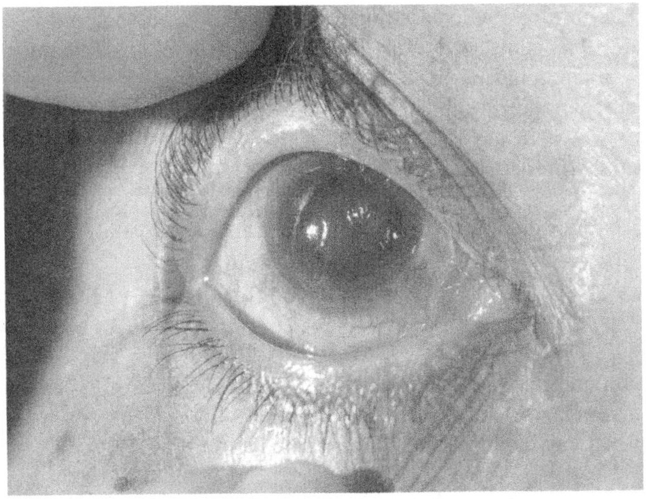

Symptoms vary depending on the advancement of the condition. Earlier stages may be relatively asymptomatic. Advanced stages can see a person develop tunnel vision, lose vision in the peripheral edges, experience headaches, nausea, vomiting, pain in the eye, and blurred vision.

***Treatments***

Treatment for glaucoma mainly focuses on reducing pressure inside the eye. Eyedrops can be prescribed that increase the amount of fluid being drained from the eye. Other eye drops may reduce the production of fluid in the eye. If these aren't useful, surgery may be performed. Laser surgery helps to open any blocked fluid draining channels. Small tubes may be put into the eye itself to help drain excess fluid.

***Contraindications***

Glaucoma is not contraindicated for massage.

## Tinnitus

*(Latin "tinnire": to ring like a bell)*

Tinnitus is the presence of a **sound** in the ear, typically **ringing**, without an external auditory source. Tinnitus is usually related to another cause, such as an injury to the ear or hearing loss. It is usually not serious, but may be somewhat irritating. Tinnitus may always be present, or may come and go. The volume and pitch of the sound may be low or high, and may be loud enough to interfere with a person's ability to hear properly.

***Causes***

Common causes of tinnitus include exposure to loud noises, such as music, machinery, and firearms, hearing loss related to aging, and Meniere's disease. Less commonly, conditions that affect the Cardiovascular System may contribute to tinnitus, such as atherosclerosis and hypertension. With these conditions, more pressure is being placed on the blood vessels, which can harm the blood vessels in the ears, making them more susceptible to developing tinnitus.

***Symptoms***

The main symptom is a sound in the ear that only the person can hear. This sound can be a ringing, clicking, humming, roaring, or buzzing sound. Depending on the cause, it may be heard in one or both ears.

***Treatments***

Treatment for tinnitus is often treating the underlying cause, which should alleviate the ringing in the ear. If a cardiovascular issue is suspected, medications may be prescribed to help treat these, which can eliminate the tinnitus. Less commonly, excessive ear wax may produce tinnitus. If this is the case, impacted ear wax may be removed. Avoiding loud noises will also help alleviate tinnitus.

***Contraindications***

Tinnitus is not contraindicated for massage therapy. However, if a client complains of ringing in the ear, other conditions should be assessed for other contraindications.

## Vertigo

Vertigo is the sensation that a person's **surroundings** are **moving** or **spinning**, which may cause **dizziness**. This can be especially prevalent if a person is looking down from a tall height.

***Causes***

Commonly, vertigo is the result of a problem with the **inner ear**. **Meniere's disease**, which causes fluid buildup that changes pressure inside the ear, is a common cause. A buildup of calcium deposits in the inner ear can alter balance. Viral infections, such as vestibular neuritis, may also cause vertigo. Less commonly, tumors in the ear may cause vertigo.

***Symptoms***

Vertigo presents with a feeling of the environment around a person spinning, moving, swaying, or tilting. A person may become unbalanced, become nauseated, vomit, or develop headaches.

***Treatments***

Treatment for vertigo is usually dependent on the cause. If calcium is present in the inner ear, certain head and neck movements may be performed to aid the calcium in leaving the inner ear, allowing it to be broken down by the body. Medications may be prescribed to aid with nausea and fluid build up associated with Meniere's disease. Surgery may be performed if there is a tumor present.

Oftentimes, no treatment is necessary, as the brain becomes acclimated to vertigo and the symptoms lessen or disappear.

***Contraindications***

Vertigo is not contraindicated for massage. The massage therapist may need to help the client on and off the table to avoid accidental falls due to dizziness.

# Psychological and Other Pathologies

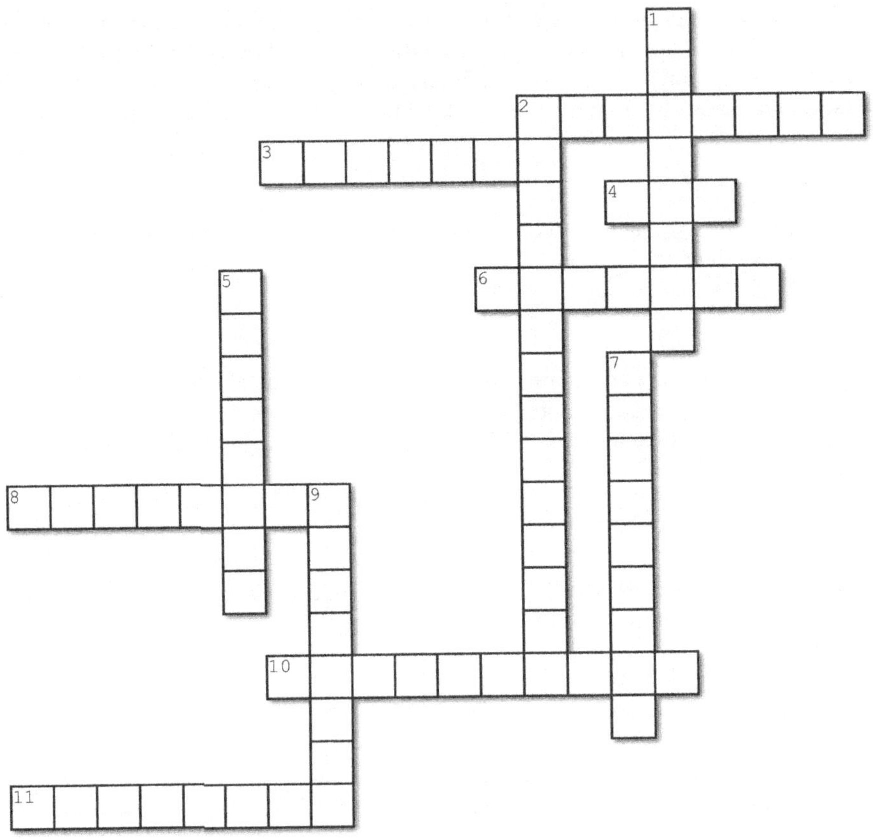

**Across**

**2.** Clouding of the eye lens
**3.** Dizziness caused by an inner ear problem
**4.** A person experiencing uncontrollable thoughts, sensations, and behaviors that they repeat constantly(abbr)
**6.** Excessive eating followed by purging
**8.** Loss of memory, social skills, and critical thinking skills over time
**10.** Mood disorder causing a person to feel unhappy over an extended period of time
**11.** Disorder causing a person to have an insufficient level of sleep

**Down**

**1.** Failure of aqueous fluid to properly drain from the eye, causing degeneration of the optic nerve
**2.** Inflammation of the conjunctiva
**5.** Constant ringing in a person's ear only audible to the person affected
**7.** The repeated use of a substance or behavior
**9.** Severe weight loss due to unhealthy calorie restriction

Answer Key on Page 288

# Psychological and Other Pathologies Quiz

1. Obsessive compulsive disorder
A. A person being unable to sleep
B. A person who experiences memory loss
C. A person who lacks adequate nutrition intake
D. A person who experiences uncontrolled thoughts and behaviors

2. A person eating an abnormally large amount of food, following by purging
A. Anorexia
B. Dementia
C. Bulimia
D. Depression

3. A person who has difficulty balancing, often experiencing a dizzying sensation due to a problem with the inner ear
A. Insomnia
B. Vertigo
C. Anorexia nervosa
D. Obsessive compulsive disorder

4. Serotonin reuptake inhibitors are useful in a person diagnosed with
A. Depression
B. Insomnia
C. Bulimia
D. Dementia

5. Self-help and recovery groups may be especially helpful for a person experiencing
A. Dementia
B. Addiction
C. Insomnia
D. Obsessive compulsive disorder

6. Inflammation of the clear membrane lining the inner eyelid, commonly caused by bacterial or viral infection
A. Cataract
B. Vertigo
C. Glaucoma
D. Conjunctivitis

7. Nervousness, increased heart rate, trembling, and digestive issues are all common symptoms of a person who experiences
A. Anorexia nervosa
B. Anxiety disorder
C. Dementia
D. Addiction

8. Glaucoma
A. Degeneration of the optic nerve due to pressure in the eye
B. Loss of balance and coordination due to an inner ear problem
C. Inflammation of the conjunctiva
D. An injury to the lens that causes it to become cloudy

9. A person having difficulty getting to sleep or getting enough sleep
A. Depression
B. Insomnia
C. Vertigo
D. Bulimia

10. Meniere's disease is a common cause of the following condition
A. Glaucoma
B. Insomnia
C. Vertigo
D. Addiction

11. A person experiencing a constant ringing sound in the ear
A. Vertigo
B. Vitiligo
C. Tinnitus
D. Insomnia

12. Of the following, which is a contagious condition
A. Glaucoma
B. Tinnitus
C. Vertigo
D. Conjunctivitis

13. Bulimia
A. A person eating excessive amounts of food, followed by purging
B. A person having difficulty balancing due to an inner ear problem
C. A person unable to get sufficient sleep
D. A person refusing to eat

14. Alzheimer's disease and strokes are common causes of
A. Dementia
B. Anxiety disorder
C. Bulimia
D. Addiction

15. Things a person constantly thinks about
A. Compulsions
B. Obsessions
C. Anxieties
D. Addictions

Answer Key on Page 289

# Answer Keys

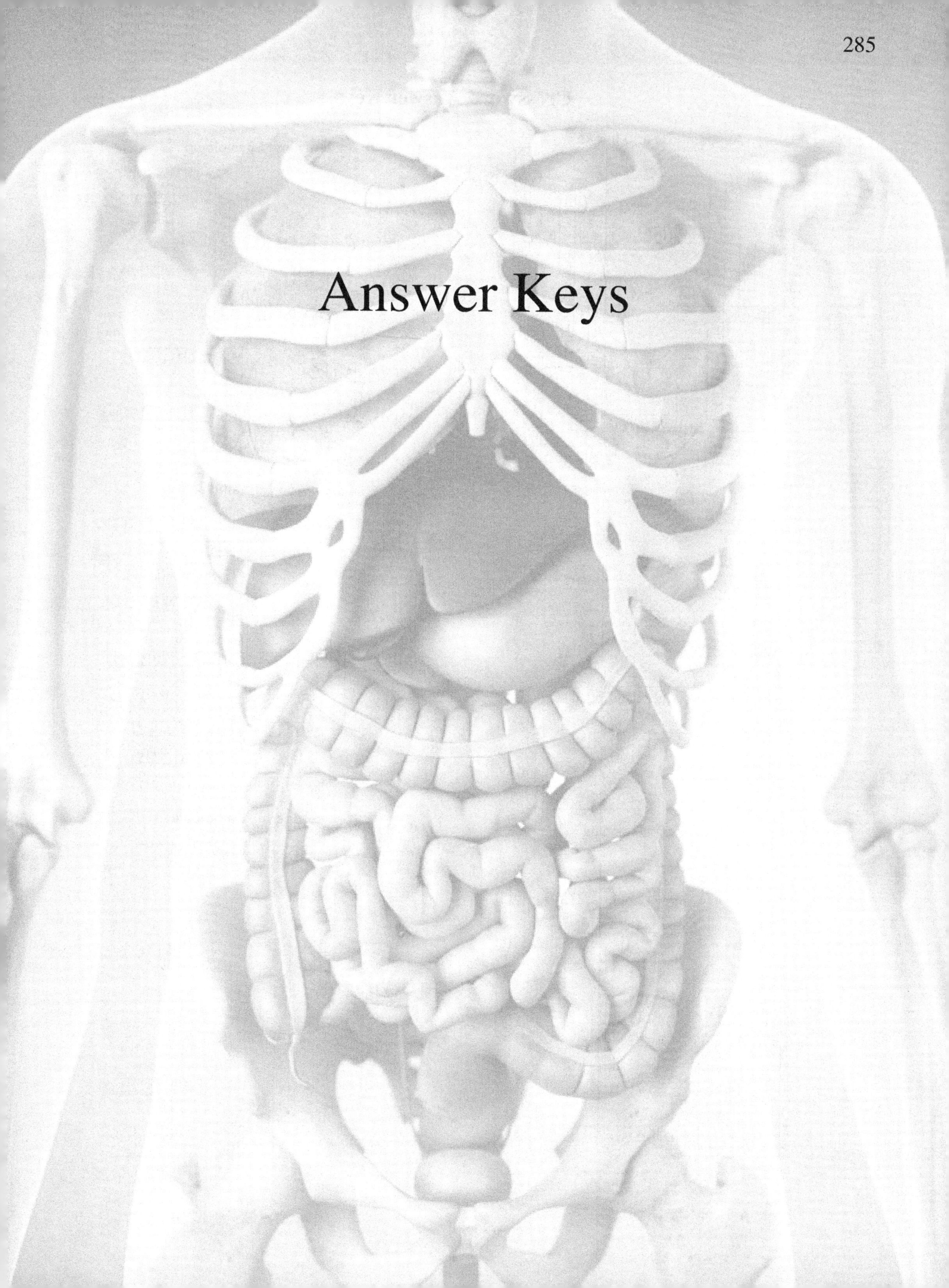

# Crossword Answer Keys

### Assessment and Intake

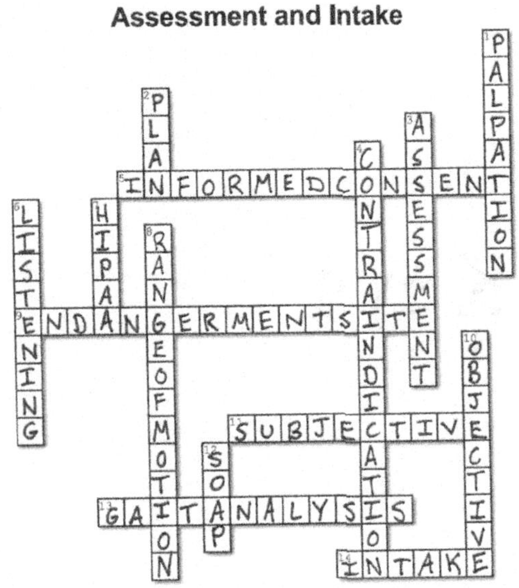


### Anatomy and Physiology

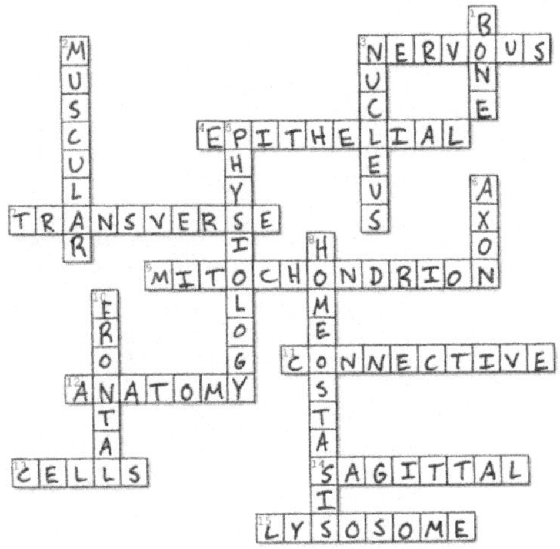


### Pathology

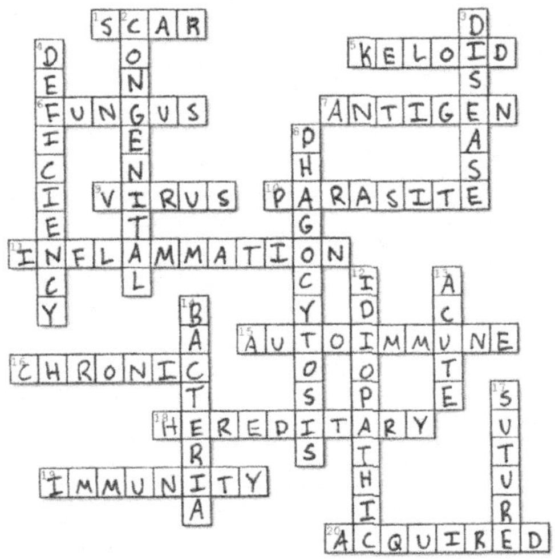


### Cardiovascular Pathologies

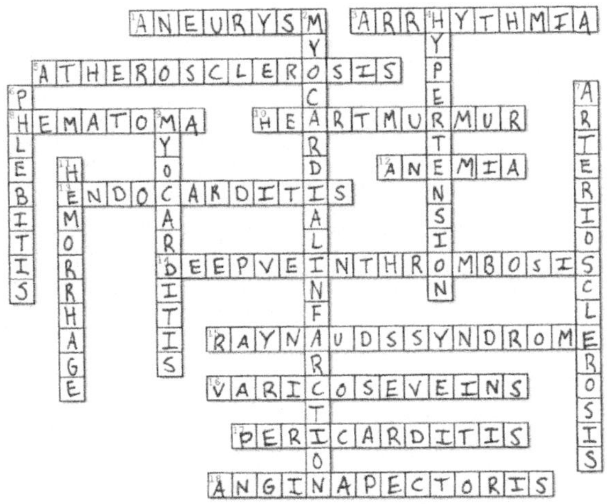


### Digestive Pathologies

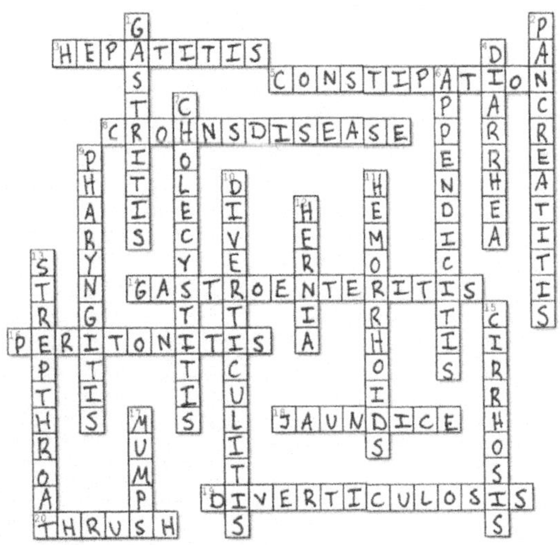


### Endocrine Pathologies

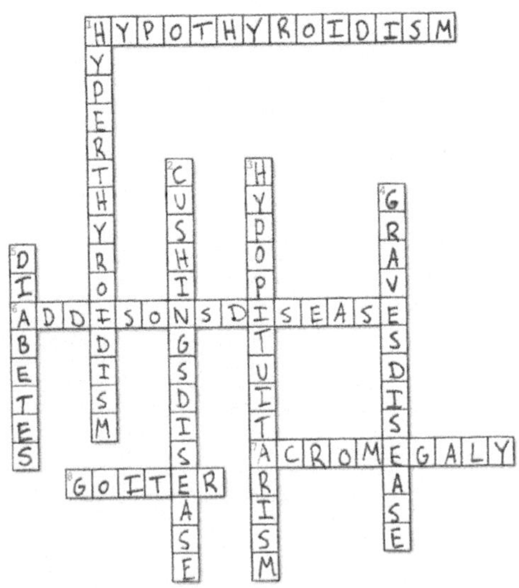

### Integumentary Pathologies

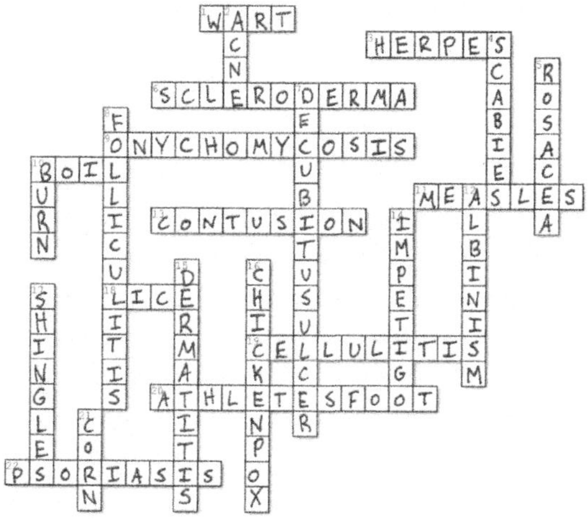


## Lymphatic Pathologies

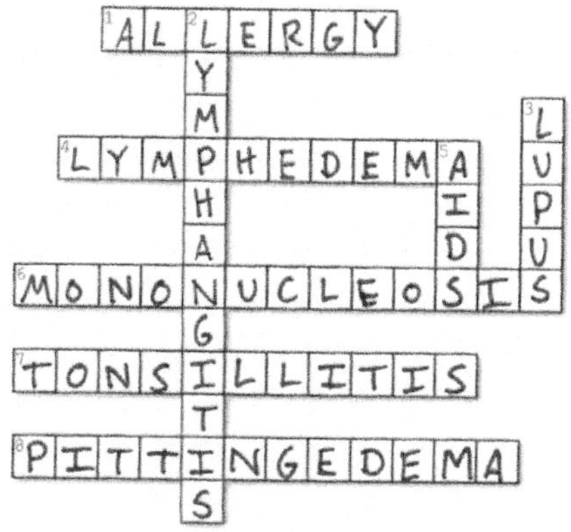


### Muscular Pathologies

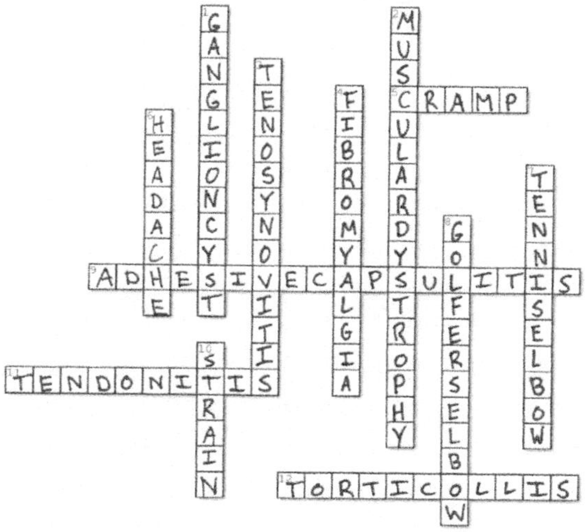


### Nervous Pathologies

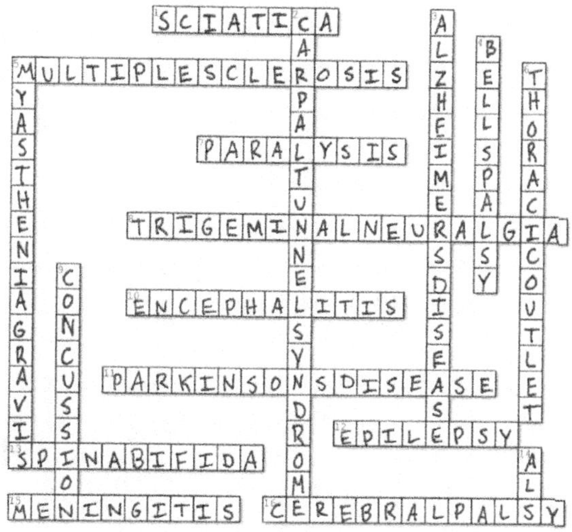


## Reproductive Pathologies

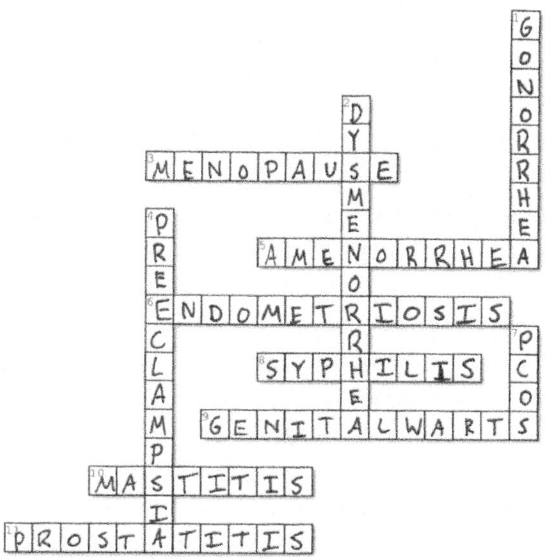


### Respiratory Pathologies

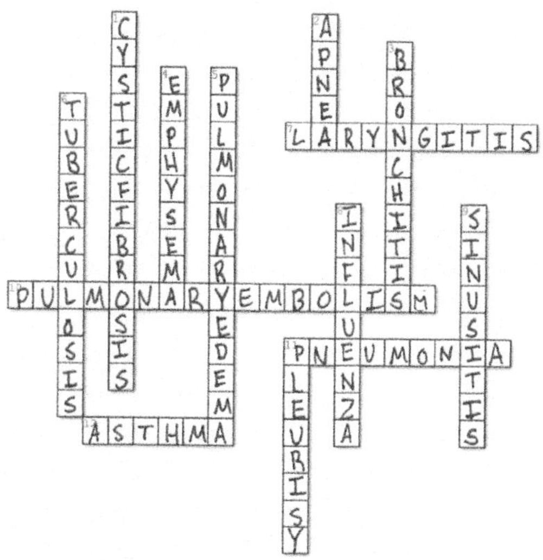

### Skeletal Pathologies

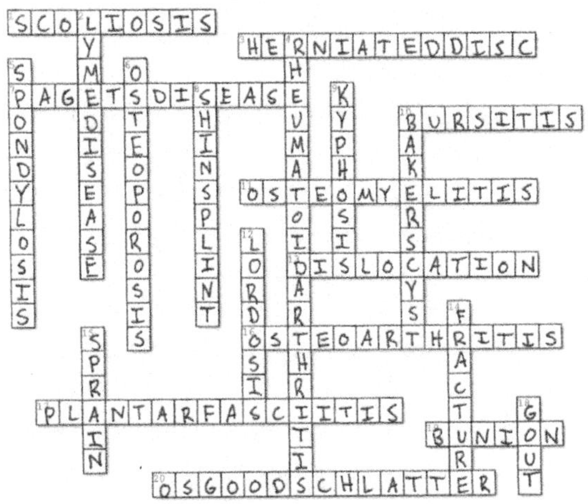

### Urinary Pathologies

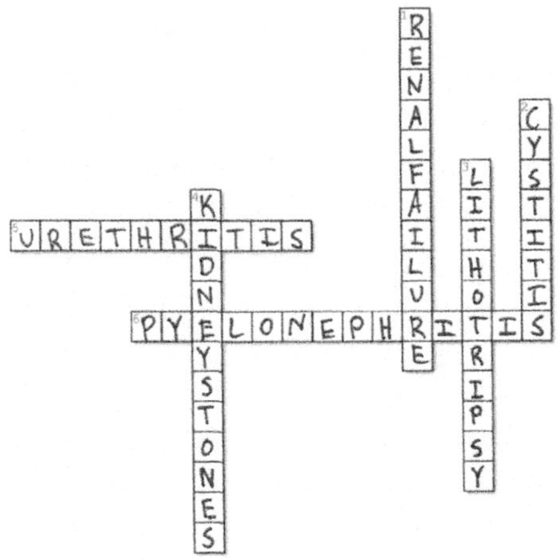

### Cancer

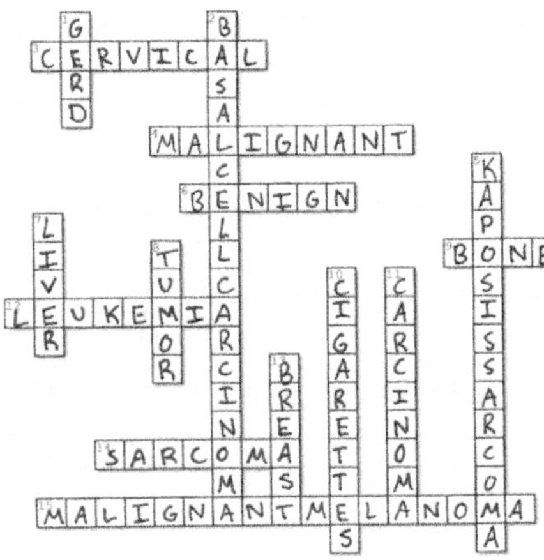

### Psychological and Other Pathologies

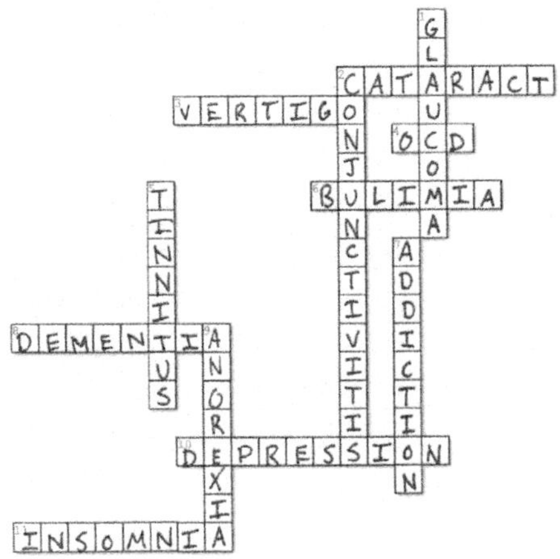

# Quizzes Answer Keys

**1. Assessment**

1. D
2. D
3. A
4. C
5. D
6. B
7. A
8. D
9. A
10. D
11. A
12. B
13. D
14. B
15. A

**2. Anatomy and Physiology**

1. A
2. C
3. D
4. A
5. B
6. D
7. A
8. A
9. D
10. B
11. D
12. B
13. C
14. B
15. D

**3. Disease, Immunity, and Medications**

1. C
2. C
3. D
4. D
5. A
6. A
7. B
8. C
9. A
10. D
11. A
12. C
13. B
14. C
15. A

**4. Cardiovascular**

1. A
2. D
3. C
4. D
5. C
6. B
7. A
8. A
9. B
10. A
11. B
12. A
13. C
14. C
15. A

**5. Digestive**

1. D
2. C
3. A
4. A
5. A
6. A
7. A
8. B
9. B
10. C
11. A
12. D
13. C
14. B
15. A

**6. Endocrine**

1. A
2. B
3. C
4. D
5. D
6. A
7. D
8. D
9. C
10. A
11. A
12. C
13. A
14. C
15. A

**7. Integumentary**

1. B
2. A
3. B
4. C
5. C
6. C
7. D
8. B
9. A
10. B
11. C
12. D
13. A
14. A
15. A

**8. Lymphatic**

1. D
2. A
3. C
4. A
5. C
6. B
7. A
8. C
9. D
10. A
11. D
12. A
13. B
14. C
15. A

**9. Muscular**

1. C
2. B
3. B
4. A
5. D
6. C
7. B
8. A
9. D
10. A
11. B
12. C
13. C
14. A
15. B

**10. Nervous**

1. C
2. A
3. A
4. D
5. C
6. A
7. A
8. B
9. B
10. B
11. D
12. A
13. B
14. D
15. C

**11. Reproductive**

1. D
2. A
3. C
4. B
5. A
6. D
7. C
8. B
9. A
10. A
11. C
12. B
13. C
14. A
15. A

**12. Respiratory**

1. C
2. D
3. A
4. A
5. A
6. B
7. B
8. A
9. A
10. D
11. A
12. B
13. D
14. A
15. C

**13. Skeletal**

1. C
2. C
3. C
4. B
5. C
6. B
7. C
8. D
9. A
10. A
11. B
12. A
13. D
14. B
15. C

**14. Urinary**

1. D
2. C
3. D
4. A
5. B
6. B
7. D
8. A
9. B
10. B
11. C
12. D
13. A
14. B
15. C

**15. Cancer**

1. B
2. B
3. C
4. C
5. C
6. D
7. A
8. D
9. D
10. C
11. A
12. A
13. C
14. A
15. C

**16. Psychological and Other Pathologies**

1. D
2. C
3. B
4. A
5. B
6. D
7. B
8. A
9. B
10. C
11. C
12. D
13. A
14. A
15. B

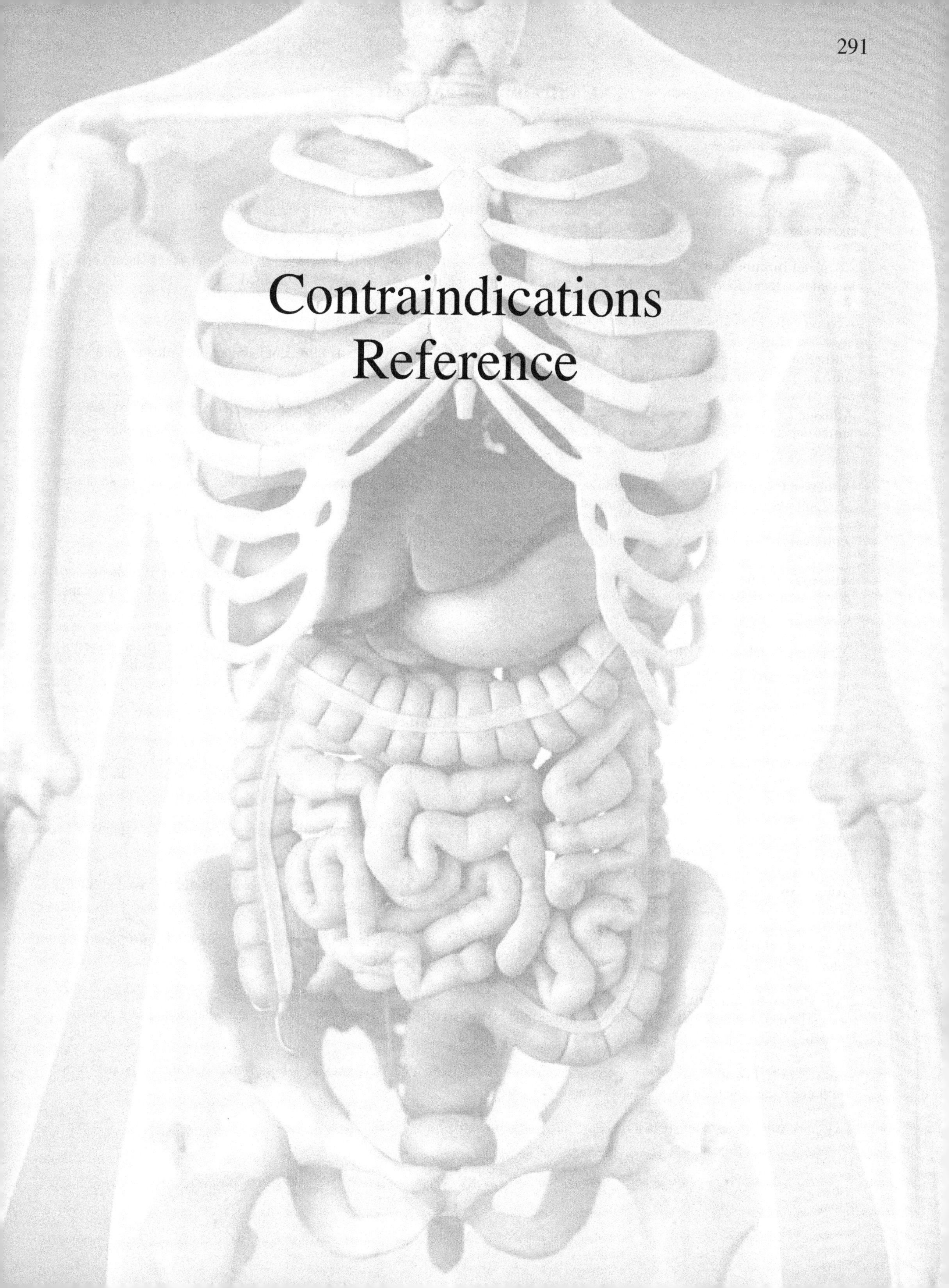

# Contraindications Reference

# Contraindications Reference

## A

**Acne**: Whiteheads are considered local contraindications. Any part of the body experiencing inflammation from acne should also be considered a local contraindication.

**Acquired Immunodeficiency Syndrome(AIDS)**: AIDS is not a contraindication to massage. Any open sores should be treated as a local contraindication. If the client isn't feeling well, massage should be rescheduled.

**Acromegaly**: Massage is indicated for acromegaly.

**Addiction**: A person suffering from an addiction may receive massage therapy. If the client is under the influence of a substance at the time of the massage, the massage should be postponed and rescheduled.

**Addison's Disease**: Massage is indicated for a client with Addison's Disease. However, the type and length of massage varies depending on how a client is feeling and their stamina. Clients with low stamina should receive shorter, lighter massages, while clients with increased stamina may receive longer and stimulating massages.

**Adhesive Capsulitis**: Adhesive capsulitis is not a contraindication. Massage may help loosen adhesions and increase range-of-motion. Stretching should be performed, as well as compression in the joint.

**Albinism**: Albinism is not a contraindication for massage.

**Allergy**: Allergies should be determined prior to massage to avoid using any allergens in massage lubricant. If a client develops any signs of contact with an allergen during the massage, massage should be stopped. If essential oils are the cause of the allergic reaction, effects can be managed with the application of vegetable oil.

**Alzheimer's Disease**: Alzheimer's Disease is not contraindicated, although precautions may be taken in advanced stages of the disease. A person the client knows and is familiar with may stay in the room to assist with the client if the client becomes forgetful regarding their location.

**Amenorrhea**: Massage is generally not contraindicated for amenorrhea.

**Amyotrophic Lateral Sclerosis(ALS)**: Massage is indicated for Amyotrophic Lateral Sclerosis. In advanced stages, the therapist may need to assist the client on and off the table. Because the muscles have atrophied, lighter pressure should be performed to avoid damaging tissue.

**Anemia**: Massage is indicated for a client with anemia. Massage helps increase circulation and oxygen intake, which provides the body with needed nutrients.

**Aneurysm**: Massage is indicated with a doctor's note. Any massage that increases blood pressure should be avoided, such as deep tissue, because it can put pressure on arteries, which may lead to bursting of an aneurysm.

**Angina Pectoris**: Angina pectoris is generally indicated for massage. During acute pain, massage should be postponed until the client is comfortable enough to continue with massage.

**Ankylosing Spondylitis**: Massage is indicated for ankylosing spondylitis. Stretching and range-of-motion exercises should be performed within the client's pain tolerance. If the client has difficulty lying supine due to kyphosis, side-lying position may be needed.

**Anorexia Nervosa**: Massage therapy is not contraindicated in clients with anorexia. A lighter massage should be performed to prevent damage to bones and other structures in the body.

**Anxiety Disorders**: Anxiety disorders are not contraindicated for massage therapy.

**Apnea**: Apnea is not contraindicated for massage.

**Appendicitis**: Appendicitis is considered an absolute contraindication for massage, and is a medical emergency.

**Arrhythmia**: Untreated arrhythmia is an absolute contraindication for massage therapy. If a client has a pacemaker, massage may be performed. A client may have discomfort while lying prone due to pressure on the pacemaker, which may call for side- lying massage to be performed, or pillows to be used to take pressure off the area. Avoid massaging the site of the pacemaker(upper left chest just below clavicle).

**Arteriosclerosis**: Massage for arteriosclerosis may be performed. Certain medications may require a lighter massage to be performed, because they may thin the blood and damage to a blood vessel can lead to increased bleeding internally.

**Atherosclerosis**: Massage for atherosclerosis may be performed. Certain medications may require a lighter massage to be performed, because they may thin the blood and damage to a blood vessel can lead to increased bleeding internally.

**Asthma**: In the acute stage, asthma is considered an absolute contraindication. Once breathing has returned to normal, massage may be performed. Tapotement may be performed on the back and chest to help loosen any excess phlegm that may be present.

**Athlete's Foot**: Because athlete's foot is contagious, it is considered a local contraindication. The feet should be avoided, and any linens the feet have come in contact with should be treated as contaminated.

## B

**Baker's Cyst**: A Baker's Cyst is considered a local contraindication. Massage may be performed, but massaging the cyst itself should be avoided.

**Basal Cell Carcinoma**: Massage is indicated for a client with basal cell carcinoma. However, the tumor is a local contraindication, and massage around the area should be avoided to prevent spreading of cancerous tissue through increased blood and lymph flow.

**Bell's Palsy**: Bell's Palsy is indicated for massage. The side of the face that is paralyzed should be massaged lightly to avoid damaging any tissue. The client may not be able to tell the therapist if the massage is too deep around facial structures, so lighter massage on the affected area should be performed.

**Bladder Cancer**: A massage therapist should obtain a doctor's note approving massage. Afterwards, massage may be performed, avoiding any tumors, lymph nodes, or other areas affected.

**Boil**: A boil is considered a local contraindication for massage.

**Bone Cancer**: A massage therapist should obtain a doctor's note approving massage. Afterwards, massage may be performed, avoiding any tumors, lymph nodes, or other areas affected.

**Brain Cancer**: A massage therapist should obtain a doctor's note approving massage. Afterwards, massage may be performed, avoiding any tumors, lymph nodes, or other areas affected.

**Breast Cancer:** A massage therapist should obtain a doctor's note approving massage. Afterwards, massage may be performed, avoiding any tumors, lymph nodes, or other areas affected.

**Bronchitis**: Acute bronchitis is considered an absolute contraindication, because it only appears as a secondary condition with another infection that is an absolute contraindication, such as influenza or pneumonia. Once these conditions resolve, the bronchitis will also resolve, and massage may be performed. Chronic bronchitis is indicated for massage. Tapotement may help loosen any excess phlegm as a result of the bronchitis, which can help breathing.

**Bulimia**: Bulimia is not contraindicated for massage. Massage may help psychologically and improve self esteem and body image. A lighter massage may be indicated, as the client may have atrophied muscles and a weakened body due to lack of nutrients.

**Bunion**: Massage is generally not contraindicated for a bunion. However, if the client is experiencing pain as a result of the bunion, massage in the area should be avoided.

**Burns**: Burns are considered local contraindications for massage. Avoid any area experiencing inflammation, blistering, or has suffered necrosis.

**Bursitis**: Bursitis is considered a local contraindication for massage. Cold packs may be used to help decrease inflammation in the area.

## C

**Carpal Tunnel Syndrome**: Massage is indicated for carpal tunnel syndrome. Cross-fiber and circular friction on the transverse carpal ligament should be performed to help loosen adhesions in the area. Application of heat can help soften the ligament, and allow more space in the carpal canal.

**Cataract**: Cataracts are not contraindicated for massage.

**Cellulitis**: Cellulitis is considered a local contraindication. Any open wounds should be avoided.

**Cerebral Palsy**: Massage is indicated for clients with cerebral palsy. Depending on severity, the therapist may need to help the client on and off the table.

**Cervical Cancer**: A massage therapist should obtain a doctor's note approving massage. Afterwards, massage may be performed, avoiding any tumors, lymph nodes, or other areas affected.

**Chickenpox**: Because chickenpox is highly contagious, it is considered an absolute contraindication to massage.

**Chlamydia**: Because massage is not generally performed on the genital area, massage is indicated for a client with chlamydia. If massage is performed on the genital region, gloves should be worn and properly disposed of after the massage.

**Cholecystitis**: Cholecystitis is considered an absolute contraindication in the acute stage. After the underlying cause has been determined, medications may be prescribed to help deal with the formation of gallstones and infection, or the gallbladder may be removed completely. This will require a hospital stay, in which massage will not be performed.

**Chondromalacia Patellae**: Chondromalacia patellae is considered a local contraindication due to pain and inflammation in the area.

**Cirrhosis**: Massage should be avoided in a client with cirrhosis, due to increased waste products being filtered through the liver.

**Colon Cancer**: A massage therapist should obtain a doctor's note approving massage. Afterwards, massage may be performed, avoiding any tumors, lymph nodes, or other areas affected.

**Concussion**: In the acute stage immediately following a concussion, massage is considered an absolute contraindication. After a few days and clearance from a doctor, massage may be performed. People who have suffered from a concussion should avoid any activity that may over-stimulate the brain, and massage may be one of those.

**Congestive Heart Failure**: Massage is indicated for a client with congestive heart failure, as massage may help lower blood pressure and increase oxygen intake, both vital in the treatment of congestive heart failure.

**Conjunctivitis**: Conjunctivitis is generally not a contraindication, unless it is caused by bacteria or a virus. If this is the case, massage is considered an absolute contraindication, and should be rescheduled until after the condition has resolved.

**Constipation**: Massage is indicated for constipation. Massaging the abdomen in a clockwise motion may help promote peristalsis and improve the likelihood of defecation.

**Contusion**: A contusion is considered a local contraindication to massage, due to the potential presence of blood clots in the contusion.

**Corn**: A corn is generally not considered a contraindication to massage. If the corn causes pain, however, it may be treated as a local contraindication, depending on the client's pain tolerance.

**Crohn's Disease**: Massage in the acute stage of Crohn's disease should be avoided, as the client may be in pain and experience symptoms such as diarrhea. In the post-acute stage, massage is indicated for Crohn's disease.

**Cushing's Disease**: Massage is indicated for Cushing's Disease, but precautions may be taken in clients with weakened bones. Lighter massage is recommended for these clients to prevent damaging bone.

**Cystic Fibrosis**: Massage is indicated for cystic fibrosis. Tapotement may aid in loosening phlegm in the lungs.

**Cystitis**: In the acute stage of infection, massage is contraindication for cystitis. Once the infection has cleared, massage may be performed.

## D

**De Quervain's Tenosynovitis**: Massage is a local contraindication for De Quervain's Tenosynovitis, as it may increase inflammation and pain. Application of cold may be performed to decrease inflammation around the thumb.

**Decubitus Ulcer**: A decubitus ulcer is considered a local contraindication if the skin has developed into an ulcer. If the skin has not opened, massage in the area is indicated to increase blood flow into the affected tissue. If the sore is present, massage up to two inches around the area is indicated to increase circulation and prevent further necrosis.

**Deep Vein Thrombosis**: Deep vein thrombosis is typically a local contraindication. Avoid the site of the thrombus, as dislodging the clot may lead to circulation being cut off in organs such as the lungs, brain, or heart. Massage that increases blood pressure may be contraindicated, and deeper massages may be contraindicated due to the use of anticoagulants and thrombolytics.

**Dementia**: Dementia is not contraindicated for massage therapy.

**Depression**: Depression is not contraindicated for massage therapy. Massage may help relax a person with depression, increase self- esteem and body image, and help manage hormone levels in the body.

**Dermatitis**: Dermatitis is considered a local contraindication, as massage to the affected area will increase inflammation.

**Diabetes Mellitus**: Massage is indicated for a client with diabetes. If neuropathy is present, lighter massage in the affected area should be performed. If ulcers are present in areas afflicted with neuropathy, ulcers should be treated as local contraindications. If a client injects insulin, the injection site should also be avoided.

**Diarrhea**: Massage is indicated for a client with diarrhea. Massage of the abdomen, if performed, should be done counter-clockwise along the path of the large intestine to help the feces from moving further along in the colon.

**Dislocation**: In the acute stage, a dislocation is considered a local contraindication. If the joint has healed, massage may be performed on the area with caution. Stretching and range-of- motion should be avoided because the joint is much weaker after a dislocation.

**Diverticulitis**: Diverticulitis is considered an absolute contraindication to massage.

**Diverticulosis**: Diverticulosis is not contraindicated for massage. If pain is present, massage of the lower back and abdomen should be avoided, but may be performed elsewhere.

**Dupuytren's Contracture**: Dupuytren's contracture is indicated for massage, although massage is unlikely to help loosen the tendon and help the finger return to its normal position.

**Dysmenorrhea**: Massage for dysmenorrhea is dependent on the symptoms being experienced. Generally, it is not contraindicated. If a client is experiencing pain and cramping, massage of the abdomen and/or lower back may need to be avoided depending on the client's pain. If the client is nauseated, the massage may need to be rescheduled.

## E

**Emphysema**: Massage is indicated for emphysema.

**Encephalitis**: Because encephalitis is contagious and a serious medical condition, it is an absolute contraindication. Massage may be performed after the condition has completely resolved.

**Endocarditis**: Endocarditis is a serious medical condition, and is considered an absolute contraindication to massage. A person with endocarditis should seek medical attention as soon as possible.

**Endometriosis**: Massage of a client with endometriosis is generally not contraindicated. However, if a client is experiencing severe pain as a result, massage should not be performed and should be rescheduled.

**Epilepsy**: Massage on a client with epilepsy is indicated, however, precautions should be taken. If a trigger is known, it should be avoided. If a client has a seizure while receiving massage, the therapist should not attempt to put fingers in the client's mouth to prevent choking on the tongue, or catch the client if they fall off the table. The therapist should stay with the client and time the seizure. If the seizure lasts for five minutes or longer, or another seizure occurs quickly after the initial seizure, medical treatment should be sought immediately.

## F

**Fibromyalgia**: Fibromyalgia is indicated for massage, working within the client's pain tolerance.

**Folliculitis**: Folliculitis is considered a local contraindication to massage.

**Fracture**: In the acute stage, a fracture should be considered a local contraindication. After the fracture has healed, massage may be performed on the area. If metal plates, rods, screws, or pins have been placed in the bone, caution should be taken in the area, but massage may still be performed.

## G

**Ganglion Cyst**: Ganglion cysts should be treated as a local contraindication.

**Gastritis**: Massage on a client with gastritis is dependent on the cause and severity. If gastritis is causing nausea and vomiting, massage should not be performed.

**Gastroenteritis**: Gastroenteritis is often caused by a viral infection, and is contagious. Therefore, gastroenteritis is an absolute contraindication to massage.

**Gastroesophageal Reflux Disease**: Unless chest pain is present, massage is indicated for Gastroesophageal Reflux Disease. Semi-reclined position may help reduce acid from moving into the esophagus.

**Genital Herpes**: Because massage is not generally performed on the genital area, massage is indicated for a client with genital herpes. If massage is performed on the genital region, gloves should be worn and properly disposed of after the massage to avoid contracting the virus.

**Genital Warts**: Because massage is not generally performed on the genital area, massage is indicated for a client with genital warts. If massage is performed on the genital region, gloves should be worn and properly disposed of after the massage to avoid contracting the virus.

**Glaucoma**: Glaucoma is not contraindicated for massage.

**Goiter**: A goiter is considered a local contraindication.

**Golfer's Elbow**: Golfer's Elbow should be treated as a local contraindication. Application of cold may help reduce pain and inflammation at the medial epicondyle of the humerus.

**Gonorrhea**: Because massage is not generally performed on the genital area, massage is indicated for a client with gonorrhea. If massage is performed on the genital region, gloves should be worn and properly disposed of after the massage.

**Gout**: Gout is considered a local contraindication.

**Graves' Disease**: Graves' Disease is generally considered not contraindicated. However, a client with Graves' Disease may be sensitive to heat, so anything that uses heat in the massage treatment should be avoided. A goiter may also be present, which would be considered a local contraindication.

## H

**Headache**: Headaches are not contraindicated for massage. If muscular tension headache is suspected, massage should be performed on areas around the location of pain to try to ease tension and reduce pain. Application of heat or cold may be performed, depending on a client's specific needs.

**Heart Murmur**: Massage may be performed on a client with a heart murmur.

**Hematoma**: Hematomas are considered local contraindications. Depending on the cause and location, the type of massage being performed may also be altered. If a client is taking blood thinners, lighter massages are indicated.

**Hemorrhage**: Massage is locally contraindicated for a hemorrhage. Personal protective equipment should always be utilized in the presence of a hemorrhage.

**Hemorrhoids**: Massage is considered a local contraindication for hemorrhoids.

**Hepatitis**: In the acute stage, massage is an absolute contraindication for hepatitis. In the post-acute stage, massage is indicated.

**Hernia**: Massage of a hernia is locally contraindicated.

**Herniated Disc**: Herniated discs are considered local contraindications. The area around the hernia may be massaged, but the disc itself should be avoided.

**Herpes Simplex**: In the acute stage, any sore caused by the herpes simplex virus is considered a local contraindication. In the post-acute stage, massage is indicated.

**Hodgkin's Lymphoma**: A massage therapist should obtain a doctor's note approving massage. Afterwards, massage may be performed, avoiding any tumors, lymph nodes, or other areas affected.

**Hyperparathyroidism**: Generally, hyperparathyroidism is not contraindicated. However, if a client presents with associated symptoms such as osteoporosis, a lighter massage may be recommended.

**Hyperthyroidism**: Generally, hyperthyroidism is not contraindicated. However, conditions such as arrhythmia that can be caused by hyperthyroidism may be contraindicated if uncontrolled.

**Hypertension**: Hypertension is generally not contraindicated for massage. Massage that increases blood pressure, such as deep tissue or hot stone, may be contraindicated if the client is not taking medication to control hypertension. Light massage, which promotes lowering blood pressure, should be performed.

**Hypoparathyroidism**: Hypoparathyroidism is generally not contraindicated, however precautions should be taken in areas such as the fingers and toes which may experience tingling or burning sensations.

**Hypopituitarism**: Hypopituitarism is generally not contraindicated.

**Hypothyroidism**: Hypothyroidism is generally not contraindicated. A client with hypothyroidism may exhibit sensitivity to cold, so an extra blanket or increasing room temperature may be welcomed.

**Hypotension**: Generally, hypotension is not contraindicated for massage therapy. An invigorating massage may help increase blood pressure.

## I

**Ichthyosis**: Ichthyosis is generally not considered a contraindication. If fissures are painful, the massage may be altered depending on the client's pain tolerance. Body scrubs and application of lotion may help soften the built-up keratin in the skin.

**Impetigo**: Impetigo is a highly contagious bacterial infection, and therefore, is an absolute contraindication.

**Influenza**: Influenza is highly contagious, and is considered an absolute contraindication.

**Insomnia**: Insomnia is not a contraindication for massage. Massage therapy may aid a person in reducing stress and helping them obtain a normal sleep cycle.

## J

**Jaundice**: Massage of a person with jaundice is considered an absolute contraindication, due to damage to the liver that may further result from the massage.

## K

**Kaposi's Sarcoma**: A massage therapist should obtain a doctor's note approving massage. Afterwards, massage may be performed, avoiding any tumors, lymph nodes, skin lesions, or other areas affected.

**Kidney Stones**: Kidney stones are not considered a contraindication for massage therapy.

**Kyphosis**: Kyphosis is not contraindicated for massage. A person with kyphosis may be uncomfortable lying supine, and may need to be placed into side-lying position for comfort. Massage of the pectoralis minor and serratus anterior muscles may help the scapulae return to their normal locations, which can help straighten the vertebrae.

## L

**Laryngitis**: Massage on a client with laryngitis depends on the cause. If the cause of laryngitis is an infection, massage should be considered an absolute contraindication. If the cause of laryngitis is trauma, such as shouting, massage is indicated.

**Leukemia**: A massage therapist should obtain a doctor's note approving massage. Afterwards, massage may be performed, avoiding any tumors, lymph nodes, or other areas affected.

**Lice**: Lice is a highly contagious parasitic infection, and is therefore an absolute contraindication.

**Liver Cancer**: A massage therapist should obtain a doctor's note approving massage. Afterwards, massage may be performed, avoiding any tumors, lymph nodes, or other areas affected.

**Lordosis**: Lordosis is not contraindicated for massage. Stretching exercises on the psoas major, iliacus, and quadratus lumborum muscles may help return the lumbar spine back to its normal curvature.

**Lung Cancer**: A massage therapist should obtain a doctor's note approving massage. Afterwards, massage may be performed, avoiding any tumors, lymph nodes, or other areas affected.

**Lupus Erythematosus**: During flare-ups, lupus may cause extensive pain over the body, and massage would likely be postponed until the condition has gone into remission. If there are no symptoms, lupus is not contraindicated.

**Lyme Disease**: Massage largely depends on the symptoms a client is experiencing. Lesser symptoms, such as aches and joint inflammation, may allow for massage while avoiding general local contraindications. If a client is experiencing flu-like symptoms, the massage should be postponed until the client is feeling better.

**Lymphangitis**: In the acute stage, lymphangitis is contraindicated for massage because massage increases the flow of lymph, and may push the infection further throughout the body.

**Lymphedema**: Lymphedema is not contraindicated for massage. Lymphatic drainage may help move lymph out of the area. When performing lymphatic draining, light strokes moving towards the trunk should be performed on the proximal end of the affected limb, then distal areas may be worked on, again with strokes moving towards the trunk.

## M

**Malignant Melanoma**: A client with malignant melanoma should obtain permission from a doctor before proceeding with any type of massage, because the cancerous cells are easily spread throughout the body through the blood and lymph. The site of tumor growth should be avoided.

**Mastitis**: Mastitis is a local contraindication for massage. If a client presents with mastitis, the client may need to be placed into side-lying position to reduce pressure on the breasts. Massage of the breasts should be avoided. If fever is present, massage should not be performed.

**Measles**: Measles, despite its rarity, is caused by a contagious viral infection, and is considered an absolute contraindication.

**Meningitis**: Because meningitis is a contagious condition, it is an absolute contraindication to massage. Massage may be performed after the condition has completely resolved.

**Menopause**: Massage is indicated for clients with menopause. If a client is experiencing hot flashes, anything that produces heat, such as heat pads, should not be used. Cold packs may be used to help with hot flashes.

**Migraine Headaches**: Migraine headaches are generally not contraindicated for massage.

**Mole**: A mole is not contraindicated for massage. Precautions should be taken with moles that rise up off the skin, which can be painful if pulled or pinched.

**Mononucleosis**: In the acute stage, massage is an absolute contraindication. In the post-acute stage, massage may be performed.

**Multiple Sclerosis**: Massage in the acute stage of Multiple Sclerosis may be performed, but it is highly unlikely a client will seek massage because of the pain involved. Modalities that do not involve touching, such as Reiki, may be recommended and performed in these instances. In the post-acute stage, massage may be performed.

**Mumps**: Massage is an absolute contraindication for mumps, because mumps is a contagious viral infection.

**Muscle Cramp**: Muscle cramps in the acute stage should be considered a local contraindication. Reciprocal inhibition should be performed to stop the cramp. After a cramp has subsided, massage may be performed on the area, bringing fresh blood and nutrients into the area. The client should increase water intake after the massage as a preventative measure.

**Muscular Dystrophy**: Muscular dystrophy is indicated for massage. Precautions should be taken regarding pressure used. The therapist should expect to help a client with muscular dystrophy onto and off of the table. Massage can help bring nutrients into tissue and eliminate waste, which may not be sufficiently achieved if the muscles aren't being used.

**Myasthenia Gravis**: Massage may be performed on a client with myasthenia gravis. If a tumor is present on the thymus, the area should be avoided.

**Myocardial Infarction**: Massage is an absolute contraindication during a myocardial infarction. After a myocardial infarction has occurred and a client has been treated, it is a good idea to get a note from a doctor before proceeding. Depending on the severity of the infarct and treatment, certain massages should not be performed due to strain they may place on the heart when increasing blood pressure.

**Myocarditis**: Massage should be avoided until myocarditis has cleared.

## N

**Non-Hodgkin's Lymphoma**: A massage therapist should obtain a doctor's note approving massage. Afterwards, massage may be performed, avoiding any tumors, lymph nodes, or other areas affected.

## O

**Obsessive Compulsive Disorder(OCD)**: Obsessive compulsive disorder is not contraindicated for massage.

**Onychomycosis**: Onychomycosis is a contagious fungal infection, and is considered a local contraindication.

**Oral Cancer**: A massage therapist should obtain a doctor's note approving massage. Afterwards, massage may be performed, avoiding any tumors, lymph nodes, or other areas affected.

**Osgood-Schlatter Disease**: In the acute stage, massage of the tibial tuberosity is a local contraindication. If the client is beyond the age of 21, and bone is no longer being produced at the tibial tuberosity, massage on the area may be performed. In the acute stage, massage and stretching techniques should be performed on the quadriceps to loosen the muscles and take pressure off the patellar tendon, which can reduce the excessive development of bone at the tibial tuberosity.

**Osteoarthritis**: In the acute stage, massage is considered a local contraindication for any form of arthritis because it can bring more blood into the area and increase inflammation. In the post-acute stage, massage should be performed on the area usually affected to bring fresh blood and nutrients into the area, and to increase production of synovial fluid in the joint. This can help reduce irritation in the joint and lessen the effects of arthritis.

**Osteomyelitis**: Osteomyelitis is an absolute contraindication, as massage may help spread the bacterium throughout the body.

**Osteoporosis**: Massage is indicated for osteoporosis. However, precautions should be taken, such as performing a lighter massage, and not performing techniques such as tapotement to avoid damaging bone.

**Ovarian Cancer**: A massage therapist should obtain a doctor's note approving massage. Afterwards, massage may be performed, avoiding any tumors, lymph nodes, or other areas affected.

## P

**Paget's Disease**: Paget's disease is not contraindicated for massage. Massage may be implemented as part of a person's physical therapy plan to help treat symptoms.

**Pancreatic Cancer**: A massage therapist should obtain a doctor's note approving massage. Afterwards, massage may be performed, avoiding any tumors, lymph nodes, or other areas affected.

**Pancreatitis**: In the acute stage, pancreatitis is considered an absolute contraindication. In a client with chronic pancreatitis, massage may be performed in the post-acute stage.

**Paralysis**: Massage may be performed on an area that is paralyzed. Because the muscles involved will be atrophied, massage should be light to avoid damaging underlying tissue. Stretching and range-of-motion exercises may be performed to help with muscle elasticity.

**Parkinson's Disease**: Massage is indicated for clients with Parkinson's Disease. In advanced stages, when a client is unable to lie on a table without the entire body trembling, a doctor's note may be requested. In these advanced stages, the therapist may need to help the client on and off the table.

**Peptic Ulcer**: Massage of a client with peptic ulcers often depends on the symptoms and their severity. If a client is nauseated, massage should be postponed.

**Pericarditis**: Massage should be avoided until pericarditis has cleared.

**Peritonitis**: Peritonitis is considered an absolute contraindication to massage.

**Pharyngitis**: Pharyngitis is commonly considered an absolute contraindication to massage during the acute stage. After the infection has cleared, massage may be performed.

**Phlebitis**: Phlebitis should be treated as a local contraindication. Because medications may be prescribed that thin the blood, lighter massage should be performed to prevent internal bleeding from damaged blood vessels. Massaging the site of phlebitis may dislodge a clot, which can result in an embolism.

**Pitting Edema**: Massage on a client with pitting edema should not be performed until the cause of pitting edema is established. If the cause is something such as pregnancy and not organ failure, massage of the limb may be performed as it would be done with lymphedema.

**Plantarfasciitis**: Plantarfasciitis is considered a local contraindication in the acute stage.

**Pleurisy**: Pleurisy is considered an absolute contraindication until the condition has completely resolved.

**Pneumonia**: Pneumonia is a highly contagious condition, and is therefore an absolute contraindication.

**Polycystic Ovarian Syndrome(PCOS)**: Massage is generally indicated for a client with Polycystic Ovarian Syndrome.

**Preeclampsia**: Massage of a client with preeclampsia should generally be avoided until after the child has been delivered and the condition resolves.

**Premenstrual Syndrome**: Massage is indicated for premenstrual syndrome.

**Prostate Cancer**: A massage therapist should obtain a doctor's note approving massage. Afterwards, massage may be performed, avoiding any tumors, lymph nodes, or other areas affected.

**Prostatitis**: Massage is indicated for a client with prostatitis.

**Psoriasis**: Psoriasis is not contraindicated for massage. Massage may be altered if the patches are painful or are scabbing, but otherwise, the patches may be massaged.

**Pulmonary Edema**: In the acute stage, pulmonary edema is an absolute contraindication, and massage should not be performed.

**Pulmonary Embolism**: In the acute stage, if pulmonary embolism is suspected, massage is contraindicated and the client should seek medical attention. If a client is taking blood thinners, lighter massage is indicated, as any damage to underlying tissue may cause significantly more bleeding than normal. If the site of a blood clot is known, that area is considered a local contraindication and should be avoided.

**Pyelonephritis**: Pyelonephritis is considered an absolute contraindication. A client who suspects a kidney infection should seek medical treatment.

## R

**Raynaud's Syndrome**: Raynaud's Syndrome is indicated for massage. Using heat should be avoided, as sensation in the affected area may be decreased and tissue damage may result. Massaging the area can help dilate blood vessels and bring blood back into the fingers and toes. Increasing the temperature of the massage room may also help dilate blood vessels.

**Renal Failure**: Because massage may increase the load on kidneys by helping rid the body of waste, massage is considered an absolute contraindication in clients with renal failure. There is debate amongst kidney specialists on this matter, though, and some believe massage therapy does not do harm in people with renal failure.

**Rheumatoid Arthritis**: In the acute stage, rheumatoid arthritis is considered a local contraindication, as the pain may be too intense for the client to receive massage on the affected area. In general, however, a client with rheumatoid arthritis may receive massage to help ease pain associated with inflammation if the body can tolerate a light-to-medium pressured massage.

**Ringworm**: Ringworm is a highly contagious fungal infection, and is considered a local contraindication. Linens should be treated as contaminated.

**Rosacea**: Rosacea may be considered a local contraindication if pain or pus-filled bumps are present in the area. Otherwise, it is not contraindicated.

## S

**Scabies**: Scabies is a contagious parasitic infection, and is considered an absolute contraindication.

**Scar**: A scar is not a contraindication, and random collagen formation may be reduced as a result of massage.

**Sciatica**: Massage is indicated for sciatica. However, if sciatica is the result of a herniated disc, the site of disc herniation should be considered a local contraindication. Stretching techniques, especially in the glutes, may help ease some pain associated with sciatica.

**Scleroderma**: Generally, scleroderma is not considered contraindicated. Massage may help loosen collagen in the skin and increase blood flow into areas that may be affected.

**Scoliosis:** Scoliosis is indicated for massage. In instances where scoliosis is caused by hypertonic muscles, such as the rhomboids unilaterally, massage may help loosen the muscles and allow the bones to realign themselves. If surgery has been performed and metal rods have been placed in the back, massage should be performed lighter on the area, and the use of cold packs should be avoided.

**Sebaceous Cyst**: Sebaceous cysts are considered local contraindications, and should be avoided to prevent damaging the cyst and allowing the fluid inside to affect the body. The area may also be painful.

**Shin Splint**: Massage is indicated for shin splints, depending on the pain tolerance of the client. If the pain is too much, do not massage the area.

**Shingles**: Much like chickenpox, shingles should be treated as an absolute contraindication until the condition resolves.

**Sinusitis**: During the acute stage, and due to being caused by a contagious viral infection, sinusitis is considered an absolute contraindication. Once the condition has resolved, a client may receive massage.

**Spina Bifida**: Spina bifida is considered a local contraindication and the area should be avoided.

**Sprain**: In the acute stage, sprains are local contraindications. If inflammation has subsided from a first degree sprain, gentle massage in the area may be performed to bring fresh blood and nutrients into the area and speed healing. Contrast therapy may be performed in addition to gentle massage to reduce any inflammation that may occur due to the massage.

**Squamous Cell Carcinoma**: A client with squamous cell carcinoma may receive massage, but the site of the tumor should be avoided due to possible spreading of cancerous tissue.

**Stomach Cancer**: A massage therapist should obtain a doctor's note approving massage. Afterwards, massage may be performed, avoiding any tumors, lymph nodes, or other areas affected.

**Strain**: Acute strains are considered a local contraindication, and should be avoided to prevent increasing pain and inflammation in the area. Contrast therapy, utilizing alternating cold and heat, ending with cold, may be performed to decrease inflammation and bring fresh blood to the area.

**Strep Throat**: Because strep throat is highly contagious, it is considered an absolute contraindication until the condition has completely cleared.

**Syphilis**: Because massage is not generally performed on the genital area, massage is indicated for a client with syphilis. If massage is performed on the genital region, gloves should be worn and properly disposed of after the massage.

## T

**Temporomandibular Joint Dysfunction(TMJD)**: Massage is indicated for Temporomandibular Joint Dysfunction. Massage of the temporalis may help the jaw realign and reduce the pain and clicking.

**Tendonitis**: Tendonitis should be treated as a local contraindication. Alternating application of cold and heat, ending with cold, can assist in decreasing inflammation and associated pain.

**Tennis Elbow**: Tennis Elbow should be treated as a local contraindication. Alternating application of cold and heat, ending with cold, can assist in decreasing inflammation and associated pain at the lateral epicondyle of the humerus.

**Tenosynovitis**: Massage is a local contraindication for tenosynovitis, as it may increase inflammation and pain. Application of cold may be performed to decrease inflammation in the tendon and reduce pain.

**Thoracic Outlet Syndrome**: Massage is generally indicated for thoracic outlet syndrome. Massaging the scalenes and pectoralis minor may assist in releasing pressure on the area, returning sufficient blood supply to the area. Sensation may return to the upper limb as a result. If thoracic outlet syndrome is the result of tumors, the area should be avoided, and massage would be a local contraindication.

**Throat Cancer**: A massage therapist should obtain a doctor's note approving massage. Afterwards, massage may be performed, avoiding any tumors, lymph nodes, or other areas affected.

**Thromboangiitis Obliterans**: The area affected by thromboangiitis obliterans is generally considered a local contraindication and should be avoided during massage due to pain and possible tissue damage that has occurred.

**Thrush**: Thrush is generally considered a local contraindication, and the face would be avoided. However, the massage therapist should determine if thrush is the result of another type of disorder that affects the immune system, and proceed based on those findings.

**Tinnitus**: Tinnitus is not contraindicated for massage therapy. However, if a client complains of ringing in the ear, other conditions should be assessed for other contraindications.

**Tonsillitis**: Tonsillitis is commonly caused by an infection that is contagious, and is therefore an absolute contraindication until the condition has resolved.

**Torticollis**: Torticollis is generally not considered a contraindication, but precautions should be taken if damage to a muscle or nerve is the cause.

**Trigeminal Neuralgia**: Massage for trigeminal neuralgia is generally not contraindicated, but everything is dependent on the severity of pain experienced by the client. If pain is severe, massage may be considered a local contraindication, or the client may not want to be massaged at all and the appointment would need to be rescheduled. If massage is able to be performed, the therapist should not use a face rest, instead opting to use a pillow for the client to rest their head upon while prone.

**Tuberculosis**: Tuberculosis is a contagious condition, and is considered an absolute contraindication.

## U

**Ulcerative Colitis**: Massage of a client with ulcerative colitis depends on the client's symptoms and how they are feeling that day. If a client presents with fever and body aches, massage should be postponed until the symptoms resolve. If symptoms are generally mild, massage may be performed.

**Urethritis**: Massage is indicated for clients with urethritis.

**Urticaria**: In the acute stage, the cause of the hives should be determined before massage can be performed. Once the cause is determined, massage on the area should be avoided, or if it's a more serious reason for hives, massage should be avoided completely.

## V

**Varicose Veins**: Varicose veins are a type of phlebitis, and are considered a local contraindication. Massaging a swollen vein may dislodge a clot, which could become an embolism.

**Vertigo**: Vertigo is not contraindicated for massage. The massage therapist may need to help the client on and off the table to avoid accidental falls due to dizziness.

**Vitiligo**: Vitiligo is not contraindicated for massage.

## W

**Wart**: Warts are contagious, and should be treated as a local contraindication.

**Whiplash**: In the acute stage, massage is considered a local contraindication for a client with whiplash. Once the symptoms have subsided, gentle massage in the area may be performed. Stretching of the neck should be avoided to prevent injuring the tissue.

**Wounds**: Wounds should be treated as local contraindications until healed.

# Index

## R



## S



## T

# Resources

This book was created with the assistance of the following resources:

- Tappan's Handbook of Massage Therapy: Blending Art with Science(6th Edition), 2015 – Patricia J. Benjamin, PhD
- 30 Second Anatomy: The 50 Most Important Structures and Systems in the Human Body, Each Explained in Half a Minute, 2013 – Gabrielle M. Finn, Judith Barbaro-Brown
- Anatomica: The Complete Home Medical Reference, 2010 – Ken Ashwell
- The Four Hour Chef : The Simple Path to Cooking Like a Pro, Learning Anything, and Living the Good Life, 2013 – Timothy Ferriss
- Gray's Anatomy – Henry Gray
- Essentials of Anatomy and Physiology(4th Edition) 2002 – Rod Seeley, Trent Stephens, Philip Tate
- Introducing Medical Terminology Specialties: A Medical Specialties Approach with Patient Records, 2003 – Regina Masters, Barbara Gylys
- Exploring Medical Language: A Student-Directed Approach(5th Edition), 2002 – Myrna LaFleur Brooks
- Basic Clinical Massage Therapy: Integrating Anatomy and Treatment, 2003 – James H. Clay, David M. Pounds
- Milady's Theory and Practice of Therapeutic Massage, 1999 – Mark F. Beck
- The Mayo Clinic
- National Institutes of Health

# Also Available!

For more textbooks, visit us online at MBLExTestPrep.com!

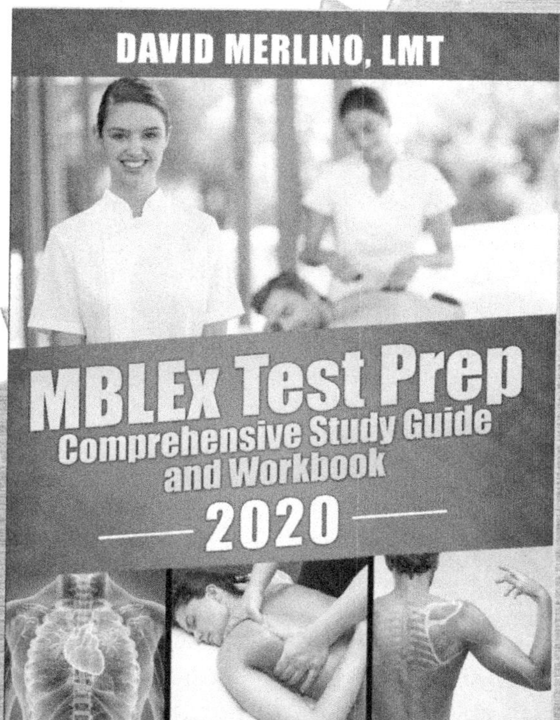


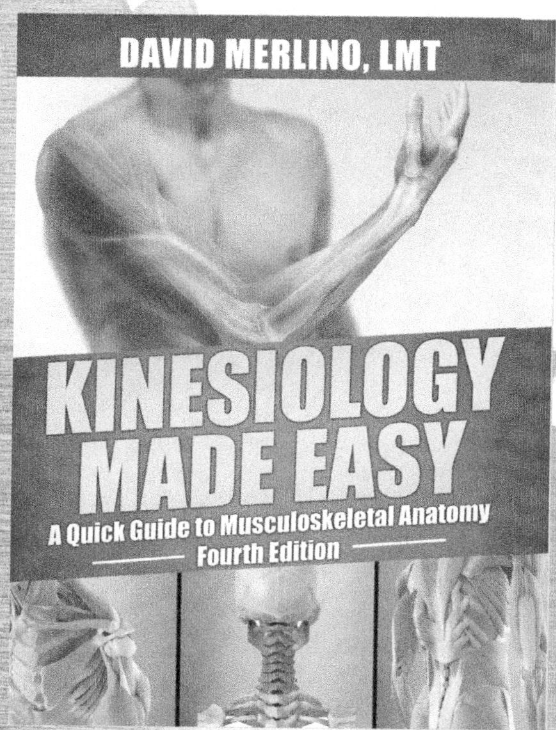


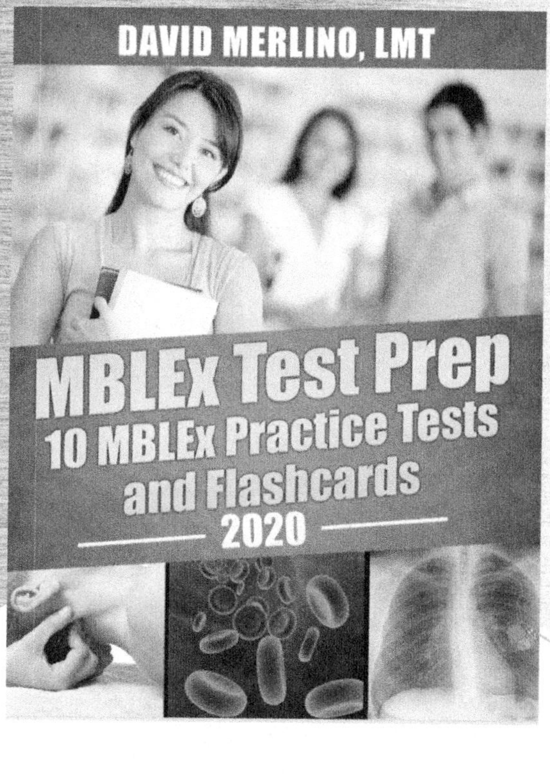

Made in the USA
Coppell, TX
08 September 2026

89396893R00175